KRIPALU YOGA

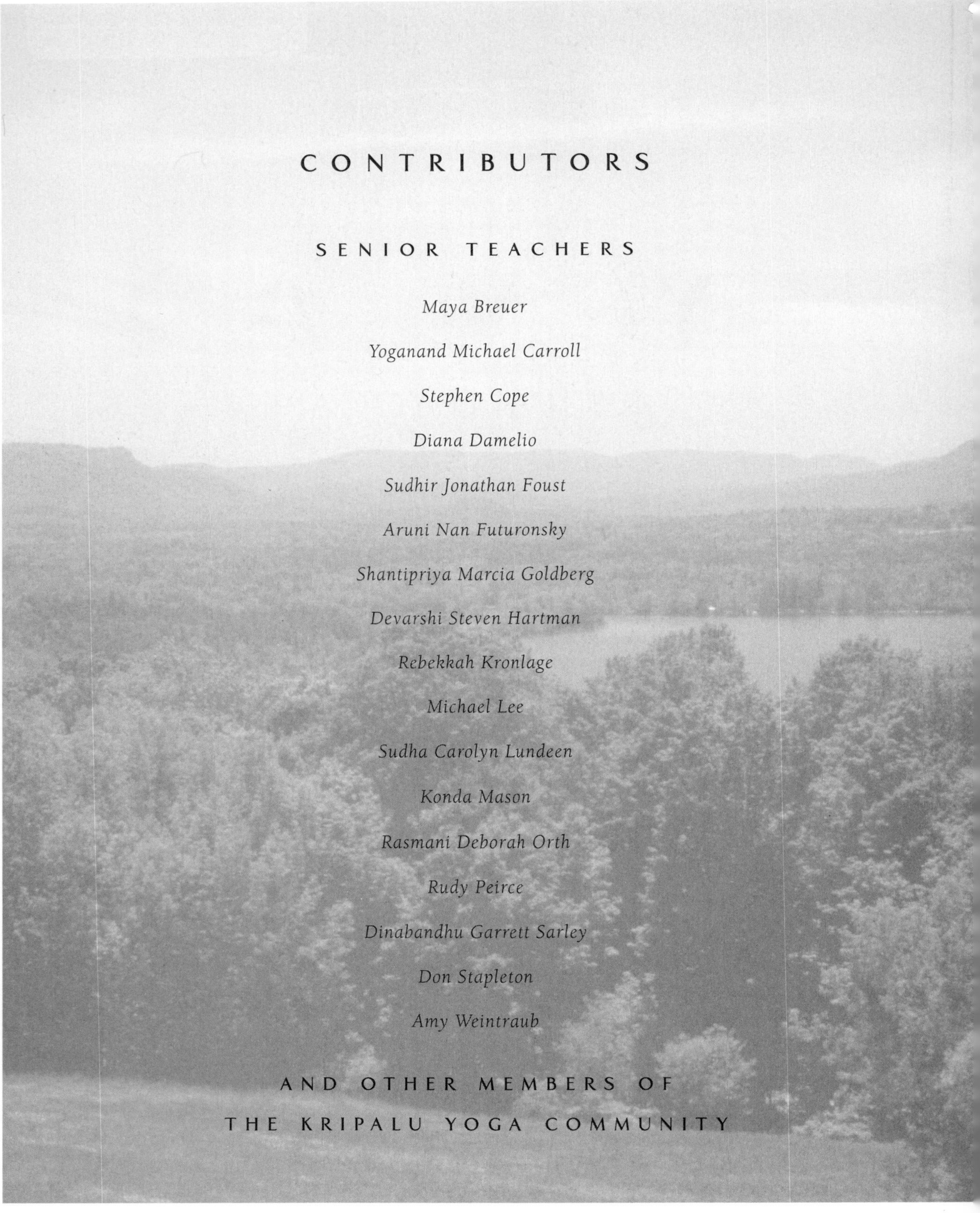

CONTRIBUTORS

SENIOR TEACHERS

Maya Breuer

Yoganand Michael Carroll

Stephen Cope

Diana Damelio

Sudhir Jonathan Foust

Aruni Nan Futuronsky

Shantipriya Marcia Goldberg

Devarshi Steven Hartman

Rebekkah Kronlage

Michael Lee

Sudha Carolyn Lundeen

Konda Mason

Rasmani Deborah Orth

Rudy Peirce

Dinabandhu Garrett Sarley

Don Stapleton

Amy Weintraub

AND OTHER MEMBERS OF

THE KRIPALU YOGA COMMUNITY

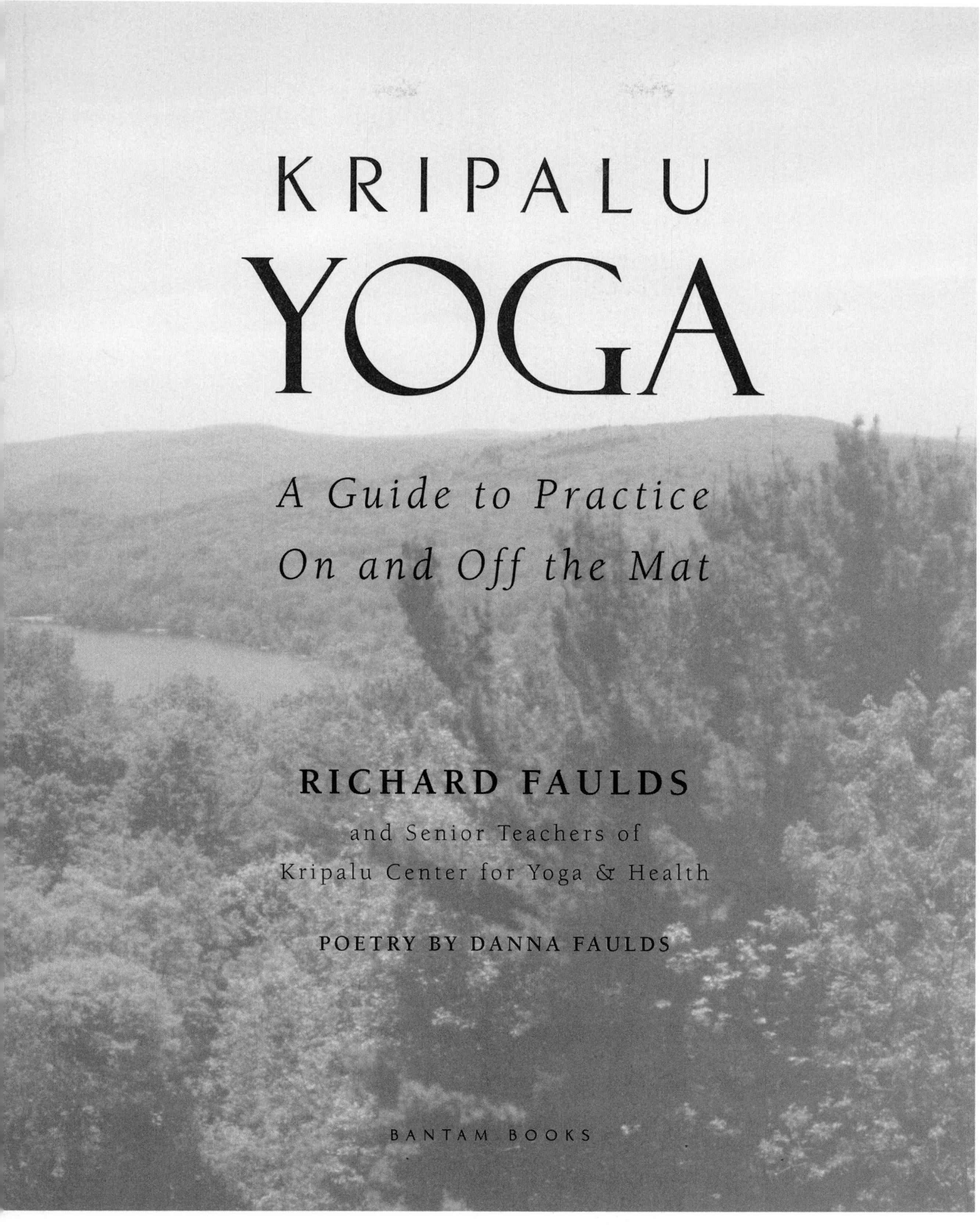

KRIPALU YOGA

A Guide to Practice On and Off the Mat

RICHARD FAULDS

and Senior Teachers of
Kripalu Center for Yoga & Health

POETRY BY DANNA FAULDS

BANTAM BOOKS

KRIPALU YOGA
A Bantam Book / January 2006

Published by
Bantam Dell
A Division of Random House, Inc.
New York, New York

Cover design by Belina Huey

Illustrations by Robert Bull
Photographs by Paul Conrath
Book design by Patrice Sheridan

Library of Congress Cataloging-in-Publication Data
Faulds, Richard.
Kripalu yoga : a guide to practice on and off the mat / Richard Faulds, and senior teachers of Kripalu Center for Yoga & Health.
p. cm.
Includes bibliographical references and index.
ISBN-10: 0-553-38097-4
ISBN-13: 978-0-553-38097-2
1. Hatha Yoga. I. Kripalu Center for Yoga and Health. II. Title.
RA781.7.F38 2006
613.7'046—dc22
2005053655

Printed in the United States of America
Published simultaneously in Canada

www.bantamdell.com

RRH 10 9 8 7 6 5

This book reflects the spiritual practice and heartfelt aspiration
of thousands of people over many years.
It is dedicated to everyone East and West
who has practiced, served, and taught
in the Kripalu Yoga tradition.

CONTENTS

PART FOUR: PSYCHOLOGICAL AND SPIRITUAL GROWTH

PART FIVE: EVOLVING YOUR PRACTICE

KRIPALU YOGA

WELCOME TO KRIPALU YOGA

In Kripalu Yoga, you learn many of the same postures as in other yoga classes, but the emphasis is not only on how you practice, but also on how you live your life.

—BRAHMANI HOLLY LIEBMAN

People come to yoga for different reasons. Most are looking for a way to improve their health. Others are interested in effective tools to manage stress. Still others seek personal and spiritual growth. Kripalu Yoga offers all these things. It's a practice that revitalizes the body, calms the mind, and deepens self-awareness.

Kripalu Yoga works its magic by bringing body, mind, and spirit into a state of harmony and balance. Focusing on the sensations that arise as you breathe and move bridges the chasm separating body and mind, allowing you to become fully present in your body. A balanced sequence of yoga postures stretches and strengthens the entire body, releasing the chronic tension that so often dulls vitality. As you conclude your yoga session with deep relaxation, energy naturally flows to the areas of your body most in need of rejuvenation and healing. You leave feeling balanced, energized to resume your life, and naturally motivated to sustain your practice.

Regular practice takes you to deeper levels, initiating a gradual process of growth and transformation. Concentration deepens, enabling you to observe the inner flow of emotion and thought with heightened awareness. Riding the wave of your moment-to-moment experience, you release trapped emotion by choosing to feel it fully. Witnessing the activity of the mind, you learn to recognize unproductive thinking and let it go. As these obstacles fall away, a joyous clarity emerges. Moments arise where you touch into the core energy underlying body and mind, expanding your sense of self.

Slowly and steadily, your experience on the yoga mat begins to overflow into the rest of your life. In touch with your body, habits fall away and your lifestyle becomes more supportive of health. Aware of deeper feelings and thoughts, your words and actions begin to express more of who you really are and the quality of your relationships deepens. With abundant energy at your disposal, life's challenges occur as opportunities for growth. On all levels, you feel more vital and fully alive. This is the experience of Kripalu Yoga.

> *Kripalu Yoga initiated a course of profound change in me: It connected me to my body in ways I had never experienced before. Through Kripalu Yoga, I have found gentleness, spaciousness, and a way to express who I really am.*
>
> —Marcia Reass

A Contemporary Approach

Kripalu Yoga is a contemporary approach to yoga practice designed for mainstream people leading active lives. Brought to America in the 1960s, the roots of Kripalu Yoga reach back thousands of years into an ancient and authentic yoga tradition. Over the last thirty years, Kripalu Yoga has been assimilated into Western culture by a large and diverse community of North American practitioners and teachers. The result is a potent spiritual practice free of unnecessary cultural trappings and dogmatic lifestyle restrictions, a yoga approach especially suited to our time and place.

Anyone can do Kripalu Yoga—it certainly isn't limited to those with a flexible or trim body. Nor does it require the adoption of any religious beliefs, as people of all faiths practice Kripalu Yoga. The theory and techniques of Kripalu Yoga can be explained in English, so you won't be faced with learning a large number of Sanskrit terms. Although the English names of yoga postures are used throughout the text, the traditional names are also listed to make it easy to cross-reference to other approaches that rely on Sanskrit.

For thousands of years, yoga has recommended a natural and wholesome lifestyle supportive of health. Building on this solid base, Kripalu Yoga integrates principles of holistic health, preventive medicine, and medical research into the traditional yoga lifestyle, augmenting age-old wisdom with contemporary health science.

Kripalu Yoga is not based on the guru/disciple relationship, a paradigm that has proved problematic in so many spiritual communities across America. In its place is an experiential model of education that empowers the learner to discover what is true based on his or her own direct experience. Yoga's traditional emphasis on transcending the ego to attain an otherworldly enlightenment has been balanced with a developmental perspective drawn from Western psychology. The result is an approach that facilitates psychological growth without negating the potential for deeper levels of spiritual awakening.

Although a group class is a great way to jump-start a practice, Kripalu Yoga can be learned in the comfort and privacy of your own home, and requires nothing more than some loose-fitting clothing and a little floor space. Perhaps best of all, Kripalu Yoga doesn't demand an excessive time commitment to bestow its gifts. This book recommends a regular practice of thirty minutes to an hour. Even a daily ten-minute dose of deep breathing and relaxation can make a real difference in your life.

While its form has evolved, Kripalu Yoga still conveys the authentic spirit of yoga and does so in a commonsense practice accessible to everyone. You don't need the body of an athlete, the mind of a mystic, or the lifestyle of a monk to benefit from Kripalu Yoga. Yet if you practice consistently, you will not only nurture your health but also experience the unity of body, mind, and spirit that lies at the heart of all mystical traditions.

> *I only recently discovered Kripalu Yoga, having practiced Bikram, Ashtanga, Jivamukti, and Anusara yoga before. While each approach has its place, I found that Kripalu Yoga speaks directly to the heart, and then flows out to work with the body. The other forms start with the body and then extend to the heart. This is a powerful twist. With Kripalu Yoga, there is an immediate acceptance of individuality, and an inherent permission to move the body as guided from within. With this approach, truly big things can happen on the mat.*
>
> —Kim Ellner

What Distinguishes Kripalu Yoga?

Although yoga traditions vary widely in their approaches, most teach the same basic yoga postures. Here are the attributes unique to Kripalu Yoga.

- **Practice begins gently with an emphasis on being present in your body, sustaining a flowing breath, and warming up.** The overall experience is one of learning to love and nurture your body, not whip it into shape.

- **It allows you to choose the level of physical intensity right for your body.** Instead of encouraging you to judge your performance today against yesterday, or compare your stretch with that of your classmate's, Kripalu Yoga teaches you how to listen to your body and honor its needs. On some days this may lead you to challenge yourself physically to work the kinks out. On others you may move more gently to relax the body and soothe the mind.

• **It recognizes that every body is different.** The goal of Kripalu Yoga is not to perfect the external form of the postures. It views postures as tools to release chronic tension, stretch and strengthen the body, and increase self-awareness. Rather than forcing the body into the classic form of the posture prematurely, postures are modified to meet individual needs.

• **It activates the life force of the body that yoga calls *prana*.** Kripalu Yoga teaches that the body is animated by an energetic life force intimately tied to the breath. Rhythmic breathing charges the system with energy. A balanced sequence of yoga postures encourages it to flow freely and evenly to all parts of the body. As practice deepens, the life force becomes more active and can be felt as warmth, tingling, and currents of energy.

• **It encourages you to create a lifestyle supportive of your health by listening to your own body.** As you practice Kripalu Yoga, you become more sensitive to the needs of your body and are naturally drawn to make healthier choices about diet, exercise, and other lifestyle habits. Kripalu Yoga considers each person's body the ultimate authority on what promotes health and teaches you how to access this *body wisdom* to live with more vitality.

• **It's a yoga you can practice "off the mat."** Being alive is a richer experience when you are connected to your body and breath. Through Kripalu Yoga, you discover that the same principles that bring out the best in you on the yoga mat can be applied to daily life. You learn how to meet challenges with a sense of relaxation, self-acceptance, strength, courage, and openness to change.

• **It offers practical tools to foster psychological and spiritual growth.** By teaching you how to fully feel strong emotion and compassionately observe the activity of the mind, Kripalu Yoga fosters emotional healing and facilitates psychological growth. As a result, your ability to express yourself, listen to others, and be in relationship deepens. Kripalu Yoga also includes sensible spiritual teachings that demystify the process of spiritual awakening and make it accessible to contemporary people living active lives.

• **It acknowledges that regular yoga practice is designed to initiate a process of personal transformation.** By nurturing the body, opening the heart, and clearing the mind, Kripalu Yoga removes the obstacles that so often stifle and stunt the natural progression of human development. Regular practice stimulates an ongoing process of positive change that inspires you to realize your full potential.

Kripalu Yoga has brought me the skills
I need to be fully alive in my life's journey.

— Karen Bentrup

Three Stages of Kripalu Yoga

Kripalu Yoga is taught in three stages that help you safely start and progressively deepen your practice. An overview of the stages appears below. As you make your way through this book, each stage is addressed in detail.

Stage One: Body and Breath Awareness

In the first stage of Kripalu Yoga, you learn how to bring yourself fully present in your body and practice the classic yoga postures with a flowing breath, proper alignment, and a mental focus on sensation. The purpose of stage one practice is to stretch and strengthen your entire body, releasing the chronic muscle tension that inhibits relaxation and underlies many health problems. During the process of stretching and strengthening the body, it is common to encounter physical limitations and emotional blocks. An attitude of compassionate self-acceptance is stressed as an essential element of practice. Each session concludes with the

A WORD ABOUT KRIPALU . . .

Kripalu (Krih-PAH-loo) means *being compassionate* in Sanskrit, the language of the yoga tradition. Both Kripalu Yoga and Kripalu Center were named in honor of Swami Kripalu, a yoga master renowned in India for the depth of his compassion and the intensity of his spiritual practice.

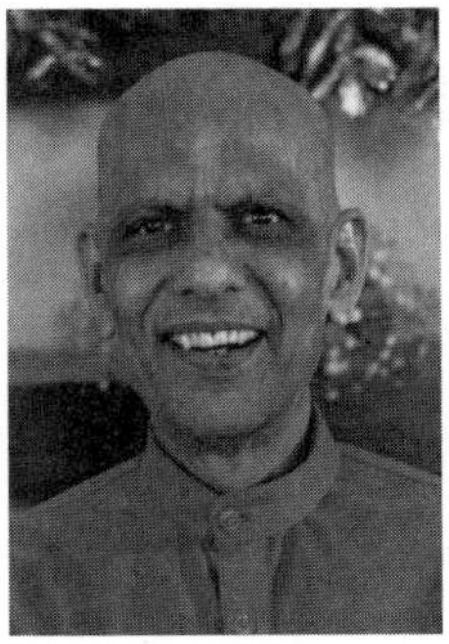

Swami Kripalu
1913–1981

The teachings of Swami Kripalu were first brought to America in the 1960s by one of his close disciples, Yogi Amrit Desai. A powerful 1970 yoga experience led Yogi Desai to adapt the teachings of Swami Kripalu into a format suited to Western students that he called *Kripalu Yoga*. Yogi Desai founded Kripalu Center in 1974 and attracted a loyal following of American students. Through their dedicated efforts, Kripalu Yoga evolved into a popular and effective approach to yoga practice and Kripalu Center quickly grew into the largest yoga and holistic health center in North America, a distinction it has held for more than twenty years.

Swami Kripalu came to America in 1977 and spent his last four years in residence at Kripalu Center, where he continued his life of intensive spiritual practice, scriptural study, and devotional music until shortly before his death in 1981. Swami Kripalu's teachings on yoga practice and supportive lifestyle still form the basis of the Kripalu Yoga approach.

rejuvenating experience of deep relaxation. Regular practice revitalizes the respiratory, nervous, endocrine, digestive, and other major systems of the body that support healthy functioning.

Stage Two: Focusing Inward

In the second stage of Kripalu Yoga, you learn how to encounter and release deep-seated emotional and mental tensions. The purpose of stage two practice is to open the heart and clear the mind. Postures are held for longer periods of time, and the mind is focused on the intensified flow of sensation, emotion, and thought that results. Holding a posture not only strengthens the physical body, it heightens self-awareness and naturally produces meditative states of introversion and introspection. Prolonged holding causes buried emotion and other unconscious material to surface, where it can be felt, seen, and let go. Regular practice restores emotional balance and mental clarity, increasing your capacities for learning and growth.

Stage Three: Meditation-in-Motion

A hallmark of Kripalu Yoga is an experience called *Meditation-in-Motion*. With the mind deeply relaxed, you allow the body to move spontaneously as guided from within. Entering this experience, you drop everything learned from external sources and respond directly to the urges and intuitive prompting of the body. Stage three is a form of moving meditation that reveals the essential mystical truth: Spirit dwells within you as the intelligent energy underlying body and mind. Kripalu Yoga's approach to meditation is unique, because it recognizes that the essence of meditation is a state of deep inner absorption that can occur in either the flow of yoga postures or in moments of physical stillness.

> *As I practice Kripalu Yoga, I am consistently reminded that I am traveling on a spiritual path. This is a path with heart for me. I feel it. I know it when I'm on it. My heart and gut, my soul if you will, feel good about it. Kripalu Yoga allows me to experience life rather than think and talk about it.*
>
> —Dean Fulco

Getting Started

The benefits of yoga come from practice, and this book is designed to get you on the mat as quickly as possible.

- *Part One* presents Kripalu Yoga's techniques of *Body and Breath Awareness,* featuring a series of guided experiences that teach you the essentials of practice in a step-by-step fashion. These experiences distill the basic principles of yoga into simple formats you can revisit again and again as your practice advances.

- *Part Two* presents the *Sun Series* and *Moon Series,* two balanced yoga sessions suitable for daily practice. Taken together, Sun and Moon Series will teach you the classic yoga postures taught in almost all yoga traditions.

• *Part Three* details the amazing *health benefits of yoga* in a way that will inform your practice, making it more supportive of health and healing. It includes practical guidance for overcoming physical challenges and creating a lifestyle based on the wisdom of your own body.

• *Part Four* presents the awareness-focusing and energy-awakening techniques that make Kripalu Yoga a potent and powerful catalyst for *psychological growth and spiritual awakening*. One of the key attributes of Kripalu Yoga is that it skillfully integrates yoga philosophy with growth psychology, and everything you need to deepen your practice is here.

• *Part Five* provides a broad menu of additional warm-ups, postures, and exercises that help you *Evolve Your Practice,* allowing you to make steady gains in strength and flexibility while keeping your experience perpetually fresh and satisfying. If you master the techniques presented here, you will be prepared to learn even the most difficult poses safely and effectively.

The only way to successfully embark on anything new is to *start where you are right now*. None of us are perfect. Most of us aren't even close! Learning happens best when we can relax and accept ourselves, whatever our level of flexibility, whatever our state of mind. Then we are ready to explore, celebrating each step of the path toward greater health and wholeness as a journey of self-discovery. All of us share a deep longing to realize our potential for full aliveness. May this book be a helpful step on your journey.

1. BODY AND BREATH AWARENESS

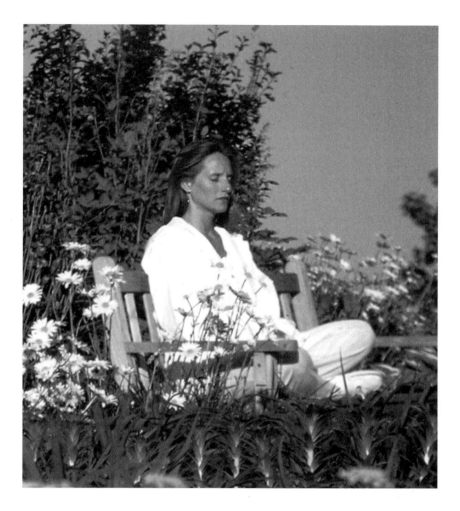

CHAPTER ONE

THE PRACTICE OF BEING PRESENT

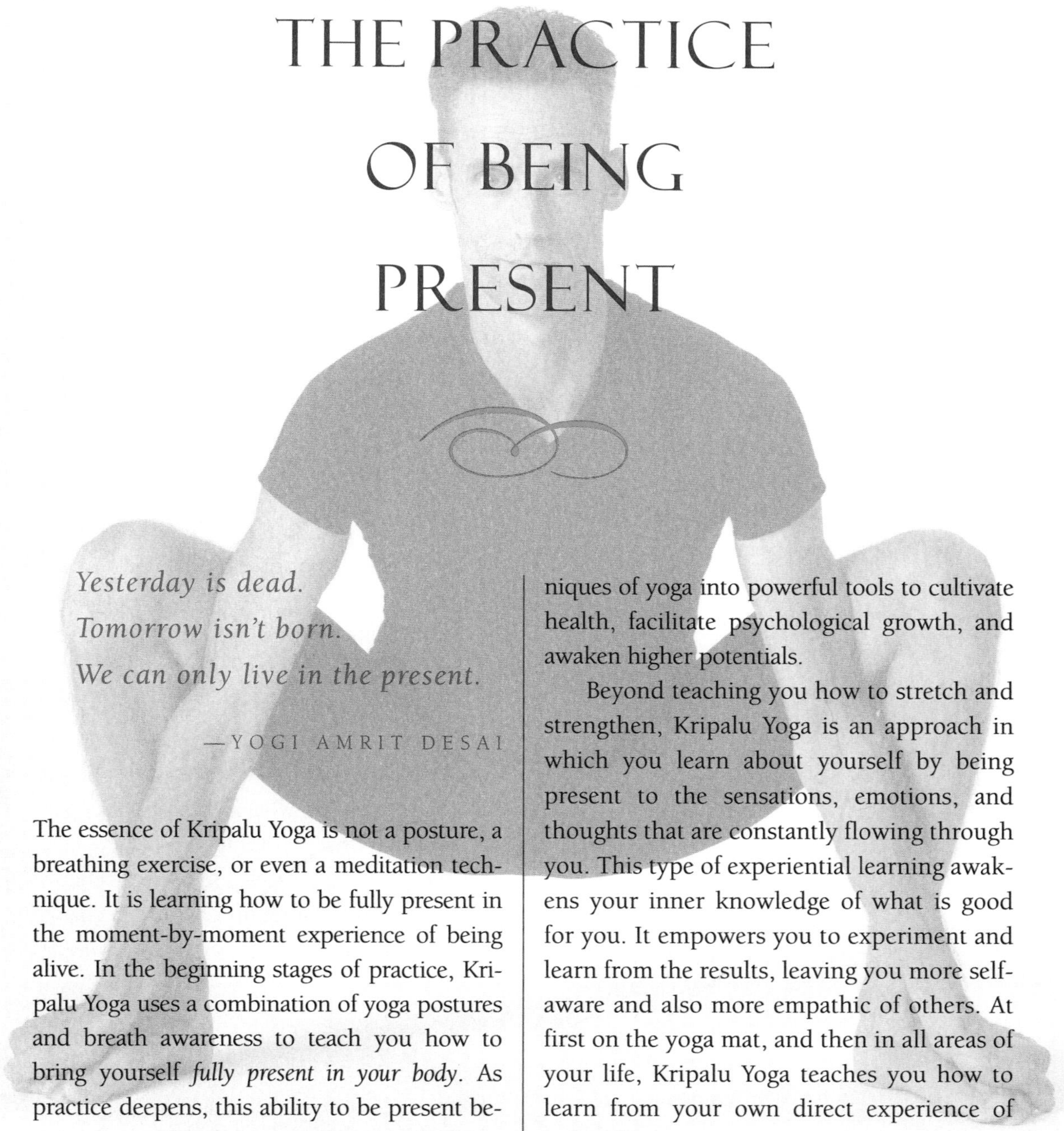

Yesterday is dead.
Tomorrow isn't born.
We can only live in the present.

—YOGI AMRIT DESAI

The essence of Kripalu Yoga is not a posture, a breathing exercise, or even a meditation technique. It is learning how to be fully present in the moment-by-moment experience of being alive. In the beginning stages of practice, Kripalu Yoga uses a combination of yoga postures and breath awareness to teach you how to bring yourself *fully present in your body*. As practice deepens, this ability to be present becomes a tangible force, transforming the techniques of yoga into powerful tools to cultivate health, facilitate psychological growth, and awaken higher potentials.

Beyond teaching you how to stretch and strengthen, Kripalu Yoga is an approach in which you learn about yourself by being present to the sensations, emotions, and thoughts that are constantly flowing through you. This type of experiential learning awakens your inner knowledge of what is good for you. It empowers you to experiment and learn from the results, leaving you more self-aware and also more empathic of others. At first on the yoga mat, and then in all areas of your life, Kripalu Yoga teaches you how to learn from your own direct experience of being alive.

Ten Feet by Ten Feet

Swami Kripalu used to tell the following story: There once was a traveler on a long and pressing journey. Night fell, and he lost his way in the dark of a thick forest. On the verge of despair, he saw a light flickering in the distance. Making his way toward the light, he found a hut in a small clearing. When he knocked at the door, an old yogi answered and said, "What is it, my friend?" "I've lost my way," said the traveler, "it is a moonless night and the path I am following is hard to see." "Come in and pass the night with me. Although my hut is humble, it is warm and I have food to share," answered the yogi. "Thank you," said the traveler, "but I must arrive at my destination by morning. Can you help me?" The yogi went into his hut momentarily and came back to the door smiling. "I cannot go with you, but take this lantern. It will illumine your way." Looking forlorn, the traveler held the lantern aloft and said, "But I cannot find my way with this lantern. Its light shines only ten feet ahead, and I have a journey of many miles to complete." The yogi replied, "Walk ten feet, and you will be able to see another ten. And when you have walked ten more feet, yet another ten will be illumined. So ten feet by ten feet, you will reach your destination."

Swami Kripalu taught that each of us is a pilgrim, a traveler on a spiritual journey that must be completed in the short span of a lifetime. Along the way, it is inevitable that we will lose our way and encounter moments of despair and confusion. Ultimately no one can complete the journey for us, or even provide shelter from its hardships and rigors. The most anyone can do is to offer a lantern, an aid to walking step by step from the known of the past into the unknown of the future.

The Practice of Being Present

On the journey of Kripalu Yoga, the practice of being present is your lantern, a core technique you can always come back to when you have lost your way, a practice you can rely on in times of challenge. It consists of the following steps:

- ***Breathe*** Let your breath flow freely in and out.
- ***Relax*** Soften your muscles, let go of mental tension.
- ***Feel*** Open to the sensations and emotions moving through you in this moment.
- ***Watch*** Observe your experience closely, neither grasping what is pleasant nor pushing away what is painful.
- ***Allow*** Accept yourself and your experience exactly as it is, dropping the need to change it in any way.

Bringing yourself present is easy. Over time it becomes second nature. Come into a comfortable sitting posture and give it a try right now.

AN EXPERIENCE OF BEING PRESENT

1. ***How freely can you breathe right now?*** For a minute or two, focus your attention on the flow of breath in and out of your body. Notice all the sensations connected to the breathing process. Then begin to take long and slow breaths, inhaling all the way down to the belly and fully filling the lungs. Exhale completely by gently squeezing the abdominal muscles toward the end of exhalation. After several deep breaths, release any conscious control and let the breath flow freely and naturally. Do not try to breathe deeply, just sustain a flowing breath and let the belly soften with each exhalation.

2. ***How could you relax just a little more right now?*** Scan your body for areas of tension and consciously soften your muscles. Relaxation does not mean going limp or slouching against the back of your chair. Relaxation is using a minimum of muscular effort to maintain an erect and balanced posture. When you have relaxed your body, soften the "muscle of the mind" and let go of any tension surrounding your mental activity.

3. ***What are you feeling right now?*** Let your awareness drop from the head into the body, permeating every cell. Feel all the sensations flowing through you in this moment. This may include internal sensations as well as those of your environment—the air touching your skin and the sounds around you. Open yourself to feel everything that is present in your experience, letting it arise and pass through you in its own time.

4. ***What are you aware of right now?*** Watch the thoughts, memories, and associations moving across the surface of your mind. Resist any tendency to grasp on to what is pleasant or push away what is painful. Be the silent witness, attending to all the details of your inner experience without getting lost in any train of thought. As the mind comes into greater focus, notice if the quality of your experience changes in any way.

5. ***Can you allow the moment to be exactly as it is?*** Just for a moment, imagine that you do not have to change anything at all about your experience in order to be happy or content. Rather than trying to make something happen, observe and feel what is naturally happening without any effort on your part. Instead of trying to understand your experience, be fully present as the experience unfolds moment to moment. Allow this moment—and yourself—to be perfect just the way it is.

Simple and Profound

The practice of being present is deceptively simple. Don't discount its potency just because it appears easy to do. Being present brings your mind and body together, creating an inner state of receptivity and focus. This receptivity acts like a magnifying glass, raising your awareness of feelings and thoughts. As you attend to whatever is present by choosing to feel it fully and see it clearly, it becomes free to pass through you. Insights naturally arise in the relaxed and spacious awareness that results, leaving you perpetually fresh to the next moment.

Learning how to be present is a somewhat paradoxical process. It begins with a compassionate self-acceptance, yet it leads to the ability to act dynamically in the face of inertia and fear. A particularly common obstacle that blocks us from being present is *self-judgment,* often reflected in a critical inner voice that constantly sees ourselves as *not enough* and may tend to blame others as well. Because self-acceptance soothes and gradually quiets this inner critic, it is an essential starting place for anyone wanting to dive deeper into their here-now experience of life. But the practice of being present doesn't stop with self-acceptance. When the time is right, it encourages you to step beyond your comfort zone and challenge yourself in healthy ways. Breaking free of habits and fears that draw their power from past conditioning, you can explore new experiences that strengthen your body and mind.

Simple yet profound, the ability to bring yourself fully present is one of life's true secrets. Grounded in the body, taking good care of your health becomes a matter of listening to the urges and feelings that give voice to its needs. With your mind focused on what is happening here and now, you can respond to life directly, free of past baggage and worries about the future. Being present empowers you to make conscious choices about what you want—and don't want—to create in your life. When you are present in your body, you live with a natural ease and grace.

CENTERING

Here. Right here, right now,
bring your mind to this place
and time. Invite it, even if it
resists, to sit and witness
what it is to be alive. Let
there be no ulterior motive
in this moment but to be.

Rest on the waves of breath
and choose to experience
all of it. Let thoughts float
through and leave again, as
the mind slowly settles like
snow inside a shaken
paperweight.

This is all there is. Here.
Right here and now.

I was in the middle of a Kripalu Yoga class in 1999. The teacher led us into a seated forward bend, giving us alignment and breathing direction. He then said, "Don't abandon your body." Well, I looked down at my leg and realized that I'd been estranged from my body for most of my life. I thought, "Who are you? What are you? How are you?" At that moment, I knew that my body had been waiting all these years for my attention and love. It was the beginning of my healing journey, and of what has proved to be a continually amazing relationship of respect for my body.

—Kim Childs

Being Present On the Yoga Mat

You may be amazed at the rich mix of sensations, emotions, and thoughts you encounter on the yoga mat. When you become present to this inner flow, you discover that body and mind naturally gravitate toward a healthy state of balance. Feeling sensation, tensions release and the body begins to heal. Being with the rise and fall of emotion, defenses drop away and emotional balance is restored. Observing the flow of thought, distractions fade and the mind calms. Kripalu Yoga teaches that underlying sensation, emotion, and thought is the flow of a life force called *prana* that can be felt as tingling currents of energy. When you attune to this energy, all these levels of your being naturally come into harmony. Over the course of a yoga session, you use the techniques of yoga to come back in touch with yourself and rest there, present and relaxed.

For many years, I have pushed aside the conference tables of our Boston law firm to teach yoga to CEOs, venture capitalists, and other busy professionals. One time a leading corporate lawyer who had worked in the same high-rise for over twenty years came up to me after class and said, "I never thought I could feel so relaxed and at peace in this building." It was a beautiful moment, and I also know he was learning a major lesson. A big part of the quality of our life experience is determined by how present we are, and not by our outer circumstances.

—Justin Morreale

Being Present Off the Yoga Mat

Yoga practice is just that—practice. The fruit of practice is being more present in your life. The next time you find yourself stuck in traffic and feel your blood pressure rising, apply the principles of breathe, relax, feel, watch, and allow. Turn an unavoidable inconvenience into an opportunity to relax and center yourself. While selecting items from a salad bar or

When I first started taking Kripalu Yoga classes, I thought it was exercise, nothing more. Having struggled with body image and weight issues all my life, it was daunting to be in classes with people in much better physical shape than myself. I spoke to my teacher, insisting I didn't belong in the class. Thankfully, he didn't agree.

Two weeks into yoga, I was aching and frustrated. Gradually I began to be present and listen to my body. I had what I'd call my first transformation. I saw myself, for a fleeting moment, as perfect just the way I was. This was astonishing. My physical body began to open up and I could breathe and stretch farther. I found I could "just be," a phrase I'd heard my teacher say over and over. It started to make sense to me, and I had moments of serenity.

Several months later, I had an incredible breakthrough in class. With no expectations, and no fears, I continually asked my body and soul, "Does this feel right? Is this what I need to do in this moment?" I knew absolutely that if I kept breathing during certain postures, I could go deeper and not feel pain. I stopped judging myself. And then, most amazing of all for me, I opened my eyes and looked at the other students in the class. For the first time I didn't see them versus me. I saw individuality on each mat. I saw the beauty in being different and unique. I began to do each posture exactly the way my body wanted. I began to feel joyful in class.

I feel as if I've given birth to a new way of being in the world. My yoga teacher taught me that by continuing to practice, day after day, things open up. At first, I wondered if I belonged in that yoga class. Now I know that yoga belongs in me, and that it will continue to be my way of moving toward greater truth, clarity, presence, and serenity in my life.

—Nina Galerstein

menu, bring yourself present. In touch with your body's needs, and awake to all the sights and smells, you can make the best possible food choices.

As your practice deepens, experiment with remaining present in the face of strong emotion. Watch what arises in your mind during a frustrating moment at work, or after a heated exchange with a family member. Closely observing your inner experience in moments of challenge reveals volumes about yourself. When you are present in moments like these, life itself becomes your teacher. Connected to your body, attuned to your emotions, aware of your thoughts, you let the moment-by-moment experience of life touch, teach, and transform you.

> *I used to spend most of my waking hours planning the next day, week, or month. Although I was driven and passionate about life, I was never satisfied with myself or my family. I read self-help books and listened to tapes, but something was missing. Then Kripalu Yoga taught me how to breathe into life, feel its wonder, and watch it unfold with all its power and miracles. As a result, my relationship with my husband and daughter has deepened. I honestly love myself, the work I perform, and the people I reach out and touch. Kripalu Yoga has given me a new lease on life.*
>
> —Barbara Templeton

Being Present Versus Being Perfect

Kripalu Yoga is not about attaining any form of external perfection. It is not about developing the perfect body, doing perfect yoga postures, or living the perfect yoga lifestyle. Kripalu Yoga is a way to be fully present to the reality of life unfolding in the moment—however it is showing up. Rather than teaching you how to get somewhere else, it helps you be fully where you are.

As you practice being present on and off the yoga mat, you learn what is for many a startling lesson. Life does not require us to be perfect. You are okay, just as you are, right now. Paradoxically, it is just this type of self-acceptance that opens the door to moments in which you glimpse the divine perfection inherent in a constantly changing and always "imperfect" life. In the sweepstakes of life, you must be present to win.

CHAPTER TWO

BREATHING LIFE INTO YOUR PRACTICE

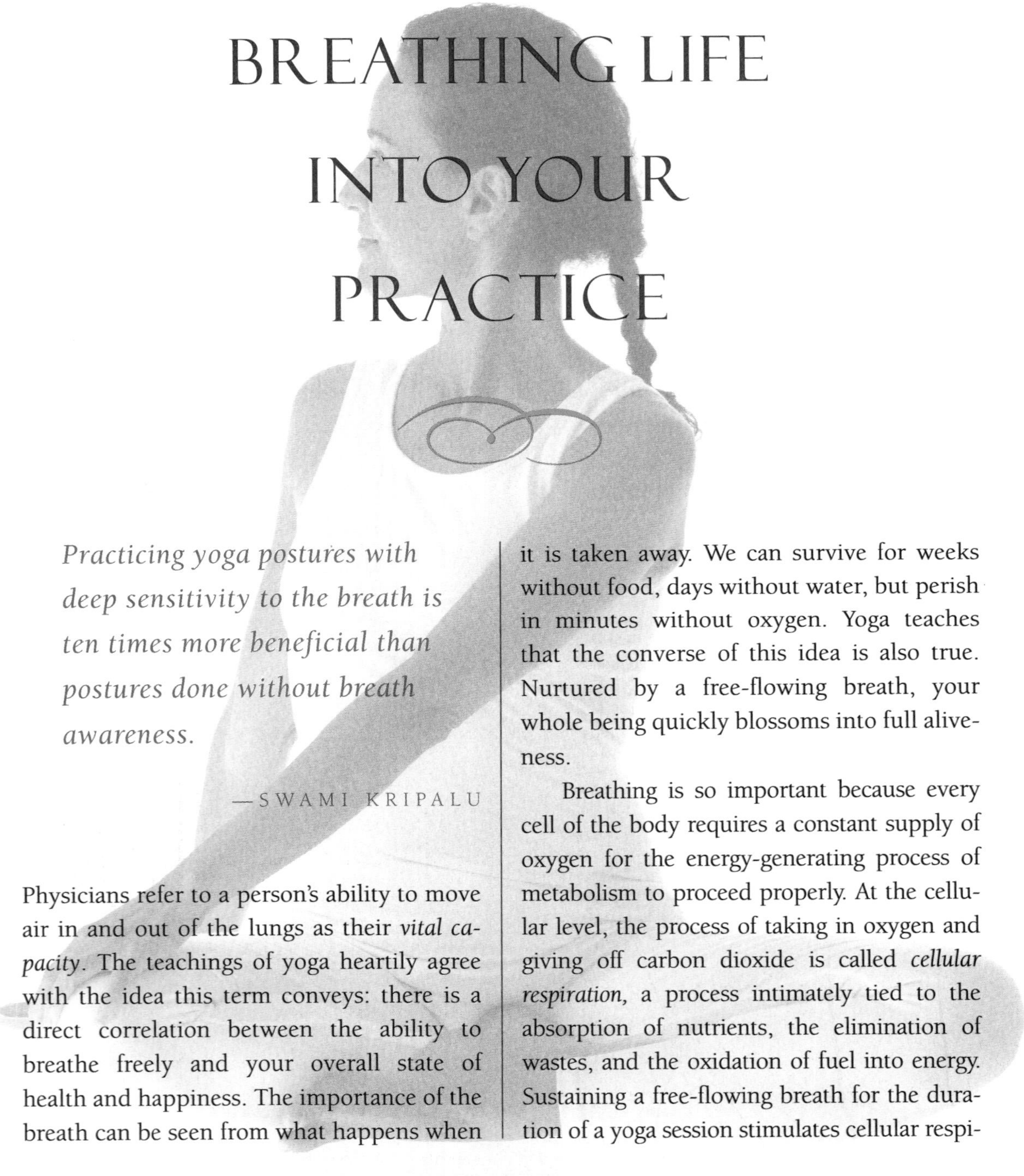

> *Practicing yoga postures with deep sensitivity to the breath is ten times more beneficial than postures done without breath awareness.*
>
> —SWAMI KRIPALU

Physicians refer to a person's ability to move air in and out of the lungs as their *vital capacity*. The teachings of yoga heartily agree with the idea this term conveys: there is a direct correlation between the ability to breathe freely and your overall state of health and happiness. The importance of the breath can be seen from what happens when it is taken away. We can survive for weeks without food, days without water, but perish in minutes without oxygen. Yoga teaches that the converse of this idea is also true. Nurtured by a free-flowing breath, your whole being quickly blossoms into full aliveness.

Breathing is so important because every cell of the body requires a constant supply of oxygen for the energy-generating process of metabolism to proceed properly. At the cellular level, the process of taking in oxygen and giving off carbon dioxide is called *cellular respiration,* a process intimately tied to the absorption of nutrients, the elimination of wastes, and the oxidation of fuel into energy. Sustaining a free-flowing breath for the duration of a yoga session stimulates cellular respiration and increases metabolism throughout the body, uplifting the health of each and every cell.

> *Deep, rhythmic breathing is the king of all exercises. Under conditions of heightened respiration, the heart, arteries, capillaries, veins, and lungs perform many days' labor in only a few hours. As blood circulation increases, basic nutrients are distributed to all the tissues in the body. Waste products accumulating in the cells are eliminated into the veins. Indeed, one can comprehend the significance of all forms of exercise by understanding this process alone. The body parts are moved merely to churn and stimulate the respiratory process.*
>
> —Swami Kripalu

The breath is also intimately tied to the mind and emotions. When the mind is agitated by anger or fear, the breath grows rapid, shallow, and irregular. When the mind is calm and focused, the breath flows slowly and smoothly. Understanding this relationship of breath and mental state is a key component of yoga practice because it works both ways. By regulating the flow and quality of the breath, the emotions can be brought into balance and the mind made calm and clear.

It seems counterintuitive that anyone would need to learn to do something as natural as breathing freely and deeply. Why do we restrict our breathing? One answer is that tightening the belly muscles is a natural short-term response to stress that dulls our ability to feel and protects us physically and emotionally. If this response becomes habitual, it creates a host of undesirable consequences. Through the practice of being

PRANA, THE LIFE FORCE

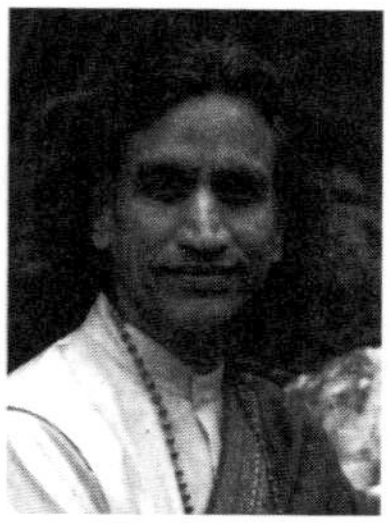

The yogis of ancient India perceived in meditation that the physical body is animated by a flow of life force intimately connected to the breath. They named this force *prana* and carefully mapped its flow through a network of pathways called the *subtle body*, which closely resembles the nervous system. Rhythmic breathing or *pranayama* acts like a pump to charge the system with life force. Postures encourage its flow through body and mind. When prana flows freely, health and well-being naturally result. Yogi Amrit Desai, the originator of Kripalu Yoga, was one of the first Indian yogis to bring a comprehensive set of teachings on prana to America.

present and breath awareness, Kripalu Yoga returns us to full feeling and releases chronic muscular and emotional tension. Unless practiced with sensitivity to the breath, yoga postures fall far short of their potential to foster healing and growth.

> *The first time I walked into a Kripalu Yoga class, I was used to feeling edgy and hard. We started in Corpse Pose and moved into some gentle warm-ups, encouraged to keep the gaze soft and feel sensation. When the teacher directed us to focus on the breath, suddenly things started changing. In all my pushing and striving, I had forgotten the breath! I began to feel the breath moving through my body, beyond my lungs. My hardness softened just a little, and I retracted my pointy edges. Not only was that okay, it was a relief. I knew then the battle I had been living was of my own making, and I didn't have to keep fighting.*
>
> —Jennifer Cann

Breathing Deeply

Most people have become accustomed to a breath pattern that limits their vital capacity. They are *chest breathers*, taking rapid and shallow breaths, often through the mouth, with a lift of the shoulders and minimal use of the diaphragm and blood-rich lower lungs. Or they are *belly breathers*, breathing more slowly and deeply but prone to have a rigid and inflexible chest due to minimal use of the intercostal muscles that expand chest capacity and inflate the upper lungs.

While breathing habits do not change overnight, the body has the innate capacity—and a hunger—to breathe deeply. The practice of Kripalu Yoga is designed to gently but steadily remove the obstacles that prevent you from breathing freely and deeply. It works in two ways to expand your vital capacity. It strengthens the abdominal muscles, diaphragm, and intercostal muscles to make full use of the lungs. It also releases physical tensions and emotional blocks that often inhibit deep breathing.

I breathe in All That Is—
Awareness expanding
to take everything in,
as if my heart beats
the world into being.

From the unnamed
vastness beneath the
mind, I breathe my
way to wholeness
and healing.

Inhalation. Exhalation.
Each breath a "yes,"
and a letting go,
a journey, and a
coming home.

EXPERIENCE: BREATHING FREELY

The ability to let the breath flow is learned through the technique of *Ocean Sounding Breath*, traditionally called *Ujjayi Pranayama*. The word *ujjayi* means *great* or *victorious sound*. Ocean Sounding Breath relaxes the body, calms the mind, and increases the flow of energy through the nervous system. You may sit in a chair, as in the instructions below, or comfortably on the floor.

1. Sit near the front edge of a chair. Adjust the feet so they are hip-width apart and parallel. Rest the hands palms up on the thighs. Elongate the spine by pressing the sitz bones down and extending through the crown of the head. Bring the chin parallel to the floor. Resist any tendency to lean against the chair back, which rounds the spine, compresses the abdomen, and restricts the free flow of breath.

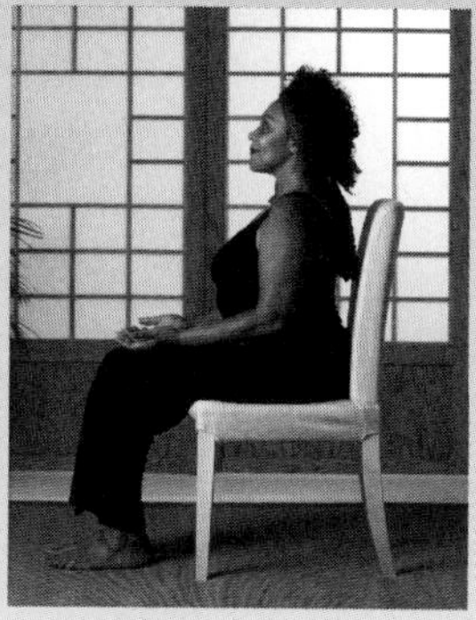

2. Close the eyes and focus your attention on the flow of the breath.

3. To come into Ocean Sounding Breath, slightly contract the back of the throat, allowing the friction of the breath against the glottis to make a sound like the rise and fall of waves against the beach.

4. If you have trouble making the ocean sound, imagine that you are holding a mirror a few inches from your mouth. Open your mouth and exhale to "fog the mirror." Repeat this several times, and then try making the same sound exhaling with your mouth closed. Then try it on the inhalation. Continue to practice until you can sustain the ocean sound inhaling and exhaling with the mouth closed.

5. Experiment with varying the volume of sound. First make the sound clearly audible, loud enough to easily be heard by a person standing ten feet away. Then let the sound soften to a volume where you can easily hear it but a person standing a few feet away from you would not. Allow the gentle sound of your breath to be a soothing point of focus that anchors the mind in the sound and sensation of breathing.

6. Smooth out the flow of breath by shifting between in-breaths and out-breaths as smoothly as possible. This creates an unbroken circle of breaths, one flowing easily into the next.

7. Sustain Ocean Sounding Breath for several minutes.

8. Release any conscious control of the breath, allowing the breath to naturally rebalance. Feel the effects, noticing if this flowing breath has left you feeling any different than when you started.

When I first started practicing, there was no way I could sustain Ocean Sounding Breath for more than a few minutes at a time. I would simply forget and when I remembered three postures later reengage the breath. Over time, I discovered that staying focused on the breath during postures was a way to deepen my attention and draw it powerfully inward. I liked that experience and it motivated me to learn how to sustain a flowing breath. Now breathing is as much a part of my practice as postures.

—Danna Faulds

Sustain a Flowing Breath

Ocean Sounding Breath is designed to help you sustain a flowing breath during the practice of warm-ups and yoga postures. Simply breathe in and out in a smooth and uniform flow, focusing on the sound and sensation of the breath. At first you may find it a significant challenge to restrain the natural urge to hold the breath as you move and stretch. Slowing down the speed of your movements and avoiding irregular or jerky motions helps keep the breath flowing in a regular rhythm.

Don't make the common mistake of straining to breathe deeply, which is unnatural when doing postures that involve the contraction or compression of the torso. Let the pace and depth of the breath be established by the type of movement or posture you are performing. In some postures, you will find it easy to sustain a longer and deeper breath. In others, the breath will naturally be shorter and shallower. When you are able to sustain a flowing Ocean Sounding Breath, you can shift your focus from breathing smoothly to breathing slowly and deeply. In the beginning, simply sustain a flowing breath.

Breathe Through the Nostrils

Learn to breathe with the mouth closed and air flowing through the nostrils. The idea is not to actively sniff the air in and out with your nose. The air is drawn into the lungs and then expelled by the large and powerful movements of the abdomen, diaphragm, and chest. En route to the lungs, it passes freely through the nostrils, which remain relaxed and passive. Breathing through the nose warms and filters that air before it enters the lungs. Yoga teaches that breathing through the nose has more subtle benefits, helping to maximize the amount of life force absorbed by the body during the breathing process. Many people find this way of breathing easy right from the start. Others have to work at it for a bit before it feels natural.

Ocean Sounding Breath is essential to Kripalu Yoga. Master this technique separately, then integrate it with your postures.

—Yogi Amrit Desai

EXPERIENCE: BREATHING DEEPLY

The ability to breathe deeply is learned in Three-Part Breathing, traditionally called *Dirgha Pranayama.* The word *dirgha* means *slow* and *deep.* The name "three-part" comes from the movement of the diaphragm, rib cage, and upper chest. Three-Part Breathing is one of the simplest and most beneficial of all yoga exercises. After a long day at work, ten minutes of Three-Part Breathing can quickly relax and rejuvenate you.

1. Lie on your back with the legs extended and symmetrically placed about a foot apart. Bring the hands to rest on the lower belly with the fingertips a few inches below the navel. Let the whole body relax and sink into the floor. If it is uncomfortable for you to lie flat on the floor, try placing a pillow beneath the knees. You can also draw the feet up toward the buttocks, about hip-width apart, and let the inside of the knees fall together to support each other.

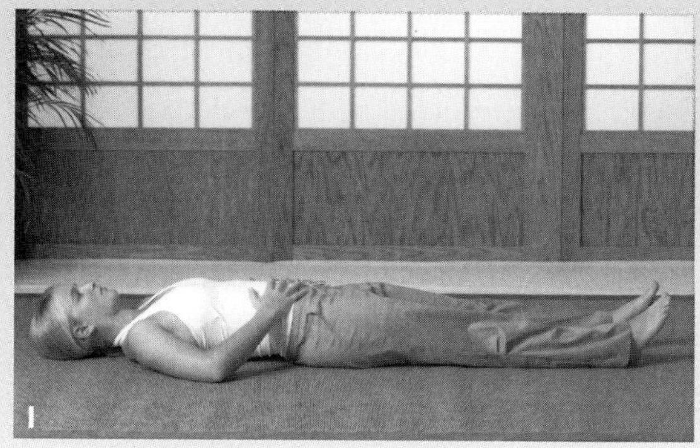

2. Close the eyes and focus your attention on the flow of the breath. Come into the Ocean Sounding Breath, and gradually smooth out the flow of breath by letting in-breaths and out-breaths flow smoothly one into the next. Let your breath flow freely for a minute or two, simply feeling and watching the process of breathing.

3. Now come into *abdominal breathing* by relaxing the belly and letting the diaphragm move freely. Feel the movement of the belly and diaphragm with your hands. The belly rises as the diaphragm descends on the inhalation, bringing air into the lungs. The belly falls as the diaphragm lifts on the exhalation. Repeat this ocean sounding abdominal breath several times.

4. Bring the fingers to rest on the ribs to come into *mid-chest breathing*. Building on the abdominal breath, let the rib cage begin to expand out to the sides, bringing additional air into the lungs. Then exhale completely, allowing the breath to flow out of the lungs in the most relaxed and natural way. As the breath flows, feel the movement of the rib cage with your hands. Repeat this ocean sounding abdominal and mid-chest breath several times.

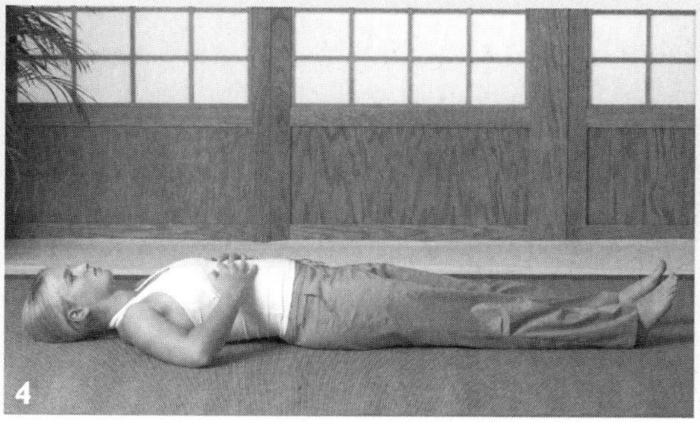

5. Bring the hands to rest on the upper chest and continue this process of deepening the breath by coming into Three-Part Breathing. Slowly take in a breath, letting the diaphragm descend and belly lift. Then let the rib cage expand out to the sides. Allow the breath to flow all the way up to lift the collarbones, feeling the movement of the upper chest with your hands as the lungs are completely filled. Then exhale completely, allowing the breath to flow out of the lungs in the most relaxed and natural way. At the end of exhalation, empty the lungs by gently contracting the abdominal and intercostal muscles, squeezing out residual air.

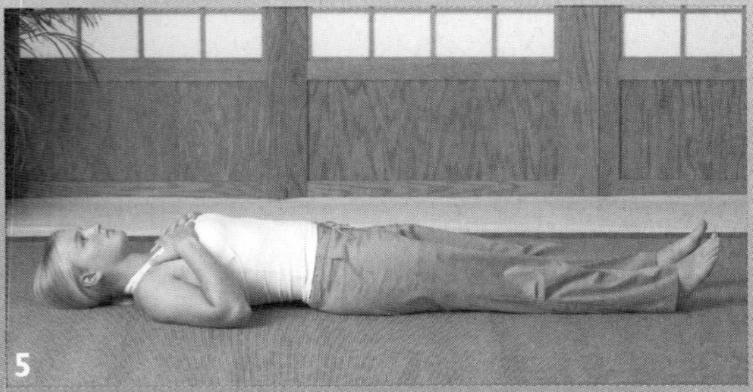
5

6. Place your right hand on your belly, just below the navel, and your left hand on the center of your chest. This hand position helps you feel all the phases of the breathing process. Repeat this slow and smooth Three-Part Breath for several minutes, filling and emptying the lungs completely, and closely attending the movement of the belly, diaphragm, rib cage, and upper chest.

7. Bring the arms to the sides with the hands palms up in what is called *Corpse Pose*. Let go of any conscious control of the breath, watching the flow of breath return to balance. Relax completely, drinking in the effects of deep breathing. Notice any sensations of openness, energy, or relaxation in the abdomen and chest. Observe any shifts in the quality of your mental awareness.

Expect Mild Resistance

Shifting your breath pattern alters your physical and mental state in significant ways. It is common to encounter momentary resistance to this process in the form of mild feelings of light-headedness, anxiety, irritation, lethargy, or mental agitation. Much like a distance runner who starts slowly and gradually finds their stride, you will learn to recognize these feelings as the sure sign that you are shifting into a more dynamic state of being. With practice, you will pass through this resistance and hardly notice it. When starting out, it can be a source of concern. If the feelings are extreme or persist, stop practice and check with your physician before continuing.

> *I've learned that I am practicing Kripalu Yoga with every breath I take. Some breaths are like the sound of the ocean and come naturally in yoga postures. Others are more mindful and meditative. Some are sighs in the shower. Others come*

as I skip along la-di-da. *And then there are those exasperated sighs of moms worldwide at four* PM, *all pooped out from mothering. Lucky moms who practice yoga know they can always come back to the breath to relax, recharge, and make it through until the kids go to sleep.*

—Diane Pomante Brav

Make Your Breathing Circular

With a little practice, you will notice that the breath tends to become unsteady at two different moments during its cyclic movement in and out of the body. The breath flutters during the pause that occurs at the end of the exhalation, just before the inhale begins. The breath flutters again, although slightly less pronounced, during the pause that occurs at the end of inhalation, just before the exhale begins.

As you notice this tendency for the breath to become momentarily unsteady at the junctures of in- and out-breaths, you can begin to consciously smooth out the breath. Allow the in-breath to flow smoothly into the out-breath, and the out-breath to flow smoothly into the in-breath. The audible sound of the Ocean Sounding Breath is helpful here. Make the sound of the breath almost constant, with just a relaxed moment of silence between in- and out-breaths that is barely perceptible. Don't strain to eliminate a natural pause between in- and out-breaths, just shift gears smoothly from one phase to the next.

The ability to sustain a smoothly flowing breath is one of the keys to deepening your ability to concentrate and remain fully present for the duration of yoga practice. Through it, you learn firsthand how closely the mind and breath are linked, seeing that the mind is prone to distraction exactly during those moments when the breath becomes unsteady. Simply by smoothing out the breath, you greatly enhance your ability to sustain mental focus.

Never a morning person, I always needed several cups of coffee to get my eyes open. Now I'm getting up forty-five minutes earlier to have time for yoga. And what a difference! I'm listening to my body to tell me what it needs to wake and limber up. I usually start right off with breathing, which really sets the stage for my practice. Somewhere near the middle I do Breath of Joy which energizes me and helps me move into the more rigorous poses. Being in menopause, the mental clarity my practice gives me is also a huge benefit, as it counters the "brainfog" that visits women in this time of life. When I use the breath, Kripalu Yoga is a body prayer that opens my mind to what is possible.

—Gail Barraco

Maintain an Even Breath

During your practice of postures, let your in-breaths and out-breaths be of equal length. In other words, take about the same amount of time to breathe in as you do to breathe out. This is called an *even breath,* which provides the oxygen and energy you need to move dynamically through a series of yoga postures. As your practice deepens, you will be able to lengthen the breath while maintaining this even ratio of inhalation to exhalation.

After postures and just before entering deep relaxation, you will be guided to lengthen your exhalations, making them roughly twice as long as your inhalations. This *relaxing breath* decreases heart rate, lowers blood pressure, and helps you enter a state of deep relaxation.

Allow Breath and Posture to Interact

You will notice that most postures enhance some phase of the breathing process and restrict another. The Sphinx, for example, makes you breathe in and out of the upper chest by restricting the movement of the diaphragm. The Bridge restricts the movement of the upper chest, allowing the belly to balloon in and out as you breathe diaphragmatically. The Twist alternately compresses the right then the left side of the chest, shifting breath flow from one lung to the other. This enhancement and restriction is a beneficial part of the practice, as a balanced series of postures isolates and strengthens all phases of the respiratory system. Just sustain a flowing Ocean Sounding Breath, breathing as deeply as you comfortably can, while entering, holding, and releasing the posture. After each posture, you may want to take a deep breath in and then let out an audible sigh to release tension. As you become comfortable in the postures, you will find yourself naturally lengthening and deepening the breath as you hold.

Coordinate Breath and Motion

Kripalu Yoga postures are always performed in coordination with the breath. This synchronization of breath and motion makes movement smooth and graceful. When coupled with an internal focus of awareness, it also makes Kripalu Yoga an experience of moving meditation.

As you practice conscious breathing and yoga postures, you will notice that the flow of breath naturally inspires and initiates movement. As you open the chest in a backward bend, the breath naturally flows in. As you fold the body to bend forward, the breath naturally flows out. As you twist to one side, abdomen and chest are compressed, making the breath flow out. As you come out of the twist, the chest opens and the breath naturally flows in. As you move through your yoga postures, remain sensitive to this natural coordination of breath and motion. All posture instructions include specific directions on how to coordinate breath and motion.

> *The beauty of Kripalu Yoga is that postures, pranayama, and meditation are all happening simultaneously—not separately.*
>
> — Swami Kripalu

EXPERIENCE: COORDINATING BREATH AND MOTION

Explore this simple flow of movements called *Sun Breath* to experience how natural it is to coordinate breath and motion.

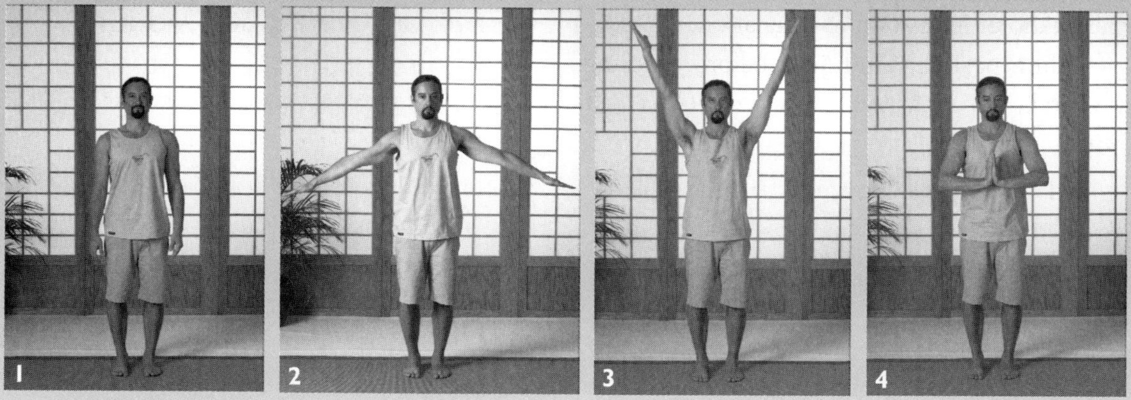

1. Stand tall with the arms at your sides and come into Ocean Sounding Breath.

2. As you begin to inhale, slowly sweep the arms out to the sides, palms facing down, and up to shoulder height.

3. Continue to inhale as the arms lift into a wide V with the palms facing up. The eyes continue to look straight ahead.

4. Begin to exhale and slowly lower the hands into Prayer Position in front of the chest. Continue to exhale as the hands return to the sides.

5. Repeat this flowing movement, synchronizing the speed of your arm motion with the length of your breath. The inhalation completes just as the palms turn upward. The exhalation completes just as the palms return to the sides.

6. If this motion is easy for you, experiment with inhaling the arms all the way overhead, palms facing and shoulder-width apart. Then exhale the hands through Prayer Position and down to the sides.

7. After a few minutes of breathing and moving, come back into stillness. Feel all the sensations present in your body. Notice the felt sense of your arms, shoulders, and chest. Did anything shift for you during this experience?

Breathing Your Way into Postures

BY SENIOR TEACHER YOGANAND MICHAEL CARROLL

Twenty-seven years later, I still remember the ease and grace with which my first yoga teacher demonstrated the postures. Still a teenager, I felt so awkward trying to emulate her flowing movement. She said the secret lay hidden in the breath and attempted to teach me Ujjayi Pranayama. Under her watchful eye, I couldn't even make the ocean sound. Her compassionate coaxing only made me more self-conscious, and the sound stuck more firmly in my throat.

I had no inkling back then that I would join the residential staff of Kripalu Center and dedicate myself to practicing and teaching yoga, especially pranayama. I soon learned that there is a split in the yoga world as to when pranayama should be taught. Some traditions consider pranayama an advanced practice meant only for those who have attained a measure of mastery in asana. As a result, they make minimal use of the breath in leading students into and out of postures. Other traditions incorporate yogic breathing right from the start. Kripalu Yoga fits into the second category. Swami Kripalu even instructed inflexible students who found it difficult to do postures to practice pranayama for one month before beginning a posture practice.

Yogic breathing brings you more in touch with your inner state. Practice begins as you sit down, close your eyes, and take a few long and slow breaths. Before even a few breaths have passed, the external world starts to fade into the background. The inner world begins to blossom. Subtle sensory input from the body that only moments ago was drowned out by the deluge of sight and sound rises into awareness. You become highly aware of sensation, of the tenseness or tiredness in your muscles, and of the emotional tugs that might be pulling you away from your present experience. Pranayama is what makes asana come alive.

Like myself years ago, you might think it would be easier to learn the postures if you just forgot about breathing. My experience is that the inner attunement that results from conscious breathing is an important quality to bring to posture practice right from the start. By increasing sensitivity to the felt sense of your body, yogic breathing provides a layer of safety that is not there when you are focused externally. This increased sensitivity also helps you feel the benefits you are deriving from the postures and drink them in more deeply.

Everyone begins posture practice aligning the body from the outside by looking at their arms and legs, or seeing someone else a little further along in their practice. While students often seem comfortable with this level of practice, as a teacher I know that something is missing. It's time to soften the gaze, breathe, and attune to the flow of energy. By adding pranayama to the mix, you will find yourself aligning from the inside out, breathing to expand fully into the pose, or adjusting slightly to bring the body into a position that feels more supported or releases tension. Pranayama brings you in touch with the body's love of stretching. It teaches you how to flow through the postures and naturally move deeper into a stretch by responding to an inner urge. As my teacher said, the secret is in the breath.

C H A P T E R   T H R E E

A MARRIAGE OF STRETCH AND STRENGTH

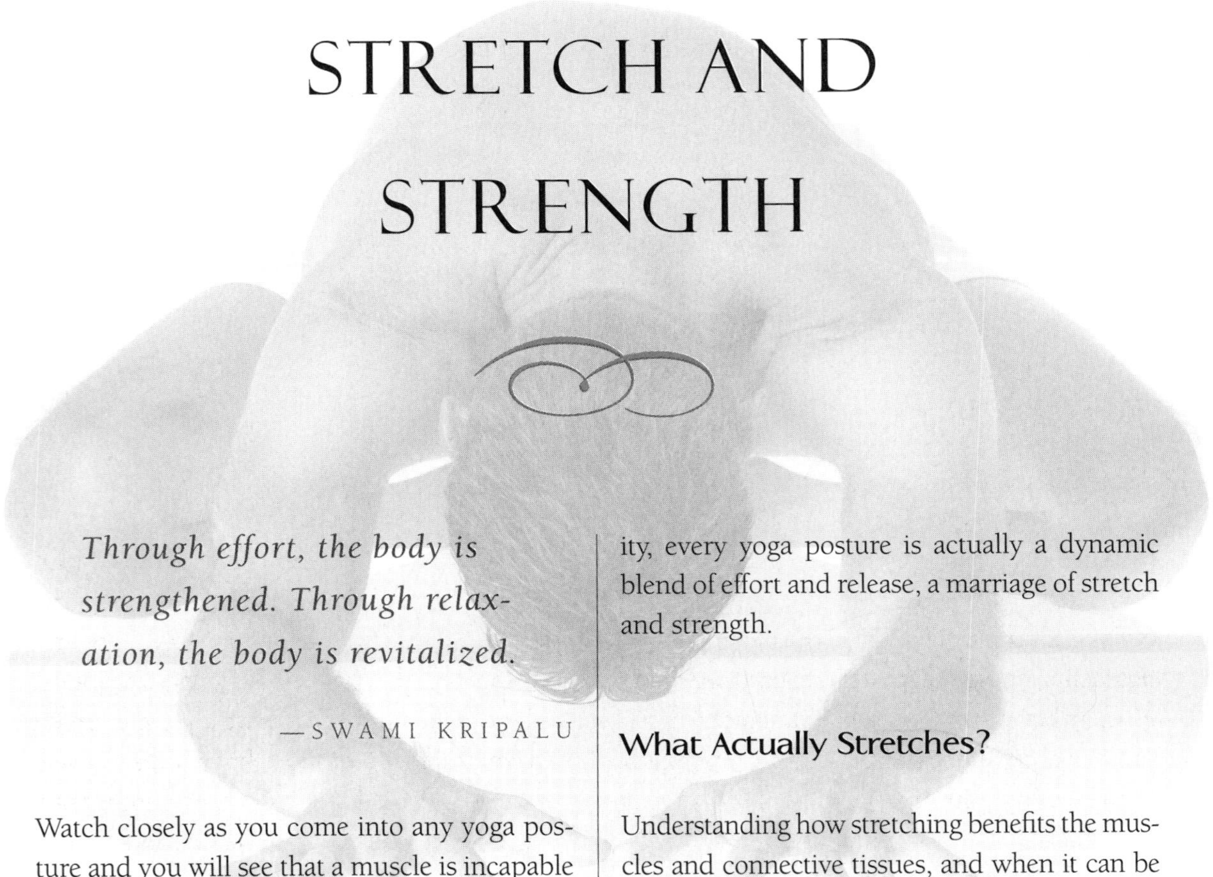

Through effort, the body is strengthened. Through relaxation, the body is revitalized.

—SWAMI KRIPALU

Watch closely as you come into any yoga posture and you will see that a muscle is incapable of stretching itself. The sensation of stretch is generated when certain muscles contract to exert a force on other muscles that relax and lengthen. It is this combination of active contraction and passive lengthening that is so beneficial to the body, simultaneously increasing both strength and flexibility. Although people equate yoga with stretching to increase flexibility, every yoga posture is actually a dynamic blend of effort and release, a marriage of stretch and strength.

What Actually Stretches?

Understanding how stretching benefits the muscles and connective tissues, and when it can be harmful, is essential to safe practice. On a basic level, you are working to stretch the approximately six hundred skeletal muscles. Skeletal muscles are composed of thousands of microscopic muscle fibers. A protective fibrous sheath called *fascia* surrounds each individual fiber, groups the fibers together in bundles, and also encases the entire muscle. What we call muscle is actually this complex of fibers, fascia, and associated blood vessels and nerves. Muscle tissue stretches easily and can be safely lengthened up to 50 percent of its resting length.

Muscles attach to the bones with *tendons,* tough cords of connective tissue that do not stretch easily. By smoothly transferring the force of muscular contraction to the bones, tendons give us the ability to move freely and easily. Designed to bear forces within a specified range, tendons begin to tear and suffer other deformities when subject to forces that stretch them beyond a mere 4 percent. Similar in composition to tendons, *ligaments* are sturdy inelastic tissues that join bone to bone. By keeping the bones aligned, ligaments protect the *joint capsule,* a bag of connective tissue that secretes and holds the synovial fluid that lubricates the joint.

Simply stated, yoga postures are intended to stretch the highly elastic skeletal muscles and fascia. Stretching should never subject the body to extreme forces that strain tendons and ligaments, cause the joints to exceed the limits of their bony structure, or risk damage to the joint capsule. Repeated trauma of this nature destabilizes a joint, compromising its strength and making movement painful.

> *My husband and I adopted a little girl in 1996. Everything was perfect, except that I grew so focused on my daughter that I gradually phased yoga out of my life. I began to experience pain in my joints, my hands refused to open jars, numbness in my feet gave me trouble walking up and down the stairs. Doing simple things became a struggle, and I felt like I was ninety-three years old. I went to an arthritis specialist, who prescribed medication. Although I seldom take medication, I eventually succumbed to its lure because the pain was unbearable. After ten months of this, I turned back to Kripalu Yoga in desperation. I began going to classes regularly and practicing at home. Gradually the joint pain and numbness melted away. A year later, I feel good and my joints are pain-free. I make time for yoga, because it continues to change my life for the better.*
>
> —Diane Pomante Brav

How Is Stretching Beneficial?

Stretching is unparalleled in its ability to maintain the health of the joints, muscles, and connective tissues on which full and free movement depends. Stretching "oils the joints" with synovial fluid and is a way to warm up for vigorous activity that is known to prevent movement-related injuries. More important, stretching helps maintain the resilient state of these soft tissues, known as *suppleness,* which allows movement to be graceful and pain-free. Soft tissues suffer from either underuse or overuse. Underuse subjects them to the stress of atrophy, which leaves muscles, tendons, and ligaments brittle and weak. Overuse causes strains, tears, and ruptures. By working the elastic muscle tissues, and applying moderate forces that pull tendons and ligaments to their full working length, stretching keeps the soft tissues healthy and supple.

Releasing Muscle Tension

Voluntary skeletal muscles are designed to contract when you need to move and take action. Task completed, the muscles relax and return to their resting muscle tone. Contrary to this natural design, people often hold parts of their body in a state of mild or moderate contraction. Almost everyone is familiar with this kind of excess muscle tension, which easily builds up over the course of a challenging day. The contraction and relaxation of the skeletal muscles is governed by the nervous system. Excess muscle tension is believed to be the result of the unconscious firing of motor neurons in the spinal cord, which produces a low-level contraction of the muscles.

Energy is required to contract any muscle, and holding a contraction is a constant energy drain that can leave you feeling fatigued and sore. If the muscle tension is in the belly or chest, it restricts breathing. Contraction of neck, shoulder, and upper back muscles constricts blood flow to the brain, one cause of "tension headaches." Contraction of the back muscles can lead to painful muscle spasms and pull the spinal vertebrae out of alignment, pinching delicate nerves and impeding their proper function. Excess muscle tension is also a known cause of insomnia, which further depletes your energy.

A delicious stretch is nature's way to turn off these motor neurons that have somehow become stuck in the ON position. When held for several flowing breaths, a good stretch gives you the pleasurable sensation of release as muscles let go and return to a resting muscle tone. A balanced routine systematically frees the body of accumulated tension. The result is an overall feeling of relaxation and a sense of coming home to your natural state of being.

> *Back in 1990, I was the mother of an eight-month-old daughter and a two-and-a-half-year-old son. My husband and I were exhausted, our finances were strained, and our relationship was flat. The kids were in day care, supper was in the Crock-Pot, and I was gone most of the time at work and school. Under the pressure of all that, I was living on caffeine and nicotine, not taking care of myself, and pretending like crazy that everything was all right in my world. When my therapist recommended yoga, I thought: "Ha . . . Like when could I fit in a yoga class?" But I managed to locate a Kripalu Yoga teacher and eventually walk into a quiet, peaceful place. We were reminded to breathe. Then we stretched and moved and sighed and softened. Something inside me melted, just a little. We were invited to release tension from our bodies, to let go of whatever we were holding, and remember that each of us was perfect, just the way we were.*

DOORBELLS AND STATIC

Frederick Matthias Alexander (1869–1955) was an Australian pioneer in body-mind integration who developed the *Alexander Technique*, a system of movement and awareness training exercises designed to help actors and artists. Alexander said that healthy nerves and muscles work like a doorbell. When the doorbell is pushed, the muscles contract. The moment the doorbell is released, the muscles return to a relaxed state. Chronically tight muscles work like a light switch. When the switch is turned on, the muscles stay contracted until the switch is turned off. Each yoga posture is an opportunity to consciously turn off the nervous system signals that lie at the root of muscular holding.

In his book *Staying Supple*, athlete John Jerome attributes the painful kernels, knots, and spasms that make muscle tissues sore in part to what he calls *neuromuscular noise*. If muscles contract in response to neural signals, Jerome reasons that they must fail to relax because they are still getting some kind of residual signals from the nervous system. Conscious stretching is a way to tune the body radio and minimize the neuromuscular static that causes excess muscle tension.

When it came time for relaxation, I drank it in. Ahhhh. That moment I woke up to the potential of taking care of myself and having a happy, loving life with my husband and children. This revelation didn't change things right away. It took time, love, consistency, and commitment. I was able to make these changes because my yoga practice kept reminding me that it was important to do this work.

—Sheila deMagalhaes

Relieving Muscle Soreness

Excess muscle tension can become so habitual and unconscious that you believe it is just the way your body feels, and it is common for people to blame aging for their increasing symptoms. A chronically tense muscle cuts off its own circulation, depriving itself and surrounding tissues of needed oxygen and nutrients. Inadequate blood flow causes lactic acids and other metabolic wastes to accumulate in the cells, resulting in the tight spots and knots that you can feel when massaging a sore muscle. Many physical therapists and sports trainers believe this kind of tightness predisposes you to muscle fatigue, aches, and pains. If the condition persists, it can cause the belly of the muscle to shorten, leaving it spindly and associated connective tissue weakened and prone to injury. Chronic muscle tension is also a suspected factor in a host of stress-related disorders and diseases such as insomnia, backaches, digestive problems, cancer, heart disease, and strokes.

Stretching is the universal prescription to remedy soreness and revitalize the soft tissues. A balanced routine done regularly addresses the underlying cause of painful symptoms: chronic tension. Within the muscle tissues themselves, the healthy pull of stretching is believed to realign the muscle fibers, fascia, blood vessels, and nerves. By working the muscles and lengthening out tendons and ligaments, stretching stimulates the tissues to eliminate their biochemical backlog of lactic acid and other residues of fatigue. This is why stretching is used therapeutically to heal injuries. It's also why stretching is done as a cooldown to minimize the negative effects of vigorous activity.

Preserving Range of Motion

Range of motion varies from person to person, even between individuals who are healthy and fit. It is dependent on your genetic inheritance and how you have used your body over the course of your lifetime. Even athletes seeking top performance do not benefit from attaining maximum or extreme joint flexibility. What constitutes ideal flexibility depends on the unique structure of your body and the activities in which you engage on a regular basis.

Kripalu Yoga does not aim to create extreme joint flexibility. It articulates the major joints of the body, helping you preserve a range of motion that allows you to feel good in your body. Practically speaking, this means that your expression of a yoga posture may be different than the photos in this book or your classmate's pose. While some forms of the classic yoga postures are safe and beneficial for the large majority of people, the degree to which individuals can do them varies considerably.

As we age, range of motion becomes a matter of "move it or lose it." Understanding fascia, and how it responds to aging and injury, makes it clear why stretching is an effective tool to maintain the body's ability to move freely and easily. Fascia does more than encase your muscles; it is literally the substance that holds the body together. Multiple layers of fascia underlie the skin, binding the body's different parts into one flexible piece. Fascia separates the body into various compartments and cavities, surrounds organs and glands, and encases bones, nerves, and blood vessels as well as muscle.

When healthy, the fascia casing of muscles is a slippery surface. By providing the lubrication needed for muscles to freely change their shape, fascia allows the forces generated by muscular contraction to be smoothly transmitted to the bones. If areas of muscular fascia lose lubrication, muscles feel tight. If fascia adheres to other tissues, extreme stiffness results, and we lose our freedom of movement.

Fascia shrinkage is a normal part of the aging process, and some associated reduction in range of motion can be anticipated. That said, most of the loss in freedom of movement experienced as people grow older is not the result of aging. It is the result of a sedentary lifestyle, which causes the fascia to respond by contracting to support a limited range of motion. If injuries immobilize body parts for prolonged periods of time, fascia shrinkage and adhesion can further aggravate the problem. In general, we don't get stiff because we get old. We get stiff because we gradually stop making full use of our bodies.

Stretching is a highly effective way to support the health of your fascia, minimize its rate of contraction, and prevent it from restricting movement in major ways by adhering to other tissues. If you are seeking to regain lost mobility, stretching gently into areas of tightness and holding there with a flowing breath is a proven way to gradually restore the flexibility of fascia and expand range of motion to healthy limits. Going too hard and fast will be counterproductive, as the fascia will respond to forceful stretching as trauma and contract even more.

Why Strength Training?

Muscular strength is not just a concern of bodybuilders; it is an essential component of a happy and healthy life. Starting in middle age, both men and women begin to lose muscle tissue and bone mass. Since muscle tissue consumes more calories than fat, the progressive loss of muscle mass lowers metabolism and is believed to be an underlying cause of the weight gain many people experience as they grow older. As muscle tissue is slowly replaced by fat, a person falls prey to creeping obesity as their body needs fewer and fewer calories to

BENEFITS OF STRETCHING

- Eases movement by "oiling the joints" with synovial fluid
- Preserves range of motion by keeping muscles and connective tissues healthy and supple
- Releases excess muscle tension and facilitates relaxation
- Relieves muscle soreness
- Is a good warm-up to vigorous activity that helps prevent injuries
- Is a good cooldown from vigorous activity that helps realign soft tissues and eliminate the chemical residues of fatigue

sustain itself. In addition, women are especially prone to bone loss and osteoporosis.

Strength training is a proven way to slow this loss of muscle tissue and bone mass. It is known to increase energy, improve stamina, make one less prone to injury, and reduce the incidence of everyday aches and pains. Where physical strength helps one feel up to a challenge, a lack of strength makes routine activities like household chores or gardening feel like a burden. Simply standing upright and walking about requires a balance of muscular strength throughout the body's system of skeletal muscles.

What Makes a Muscle Get Stronger?

Muscular fitness is actually a combination of *strength* and *endurance*. Strength is the force a muscle can exert in a single effort. Endurance is the muscle's ability to make repeated or prolonged efforts at less than full exertion. Muscles gain strength and endurance when subject to increasing demands that systematically challenge them to perform beyond existing limits.

Progressive overloading is the term for the process that builds muscle mass and strength. Overloading a muscle within healthy limits is believed to cause microscopic tears in the muscle fibers, which the body repairs by attracting proteins that build muscle mass. There are many approaches to strength training, the most common being weight lifting or working with resistance-training machines. Yoga postures use the resistance generated by the weight of the body. Endurance is built as postures are held for longer periods of time. Strength is increased by doing more challenging postures.

When practiced with body alignment, yoga tones the musculature, developing a balanced strength throughout the abdomen, chest, back, and limbs. This kind of strength holds the spine and skeleton in good posture and provides a coordinated impetus for graceful movement. Although you will probably not "bulk up" through Kripalu Yoga, regular practice will define your musculature. Because it is produced by doing postures that are always shifting the body's relationship to gravity, yoga can also help prevent the falls that can prove so devastating as we age.

I began practicing yoga for its well-known benefits of flexibility and health. Before long, I discovered that I was getting physically stronger. I was certainly stretching as I held yoga postures like the Warrior and Bridge, but parts of my body that had always been chronically weak were also gaining strength. That was an aspect of yoga practice I never anticipated. Later, I realized that these physical benefits were mirrored by emotional and mental shifts as well. My inner resolve grew stronger. My ability to stretch past perceived limits of fear or doubt noticeably increased. I stopped viewing myself as helpless and felt more substantial in the world. Now I actively embrace both the stretch and strength that come from yoga.

—Danna Faulds

BENEFITS OF STRENGTH TRAINING

- Increases energy
- Builds strength, stamina, and endurance
- Improves balance, making you less prone to falls and other injuries
- Increases metabolism, helping you burn more calories
- Helps prevent osteoporosis
- Makes it easier to enjoy both routine and recreational activities

Practicing for Flexibility and Strength

All of the above principles are reflected in the way that Kripalu Yoga postures are entered, held, and released. Flowing into the posture, you isolate the muscles necessary to hold the body in proper alignment. This process takes mental focus and body awareness, as you tease out the effort from the "let go." Completely engage those parts of the body essential to the posture to maximize your gain in strength. Let the rest of the body be passively stretched to maximize your gain in flexibility.

Some people have a tendency to overemphasize the effort, contracting many more muscles than necessary. As a result, they do not progress in terms of flexibility and tension release. Others have a tendency to overemphasize relaxation. They do not engage the active muscles sufficiently to generate a deep stretch or build strength. As you hold the posture, use sensation as a guide to walk the fine line between these two extremes. After holding, release the posture slowly and with full awareness of all the sensations flowing through you. Consciously invite both the muscles that were stretched, and those that were contracted, to let go completely, releasing muscle tension and returning to a state of relaxation.

Flexibility, strength, and endurance are often touted as the key elements of physical fitness. Feel an increase of all three in the experience on page 38.

Criticisms of Yoga

Exercise regimens are often critiqued by various health professionals, and yoga is not without its critics. Here are some common criticisms and Kripalu Yoga's responses.

EXPERIENCE: STRETCHING YOUR WAY INTO DOWNWARD DOG

1. Come onto your hands and knees. Place the hands directly under the shoulders, fingers spread wide. Place the knees directly under the hips, shins, and the tops of the feet on the floor behind you. This is Table Pose.

2. Inhale into the Dog Tilt by lifting the tailbone, letting the belly and mid-spine fall toward the floor, lifting the chin, and looking straight ahead.

3. Exhale into the Cat Stretch by tucking the tailbone under, arching the mid-back up like an angry cat, and tucking the chin into the chest.

4. Begin to flow slowly and smoothly from one stretch to the other, coordinating breath and motion. Initiate the movement with the tailbone and let it ripple through the spine, neck, and head to create a fluid and undulating movement of the spine. Notice where the spine flexes easily, and where it doesn't flex so easily. After several repetitions, come back to Table Pose.

5. Spread the fingers wide apart and curl the toes under. Take a deep breath in. Exhale as you press into the roots of the fingers and balls of the feet to lift the hips up. Keep the knees bent, the back of the neck relaxed, and the spine long. Breathe deeply, giving your body a moment to adjust to this position.

6. Begin to "walk the dog" by bending the left knee and pressing the right heel toward the floor. Repeat on the other side, bending the right knee and pressing the left heel toward

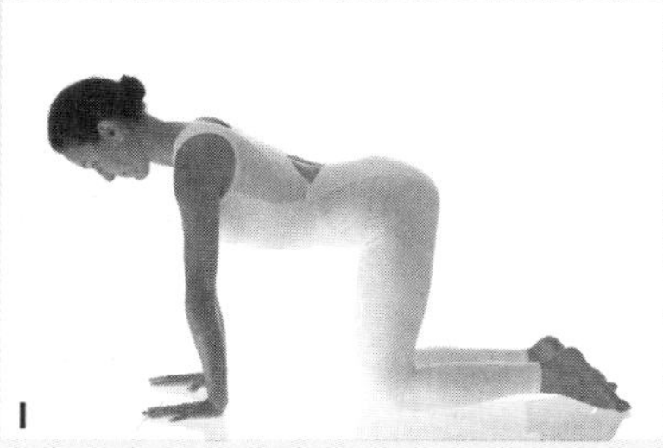
1

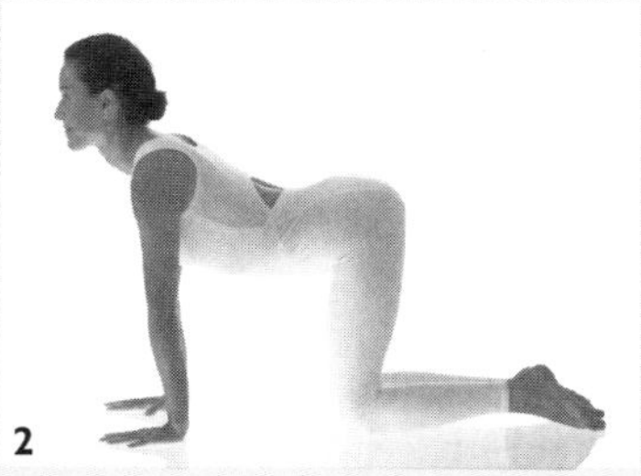
2

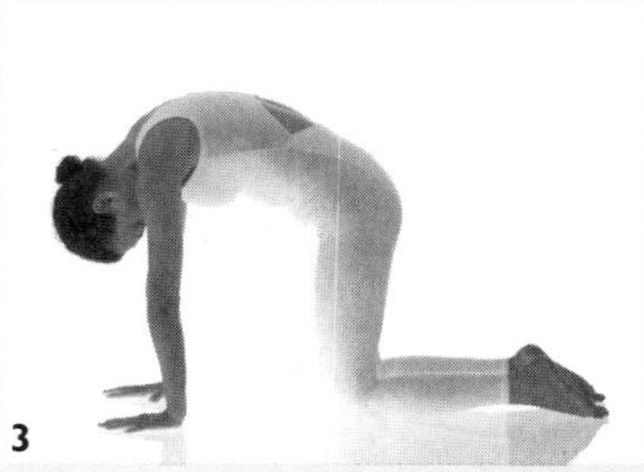
3

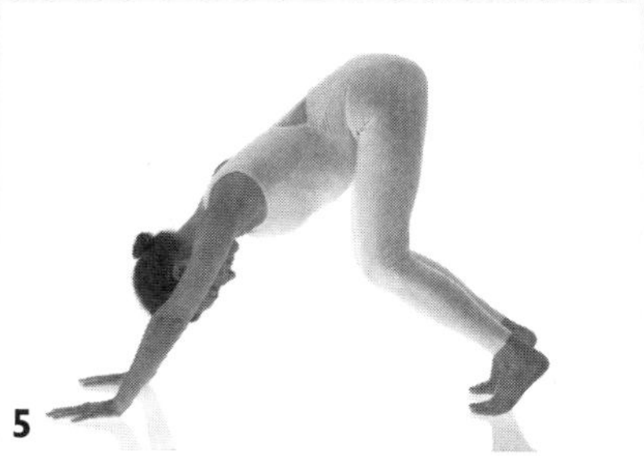
5

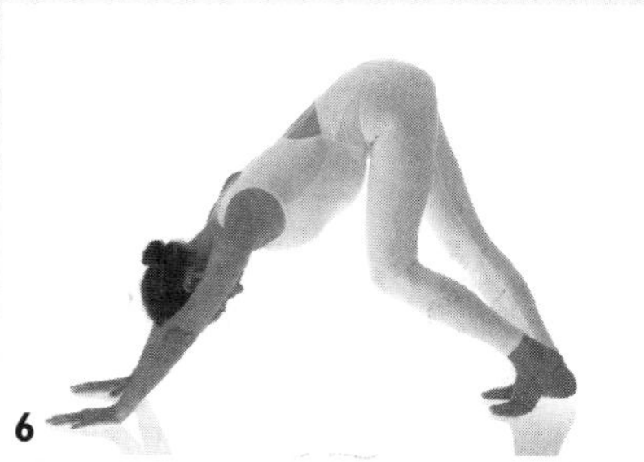
6

the floor. This motion stretches the back of the legs and the muscles diagonally across the back. Flow side to side several times, stretching the legs and letting the hips swivel slightly.

7. Return to Table Pose to rest and catch your breath.

8. Take a deep breath in. Exhale as you once again press into the hands and balls of the feet to lift the hips up. Keeping the knees bent, lift the tailbone toward the ceiling.

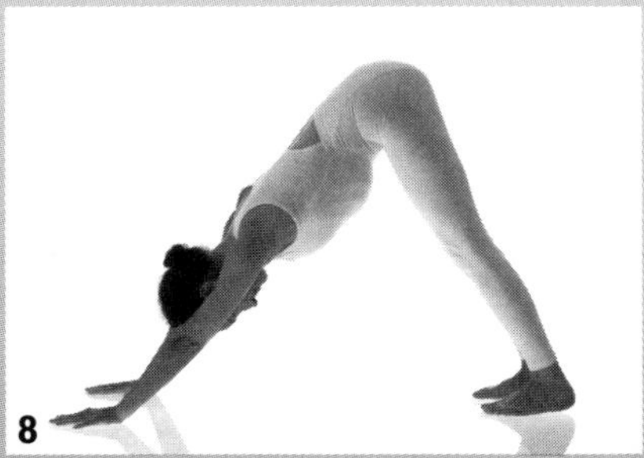
8

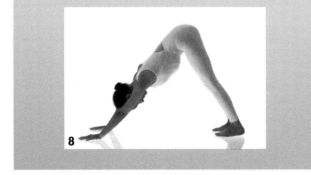

Press the roots of the fingers into the floor, engaging the arms and shoulders. Press the buttocks back toward the wall behind you, straightening the legs and bringing the heels toward the floor. Keep the neck in line with the spine and extend through the crown of the head. Feel the spine being elongated by these movements.

9. Hold the posture with a flowing breath, relaxing everywhere possible, and fully engaging the muscles necessary to keep you in the posture. Feel both the stretching and the strengthening. Stay with the posture, breathing freely and remaining present in your body.

10. To come out of the posture, bend the knees and return to Table Pose. Come onto your back and relax for a minute or two, drinking in all the sensations.

Yoga underemphasizes the need to build strength. Kripalu Yoga aspires to a balance of stretch and strength. It especially focuses on strengthening the core muscles of the torso—belly, chest, and back—that are chronically weak in many people and frequently result in back pain and other common structural problems.

Yoga overemphasizes flexibility. It is true that people new to yoga can strain their lower back with excessive backbending and improper forward bending. Kripalu Yoga teaches you how to use backbends to open the chest and stretch the upper spine without straining the low back or neck. In forward bending, Kripalu Yoga teaches you how to bend forward safely by hinging at the hips rather than round forward from the lumbar spine.

Some yoga postures are dangerous. It is true that the Headstand, Full Shoulderstand, Plough, and Lotus are classic yoga postures that pose a real risk of injury. The Headstand, Full Shoulderstand, and Plough can compress the cervical vertebrae and injure the neck. Lotus requires significant hip flexibility and when forced can result in knee injury. These advanced postures are beneficial when practiced by a person with a high degree of flexibility and overall fitness. None of these postures are presented in this book. If you desire to practice them, work one-on-one with a certified yoga professional.

> *"Pull yourself up by the bootstraps." "Keep a stiff upper lip." These were familiar phrases in my childhood that created a strength of will, fortitude, and a sense of control when times got tough. Although they served me well for many years, these beliefs also brought guilt and low self-esteem when situations became too much for me to handle. I found Kripalu Yoga rather late in life, but it gave me another way to be strong. I not only gained strength physically, but found a way to access my inner strength in a gentler, more forgiving way. When I discovered Kripalu Yoga, a door opened to a place that allows self-expression and an exploration of doubt, physical limitations, and intellectual shortfalls without judgment. Kripalu Yoga helped me discover how to be strong without having to fear being "less than."*
>
> — Gwen Fuller

CHAPTER FOUR

PRACTICING AT THE EDGE

Things really start to happen when you learn how to hold a yoga posture at the edge—a place of neither too much nor too little stretch. Too far back from the edge is boredom and atrophy. Too far out is injury. Unless you find your edge, there is no growth, no learning, and no change.

—MICHAEL LEE

Entering, holding, and releasing the posture. This little sequence is the DNA of any yoga practice. Learn how to do a simple posture as taught in this chapter, and the doors to a fulfilling yoga practice will swing open to you. Many of these principles are distilled in the concept of practicing at the edge.

In Kripalu Yoga, the body moves smoothly and with a pace that is neither hurried nor halting. *Flowing* is a good word to keep in mind as you practice. You are not trying to move in slow motion, a discipline that only leads to mental tension. You are moving consciously, and movement naturally slows down a bit as you breathe, relax, and attune to sensation. Body and breath awareness may lead you to enter a challenging posture in stages, working yourself into a deep stretch gradually by gently pulsing in and out of the posture a few times before entering it fully. This is not "ballistic stretching," a technique that is frequently criticized as a source of stretching injury in which you rhythmically bob and bounce to apply force to the tissues. This is listening to your body, taking a little time to acclimate to the stretch you are about to experience. You may come one-third of the way into the posture, and slowly back out, and then two-thirds of the way in, and slowly back out, and only then move fully into the posture. This approach will take you deeper into the posture, and with better alignment, than if you charge right in.

Finding the Edge

The *edge* marks the healthy limit of your body's flexibility, and the place where your mind is naturally focused. Coming into a stretch, you subject the muscle tissues to a force that pulls their component parts back into alignment. As the stretch culminates, you place the tissues under a healthy stress that releases muscle tension and stimulates the body to expand its range of flexibility. At this point there are paradoxical feelings of pleasure and discomfort, and your kinesthetic awareness is naturally heightened. This is your edge, and stretching beyond it begins to strain tissues and joints. If you stop short of the edge, the stretch does not release deep-seated tension and feels less than fulfilling.

Going over your edge brings pain, which is a clear signal from the nervous system that damage is occurring. Habitually going beyond your edge is often the result of a psychological need to achieve and excessive goal-orientation. If you force yourself into stretches beyond your body's capacity to tolerate, your practice will create tension instead of releasing it, and you may injure yourself in the process. Habitually practicing well short of your edge often reflects an unwillingness to put out energy and fully feel whatever is there for you in the stretch. You may avoid discomfort, but your progress quickly plateaus and you find yoga boring. Practicing at the relaxed side of your edge, you can breathe deeply and safely explore the posture with a level of intensity that makes it an enjoyable challenge. Over time, your body's limits expand and your edge moves steadily forward until you reach a healthy range of motion.

> *I had already been practicing yoga when I took a workshop about playing the edge with Michael Lee. When he described the edge as a place "where any more stretch would be too much, and any less would not be enough," it hit home in a visceral way. I am a Type A personality, and the challenge for me is to hold back just a bit and be okay with that. I don't have to look perfect in the posture, hold it longer, or be better than I am. This was a great gift to my yoga practice and my life.*
>
> — Martha Chabinsky

Hold the Posture

All postures are not created equal. Some you will be able to hold for only a few breaths, and some for much longer. Resist the tendency to "endure the posture" and instead explore and

Discovering the Edge

BY SENIOR TEACHER MICHAEL LEE

I came to Kripalu Center from my home in Australia in the early 1980s to deepen my yoga practice. When I arrived, the staff was focused on "holding the pose," a practice in which various postures were held for significant periods of time. I could endure the pain of holding a posture for a short time, but the level of discomfort I was encountering in the longer holdings was intolerable. I found myself coming out of the postures ahead of the group and feeling frustrated. It was clear to me that this was meant to be a willful practice. I was supposed to push a little and experience the discomfort. I was trying to be willful, but it was just not working. So I backed off and began to take it easy. After a while of doing this, I began to feel guilty that I was not doing my best.

One morning, I had a flash of inspiration. How about finding some place in between? Excited by this new possibility, I eased my body into the next posture. At first it was hard to find. I had to resist the tendency to try harder, and then the temptation to back off too much. After practicing this for a while, I began to find my "edge" and hold the posture there. The results were amazing. I was able to hold longer and witness the discomfort with awareness. I began to enter a state similar to what I had previously experienced in meditation, where powerful images and insights would come to me. Within days my yoga practice began to take on a whole new meaning. Only later did I realize that I had made a significant discovery, one that would open up my yoga practice and my life.

Kripalu Yoga teacher Michael Lee went on to develop Phoenix Rising Yoga Therapy, a body-centered form of psychotherapy recognized by the American Psychological Association. The edge became a core component of Kripalu Yoga, and the term is now used widely in American yoga.

embrace what occurs when you relax and breathe while holding. Rather than finding a way to collapse comfortably into the posture, breathe into the dynamic tension the pose is intended to create. Holding a steady stretch for a half minute is sufficient to maintain flexibility. Extending your holding time to one minute or longer allows you to grow in flexibility and strength.

As a rule of thumb, work up to where you can hold your postures for at least five full and flowing breaths. It takes that long for the body to recognize that the stretch is not a threat but an opportunity to let go and be nurtured. In

EXPERIENCE: FINDING YOUR EDGE IN QUARTER MOON POSE

Use this experience to help you find your edge by moving into Quarter Moon slowly and consciously. Make sure to come into an easy stretch first, so you can gradually deepen the side bend as you hold. When you find your edge, stay there with a flowing breath, noticing how the body responds.

1. Stand tall with the feet parallel, hip-width apart, and hands on the hips. Let your breath begin to flow freely in and out.

2. Inhale as you sweep the right arm out to the side in a wide arc and raise it overhead. Lengthen the whole right side of the body by pressing the fingertips toward the ceiling. Take a few breaths, feeling all the sensations as the body adjusts to this position.

3. To come into an easy Quarter Moon, take a deep breath in. As you exhale, gently press the right hip out to the side and left hand into the left hip. As the torso slowly bends to the left, come about one-third of the way into a stretch. Keep the hips and shoulders facing forward so the body stays in one plane.

4. Relax into this easy stretch for a few breaths. Resist any tendency to push deeper. Notice what it is like to hold at a place of minimal stretch.

5. Come a little deeper by gently pressing the right hip a little farther out to the side, coming about two-thirds of the way into the stretch. Extend through the right fingertips to keep the right side elongated. Hold there for a few moments, breathing into the stretch.

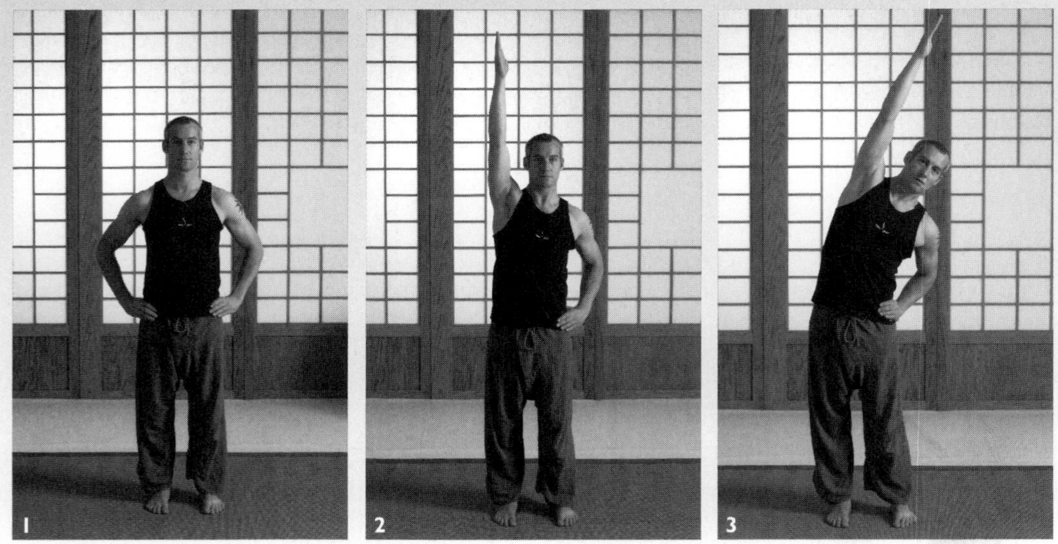

6. Now come to your edge by continuing to press out on the right hip. This is the place where any more stretch would be too much, and your body would experience it as a strain. But anything less would be less than enough. If you go over your edge, just back off the stretch, catch your breath, and then come forward again. Play with the full spectrum of stretch until you find your edge.

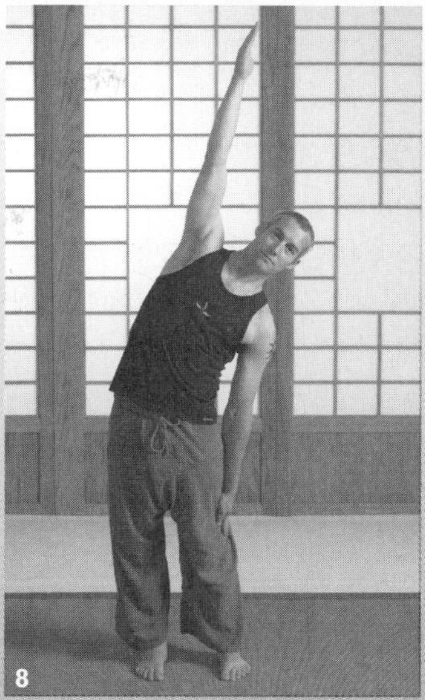

8

7. Hold the posture on the relaxed side of your edge, breathing freely and noticing what happens. Feel the intercostal muscles stretching to open the spaces between the ribs. As you hold, stay present in your body and notice if your edge shifts or changes. If you can, stay at your edge for five flowing breaths.

8. If your body wants more stretch, you can slide the left hand down the thigh. Lengthen the left fingertips toward the floor, and the right fingertips up and to the side. Don't fall off the edge!

9. To release, bring the left hand back to the hip. Inhale as you slowly bring the torso back to center. Then lower the right arm to the side, and release the left hand from the hip so both arms are at the sides. Take a moment to really feel your body. What was your experience? Were you able to stay on your edge? What were the effects of holding the posture there?

10. When you feel ready, repeat on the opposite side.

the beginning, there might be postures you cannot hold this long. Rather than forcing, accept where you are and simply be present, allowing your body to gradually grow stronger and more flexible.

The edge is not a static place. As you hold and breathe, you will often find your edge moving forward, allowing you to come deeper into the posture than initially possible. Many students find that if they can make it through five flowing breaths, their experience of the effort involved noticeably shifts in a way that makes more extended holding possible and even pleasurable. Over time, your body's limits will steadily expand and you will gain an intuitive sense for how long to hold each posture.

Allow Micromovements and Sounds to Emerge

Micromovements are small, slow-motion movements that naturally emerge from the body as you ease into and hold a yoga posture. These minor variations of the posture modify or accentuate the stretch, allowing you to explore sensation and move in ways that release tension from a broader area of the body. Some posture descriptions include possible micromovements, but don't limit yourself to the movements suggested there. Listen to the prompting of your body, and it will guide you into micromovements specifically designed for you. Micromovements are an important part of the Kripalu Yoga technique, the first step in learning how to move as guided from within.

While holding a good stretch with a flowing breath, you are quite likely to feel the urge to exhale out a sigh or other sound. Let it happen! This is one way the body releases tension, and it is entirely natural to moan or groan as you work your way through a series of yoga postures. This is not so much a technique, as permission to break the sound barrier and allow your body to express itself.

> *I've been practicing Kripalu Yoga since the '70s. At times, I like to close my eyes and focus on the sound of my breath as I flow from pose to pose. This helps me let go of distractions and notice where the muscles are being stretched, and how energy is moving or blocked in each posture. I love the freedom to respond to the needs of my body that I learned in Kripalu Yoga. The micromovements that naturally happen add a dimension to my practice that feels so organic and right. So does letting out the sighs and ahhhs that come from deep within as I let go of a clenched jaw, tense chest, or furrowed brow. This kind of practice leaves me feeling fully alive in body and soul . . . and very blessed!*
>
> —Vandita Kate Marchesiello

Working with Pain and Discomfort

"No pain, no gain" is not a maxim that applies to Kripalu Yoga. Pain is a clear signal from the body that you are exceeding healthy limits and risking injury. The joint capsule and surrounding area are rich with nerve endings designed to send clear signals to help avoid movement-related injuries. Learning to distinguish between pain and discomfort is essential for safe practice. Pain's message is to be respected, and movements that bring pain should not be performed. The onset of pain is usually sudden, often described as shooting, sharp, or searing. After injury, pain may take the form of a throbbing or aching sensation.

Discomfort, on the other hand, is a dull and slower sensation. Discomfort is often the result of inertia and resistance to moving parts of the body that have become stiff and energetically sluggish. Encountering and gently moving through discomfort is a positive aspect of

EXPERIENCE: COMPENSATORY MOVEMENTS

Compensatory movements help you stretch and strengthen without strain. After a challenging posture, doing easy movements that release tension helps the body rebalance and happily move on to the next posture. Standing Twists are a great compensatory movement for vigorous standing postures. Other compensatory movements are built into the Sun and Moon Series.

1. Stand with the feet parallel, a little wider than hip-width apart, arms at your sides.

2. Begin to slowly rotate the hips and shoulders from side to side, allowing the relaxed arms to gently flap against the sides like empty coat sleeves. Coordinate breath and motion, exhaling as you twist and inhaling back to center.

3. Let the head join in the motion, turning to look over one shoulder, and then the other. Keep the spine erect and the hips and shoulders turning as if in a barrel—versus swaying from side to side.

4. As you twist to the right, lift the left heel slightly to allow the hips a greater range of movement and release any tension in the left knee. As you twist to the left, lift the right heel slightly.

5. Repeat ten or more times, coordinating breath and motion. Let the motion gradually slow down and return to center. Take a few breaths in stillness before moving on to the next posture.

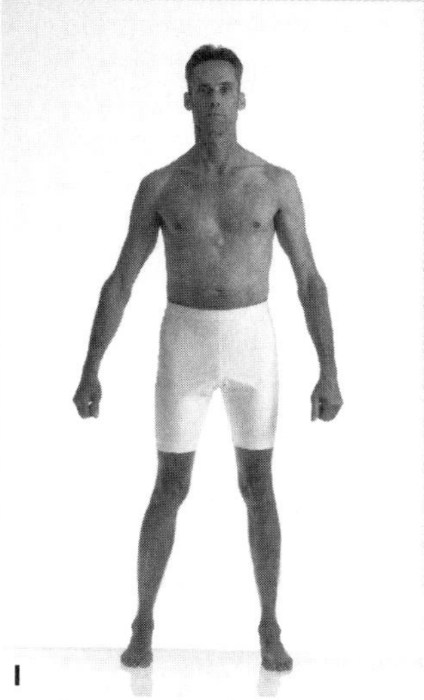

1

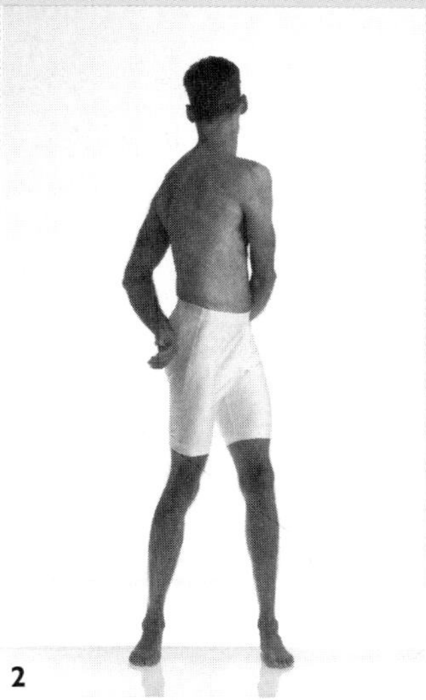

2

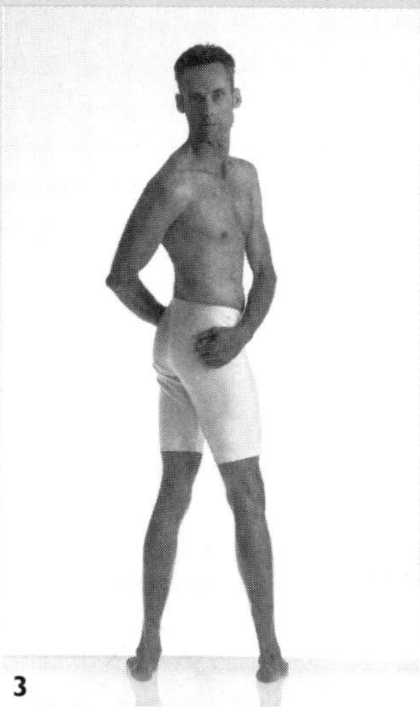

3

yoga practice, something you do every time you practice. To let go of chronic tension and heal the body, you must bring awareness to areas that feel less than good. Similarly, the process of emotional release and mental clearing always involves encountering uncomfortable feelings and thoughts.

Especially when beginning a practice, it is natural to encounter both pain and discomfort. Learn to listen to the body and hear the messages underlying these sensations. Heeding pain and exploring the edge of discomfort, you avoid injury and systematically free the body of chronic tension. While learning how to encounter, move through, and release discomfort, don't get stuck there by forming a habitual stance that yoga is about "feeling your pain." Feel all the pleasurable sensations that arise in practice, and celebrate the joy of movement and embodiment too.

Consciously Release the Posture

Move out of the posture slowly and with full awareness of all the sensations flowing through you. Each posture has an energetic echo, a reverberation that can be felt in the moments after release. Instead of moving directly into the next posture, pause for a moment to listen to this echo and allow all the muscles to return to a relaxed state. After a vigorous posture, or a cluster of postures done from the same basic position, your body may guide you to pause and catch your breath or do simple movements that relieve stress and prevent strain. These pauses are not "time out" from your practice. They are a way to remain sensitive to your body's needs and allow it to rest or lead you into compensatory movements that help avoid strain and injury.

I've noticed that unless I keep a palpable edge in my practice, it becomes rote, dry, and largely unfulfilling. What this looks like changes over time. There's the physical edge of going as deeply into a stretch as my body can in that moment without strain. This is always an exploration, different every day, and it keeps my mind engaged even when I'm entering a posture I've done a thousand times before. Then there's the inner edge, the place where my self-awareness is constantly evolving. Sometimes the inner edge leads me to let go into an ocean of energy, or make each posture an offering of myself to the Divine. This subtle edge reveals itself only if I listen closely, choosing to be so attuned that a message from beneath the surface mind can make itself known.

—Danna Faulds

C H A P T E R   F I V E

AWARENESS THROUGH ALIGNMENT

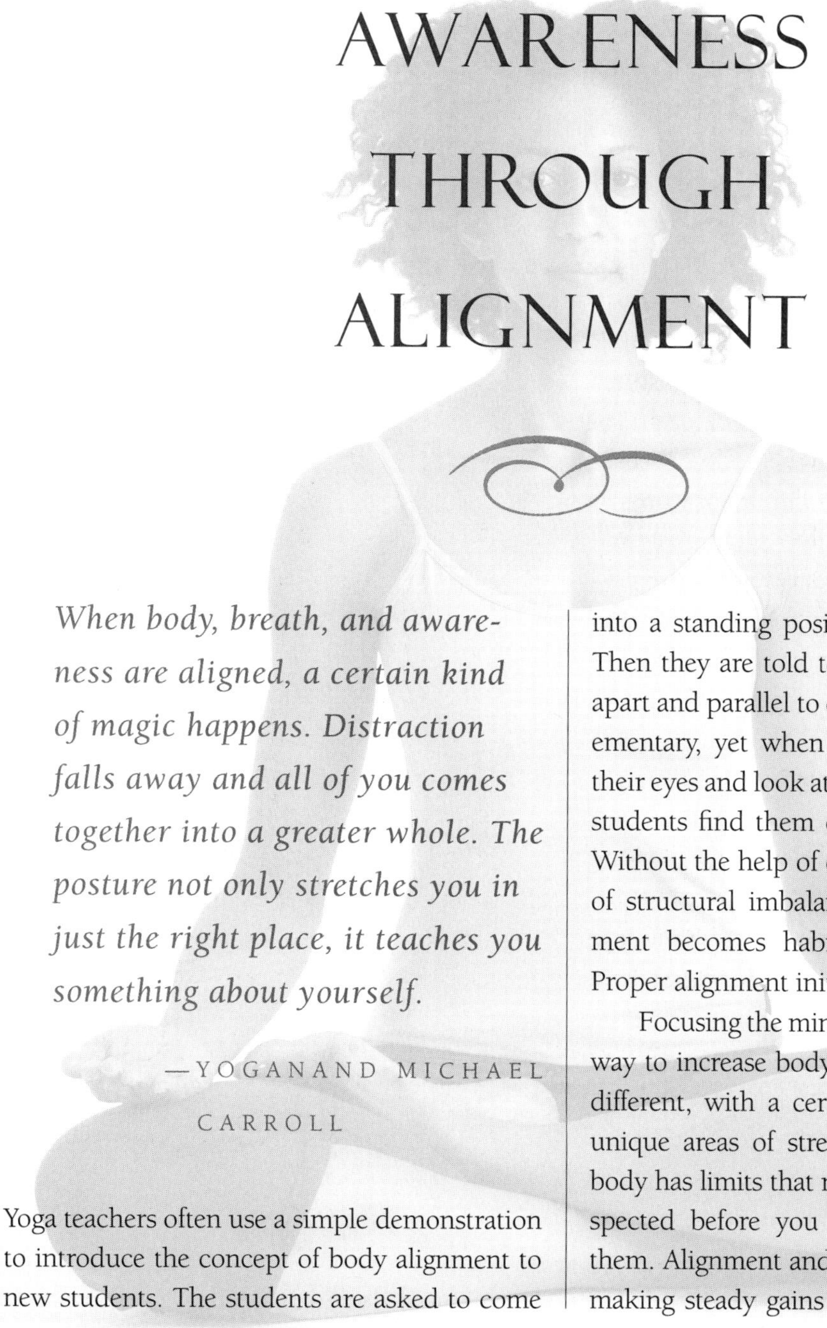

When body, breath, and awareness are aligned, a certain kind of magic happens. Distraction falls away and all of you comes together into a greater whole. The posture not only stretches you in just the right place, it teaches you something about yourself.

—YOGANAND MICHAEL CARROLL

Yoga teachers often use a simple demonstration to introduce the concept of body alignment to new students. The students are asked to come into a standing position and close their eyes. Then they are told to bring the feet hip-width apart and parallel to each other. It sounds so elementary, yet when they are invited to open their eyes and look at their feet, more than a few students find them considerably out of place. Without the help of eyesight, the phenomenon of structural imbalance is revealed. Misalignment becomes habitual and feels "normal." Proper alignment initially feels "awkward."

Focusing the mind on alignment is a proven way to increase body awareness. Every body is different, with a certain range of motion and unique areas of strength and weakness. Your body has limits that must be discovered and respected before you can safely move beyond them. Alignment and awareness are the keys to making steady gains in flexibility and strength while avoiding the injuries that result when the healthy limits of joints, connective tissues, and muscles are exceeded. While the alignment sought through Kripalu Yoga is a harmony of body, mind, and spirit, the path forward begins in a very tangible way by learning how to position the bones, joints, and muscles.

Press Points

Kripalu Yoga makes alignment easy with *press points,* guiding you in and out of the postures by instructing you to press into specific parts of the body. The press point methodology uses everyday language and a minimum of words to bring the body quickly into alignment and keep it there as you hold and release the posture. During holding, the press points remain engaged to support the active work that takes place in a posture. This requires the active muscles to make a sustained effort. It also subjects the passive muscles to a sustained stretch. The end result is the ability to stretch to your healthy limit without strain, safely increasing both strength and flexibility.

Simple language is not only easy to follow, it leaves the mind free to feel what is going on in your body. For example, the instruction *Press firmly into all four corners of your feet* guides you to engage the muscles of the legs and position the joints of the lower body properly. If you closely attend to how your body responds to this and other press point instructions, you will discover a world of anatomical detail. The leg muscles contract, hugging the leg bones. As the quadriceps or thigh muscles engage, the kneecaps lift slightly. The legs straighten, but the knees do not hyperextend. Simply as a result of pressing into the feet, the lower body grows grounded and stable. Rather than holding in mind a jumble of anatomical details, Kripalu Yoga encourages you to fully feel what happens as you engage the press points.

• **Crown of the Head:** The top center of the skull or *fontanel*. Pressing into the crown of

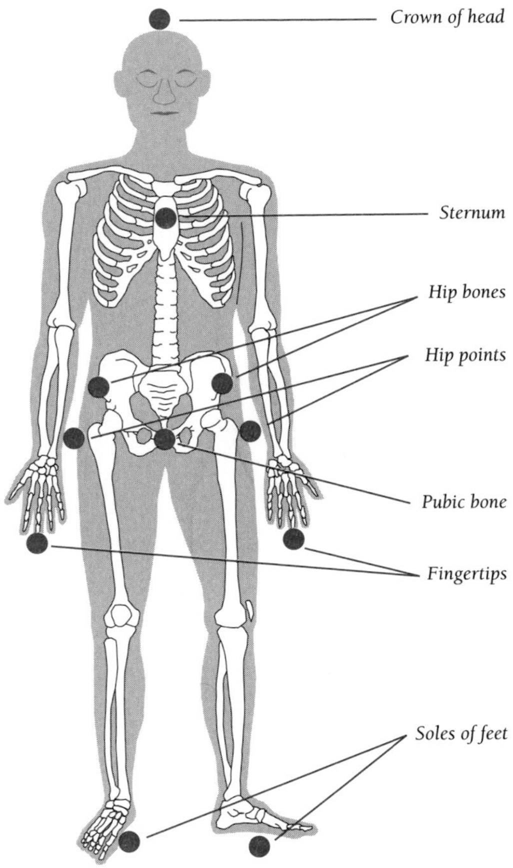

FRONT

the head elongates the upper spine and neck. The chin remains parallel to the ground as the back of the neck elongates, lifting the ears away from the shoulders.

• **Back of the Head:** The back center of the skull, which rests solidly on the floor when lying on your back.

• **Sternum:** A flat area of bone in the center of the chest several inches below the throat. Lifting the sternum without arching the spine backward keeps the spine erect, the muscles of the torso engaged, and the shoulder blades in proper position. It also helps open the chest, allowing the lungs to fill more fully with breath. Pressing the sternum forward is an effective way to initiate or deepen backbends.

• **Tops of the Shoulders, Shoulder Blades, and Wing Points:** Allowing the tops of the shoulders to relax down and away from the ears is the first step in positioning the shoulders. The shoulder blades or *scapulae* are the triangular bones that ride on the upper back. Pressing the shoulder blades back and down stretches the pectoral muscles and opens the chest. Drawing the wing points together helps position the shoulder blades deep in the shoulder girdle, providing maximum support for the arms.

• **Hip Bones:** These are the front-facing protuberances of the pelvis, anatomically called the Anterior Superior Iliac Spine, or ASIS bones. To locate the hip bones, bring the thumbs onto the top of the buttocks and pinch the front of the body with the fingers. The hip bones are two noticeable bony knobs on the front of the pelvis. Pressing the hip and pubic bones into the floor stabilizes the core of the body in belly down postures.

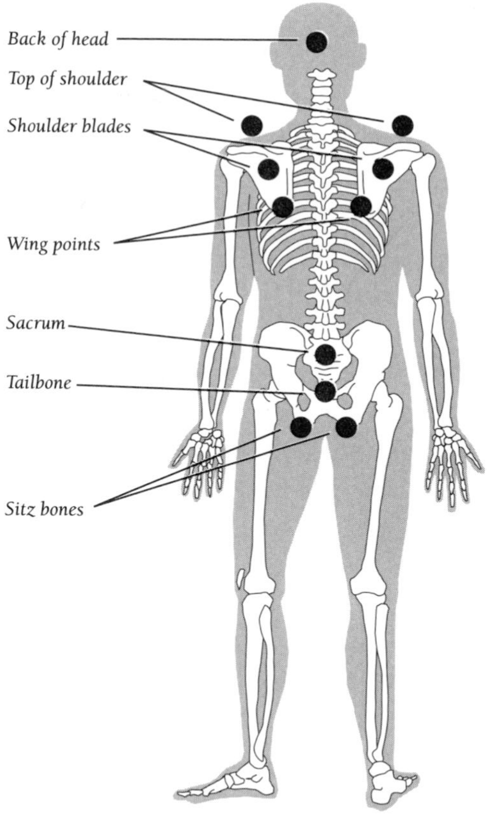

BACK

• **Hip Points:** The word *hips* is commonly used to refer to a broad area of the body including the upper thighs, pelvis, and buttocks. The hip point is the greater trochanter, the spot at the top and outside of the thigh close to where the thigh bone inserts in the hip socket. Pressing the right hip point away to the right causes the torso to bend to the left, stretching the right side.

• **Pubic Bone:** Located just above the genitals, where the two sides of the pelvis meet in front. Pressing the pubic bone forward engages the abdominals and helps initiate a backbend from the hips and sacrum versus the low back. When pressed into the floor, it helps stabilize the core of the body in belly down postures.

• **Tailbone and Sacrum:** Technically the coccyx, the tailbone is the bony tail on the end of the triangular sacrum located at the base of the spine. "Lifting the tailbone" acts like a lever that tilts the torso forward with the spine elongated, hinging from the hip joints rather than bending at the waist and rounding the low back. When lying on your back, pressing the tailbone down allows the sacrum to rest solidly on the floor, stabilizing the low back.

• **Sitz Bones:** To locate the sitz bones, sit on the floor with the legs outstretched and bring the hands under the buttocks. Rock from side to side, and you will feel two pointed bones lying beneath the flesh of the buttocks. Pressing both sitz bones down in seated postures stabilizes the core of the body and provides a base for spinal elongation. Pressing the sitz bones down in forward bending postures helps rotate the pelvis and hips forward, keeping the low back straight and focusing the stretch in the hamstrings.

• **Fingertips:** The fingertips are pressed down to lengthen the arms and lower the tops of the shoulders away from the ears. Pressed up, they help elongate the spine. They are also used to encourage the chest and torso to stretch in various ways.

• **Soles of the Feet:** Pressing all four corners of the feet evenly into the floor grounds the body, increasing stability and balance in a wide array of postures. It also engages the leg muscles and positions the bones and joints of the lower body properly. In some postures, the press is stronger in the toes or heels.

My students say that I am a stickler on alignment, paying more attention than most teachers to all the details of the postures. While this may be true, I have found that focusing on alignment does more than help students feel stable and strong in their postures. It increases their body awareness, which helps them feel good about themselves physically and mentally, both on and off the yoga mat. In Kripalu Yoga, the body is seen as the temple of the spirit. What is happening inside a person is considered more important than what is happening on the outside. As a teacher, my intention is to find just the right balance between assisting students in moving toward "correct" alignment and encouraging them to open to a deep inner experience of themselves.

— Mary Lou Buck

Principles of Alignment

As you work with the press points, the basic principles of alignment will become part of the felt sense of your body.

- Build the posture from the ground up
- Stabilize the core
- Elongate the spine
- Open the chest, position the shoulders
- Keep the neck an extension of the spine
- Position the limbs
- Hold and release with awareness

• Build the Posture from the Ground Up

Each and every moment, your body is being pulled toward the earth by the force of gravity. Gravity is an organizing principle of the physical world, and alignment is the dynamic interplay between anatomy and the force of gravity. The press points sensitize you to this ever-present pull of gravity, making you aware of the parts of your body in touch with the floor. In every posture, the weight-bearing parts of the body are pressed firmly into the floor to establish the strong foundation necessary to align, stretch, and strengthen the body.

Instructions That Ground the Body:

Standing postures: *Press all four corners of the feet evenly into the floor to engage the muscles of the legs.*

Belly down postures: *Press the pubic bone, hip bones, and lower abdomen into the floor.*

Supine postures: *Press the sacrum into the floor. Allow the shoulder blades and back of the head to rest solidly on the floor.*

Kneeling postures: *Press the knees into the floor.*

Sitting postures and twists: *Press both sitz bones into the floor and allow any other parts of the body touching the floor to rest there solidly.*

When the hands are bearing weight: *Spread the fingers wide and press the roots of the fingers into the floor.* **Or:** *Bring the thumbs and fingers close together and press the heels of the hands into the floor.* **Or in cases of wrist sensitivity:** *Make your hands into fists and press the knuckles firmly into the floor.*

Kripalu Yoga does not instruct you to lock the knees in standing postures. For some people, this hyperextends the knee joint and leaves it prone to injury. Stability in the lower body is created by firmly pressing both feet into the floor and engaging the muscles of the legs. Pressing the feet naturally straightens the leg. Engaging the muscles of the legs above and below the knee stabilizes the knee joint. In certain postures, the instructions may encourage you to keep the knees slightly flexed or "soft" to prevent knee or low back strain. Simply continue to press the feet into the floor and keep the leg muscles engaged as much as possible.

- **Stabilize the Core**

After the body is grounded, the pelvis, hips, and sacrum are brought into proper alignment. These parts of the skeleton, along with the associated musculature of the groin, pelvis, abdomen, and torso, are the body's core. The sacrum is the base of the spine. Just as strong roots anchor a tree in the earth, stabilizing the core anchors the sacrum in the pelvis. When the sacrum and pelvis are aligned, the spine has the strong foundation it needs to safely move through a full range of motion and support the weight of the limbs when they are extended away from the body. Learning how to stabilize the core protects the entire spine, and especially the low back, from movement-related injuries. It also gives you a feeling of solidity and the ability to move gracefully from your center.

The body's core is stabilized by a series of subtle movements and muscular contractions that build upon the press of the feet and the contraction of the leg muscles. First the tailbone is pressed down and the pubic bone is pressed slightly forward to bring the pelvic bowl level with the ground. This movement slightly reduces the curve of the lower back and brings the spine into an optimal position to enter the majority of yoga poses. Next the

WHY CARE ABOUT ALIGNMENT?

There is a natural tendency to compromise alignment to "look like the picture," avoid discomfort, or feel like you are "going deeper" in the posture. Compromising alignment is always counterproductive because it allows you to:

- Avoid stretching tight areas
- Overstretch areas that are already flexible
- Rely on muscles that are already strong instead of developing strength in those that are weak
- Reinforce structural imbalances

The principles of body alignment are not artificial or arbitrary; they emerge from the anatomical structure of the body. Accept the need for alignment, and a balanced routine of postures will steadily stretch and strengthen your entire musculoskeletal system.

EXPERIENCE: MOUNTAIN POSE (*Tadasana*)

The principles of proper body alignment and balance are traditionally learned in Mountain Pose and then applied in all other postures. The Mountain teaches you how to build the posture from the ground up, stabilize the core, and elongate the spine. Take a few minutes to come into Mountain Pose and get a feel for what alignment is all about.

1. Stand with your feet parallel, hip-width apart, and arms at the sides.

2. Lift the toes off the ground, spread them wide, and place them back on the floor. Balance your body weight between the heels and toes, and then between the right and left legs. Press down evenly into all four corners of the feet, engaging the muscles of the legs without locking the knees. You may feel a natural lift in the arches of the feet and a slight contraction of the quadriceps that lifts the kneecaps.

3. Stabilize the core of your body by pressing the tailbone down and pubic bone forward to level the pelvis, and gently contracting and lifting the muscles of the pelvic floor.

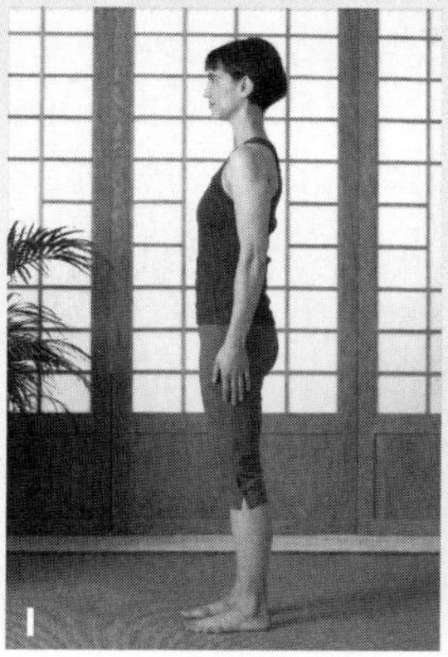

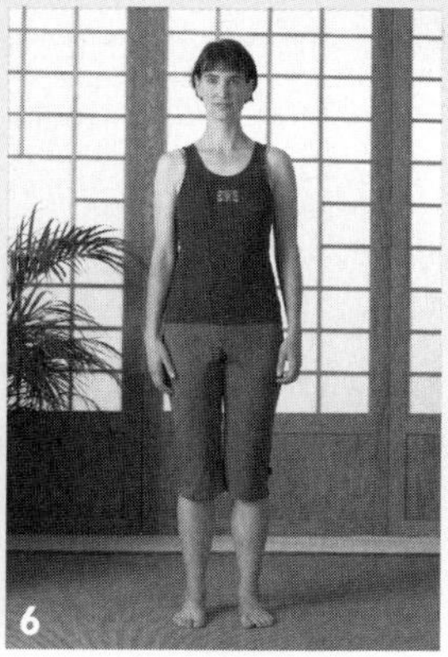

4. Elongate the spine by lifting out of the waist. Gently press the sternum forward without arching the spine back or puffing the chest out military style.

5. Allow the tops of the shoulders to relax down, away from the ears. Draw the wing points together, pressing the shoulder blades down. Press the fingertips toward the floor to lengthen the arms and further lower the tops of the shoulders.

6. Bring the chin parallel to the floor and extend through the crown of the head to elongate the neck. This is Mountain Pose.

7. Hold the posture for a minute or two, letting the breath flow freely. While remaining sensitive to the details of alignment, allow the body to relax as much as possible without compromising alignment.

8. Take a deep breath in and release the posture as you exhale. Notice how it feels for your body to resume its "normal" alignment.

muscles of the pelvic floor are gently pulled in and up. The pelvic cavity is a bowl-shaped hollow surrounded by a complex of muscles. These muscles play an important role in safeguarding the abdominal and reproductive organs while allowing free movement of the legs and upper body. Engaging these muscles, you feel a slight inward and upward pull just above the pubic bone, but the diaphragm remains able to move freely in and out with the flow of breath, and the upper buttocks remain soft.

The muscles of the pelvic floor are often weak and the neural pathways that control them underdeveloped. Many women experience a dramatic weakening of these muscles in the process of childbirth, and they can remain weak without an intentional period of conditioning. Learning how to stabilize the core takes some practice as you refine nervous system sensitivity and gradually strengthen pelvic muscles. Along the way, it is common to overly contract the large muscles of the upper thighs and buttocks, as well as the surrounding small muscles of the anus and genitals. This is a normal part of the learning process, but take care not to contract these muscles to the extent that it creates mental tension or restricts the free flow of the breath. Don't "overthink" the elements of core stabilization. These are simply small and subtle movements designed to foster pelvic, sacral, and lumbar alignment.

Instructions to Stabilize the Core:

Standing postures: *Press the tailbone down and the pubic bone forward, leveling the pelvis. Gently contract and lift the muscles of the pelvic floor.*

Belly down postures: *Press the pubic bone, hip bones, and lower belly into the floor.*

Supine postures: *Press the tailbone into the floor and allow the sacrum to rest solidly on the floor.*

Sitting postures and twists: *Press both sitz bones into the floor and level the pelvis. Gently contract and lift the muscles of the pelvic floor.*

It was in Warrior Pose that I understood that my role as a mother must include both deep-rooted stability and openhearted freedom. Practicing the Warrior, my feet press firmly into the earth. My core is stable. I am grounded while my torso floats free, vulnerable, open and welcoming to the fates. The morning after sending my twenty-year-old daughter back to college, I went to my yoga mat and realized that this is precisely the balance I was seeking with her quest for independence and my desire to support and protect her. Instead of a tug-of-war between protecting and letting go, I saw that practicing the union of these two essential qualities is the way to love my daughter completely.

—Sandy Cyrus

• Elongate the Spine

Maintaining flexibility of the spine is often touted as a primary benefit of yoga. All schools of yoga recommend a series of postures that flex the spine forward and back, bend it side to side, and twist it left and right. Before doing these movements, it is essential to ground the body, stabilize the core, and then use the solid base established to elongate the spinal column. Elongation creates maximum space between the vertebrae, allowing room for the spine to move freely as you come into postures, without compressing the vertebral disks or putting pressure on delicate spinal nerves.

The spine is a column of vertebrae stacked one on top of the other. This design meets the contrasting needs of dynamic and static movement. In dynamic movement such as walking or running, the vertebrae assume an S shape that flexes easily and uses the vertebral disks to cushion impact and protect the spinal cord from injury. When standing and performing static movements of the upper body, such as bending forward or backward, turning left or right, or reaching out with the arms, the spinal column elongates, decreasing the degree of its S curve. This markedly increases stability and strength by allowing the spine to work as a single unit and to brace movement.

Most yoga postures are static movements that require the stable base of an elongated spine to perform safely and properly. Forward bending is a good example of this. When the spine is elongated, it is easy to hinge at the hips and bend forward with a straight spine. If the spine is not elongated, we round from the waist, compressing the front side of the lumbar

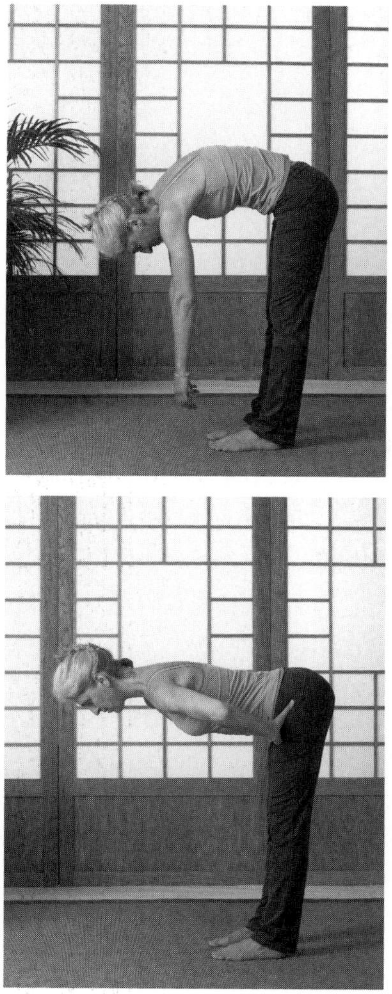

Rounding forward from the lumbar spine is a common cause of low back pain. Hinging from the hips allows you to bend forward with a straight spine and protects the low back.

EXPERIENCE: USING THE FLOOR TO ELONGATE THE SPINE

Any time you come onto your belly or back for a series of postures, start by using the support of the floor to elongate the spine. This ensures safety, while offering a great stretch for the entire body.

ON YOUR BELLY

1. Come onto your belly with the forehead, mouth, or chin on the floor. Reach your arms overhead.

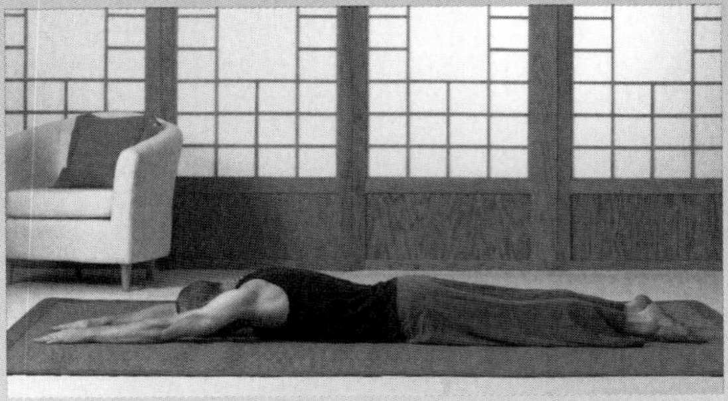

2. Wriggle the upper body from side to side, stretching one arm and then the other overhead, walking the rib cage upward to elongate the spine, shoulders, and arms.

3. Lift one foot and leg, and then the other, pressing the toes away to lengthen the sacrum, hips, and legs.

4. Come back to center. As you inhale, press the fingers and toes away from one another, stretching your body to its full length along the floor.

5. Exhale and relax completely, letting the entire body sink into the floor.

ON YOUR BACK

1. Roll over onto your back, keeping your arms overhead.

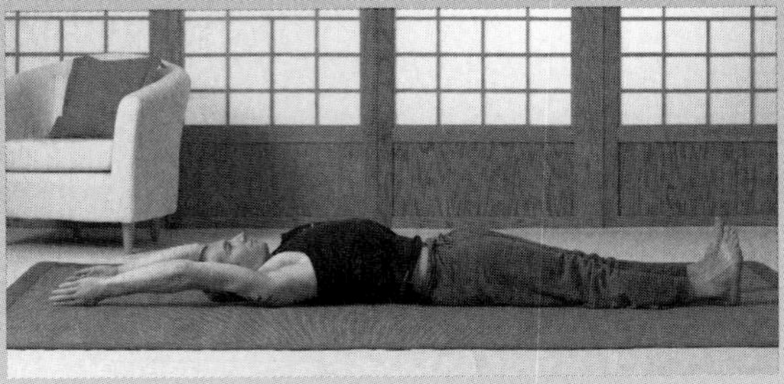

2. Wriggle the upper body from side to side, stretching one arm and then the other overhead, walking the shoulder blades up to elongate the upper spine, shoulders, and arms. Then press the mid-back and especially the area between the shoulder blades down into the floor.

3. Flex the feet and press one heel away, and then the other to lengthen the sacrum, hips, and legs.

4. Come back to center. As you inhale, press the fingers and heels away, and the sacrum and mid-back down, stretching your body to its full length.

5. Exhale and relax completely, letting out an audible sigh as the entire body sinks into the floor. Bring the arms back to the sides and rest for a moment or two in Corpse Pose.

disks. Gaining the core strength and muscular control required to elongate the spine is one of the secrets to safely realizing the many benefits that yoga has to offer.

> *By freeing up the inner flow of energy, alignment increases sensitivity and actually creates body awareness. Areas that were cut off and forgotten come back into conscious awareness.*
>
> —Rudy Peirce

Instructions to Elongate the Spine:

Standing postures: *Lift the spine out of the waist. Lift the sternum without arching back. Tuck the chin slightly and extend through the crown of the head.* When standing with arms overhead: *Press up through the fingertips.*

Belly down and supine postures: *Use the support of the floor to elongate the spine to its full length. (See experience on page 58.)*

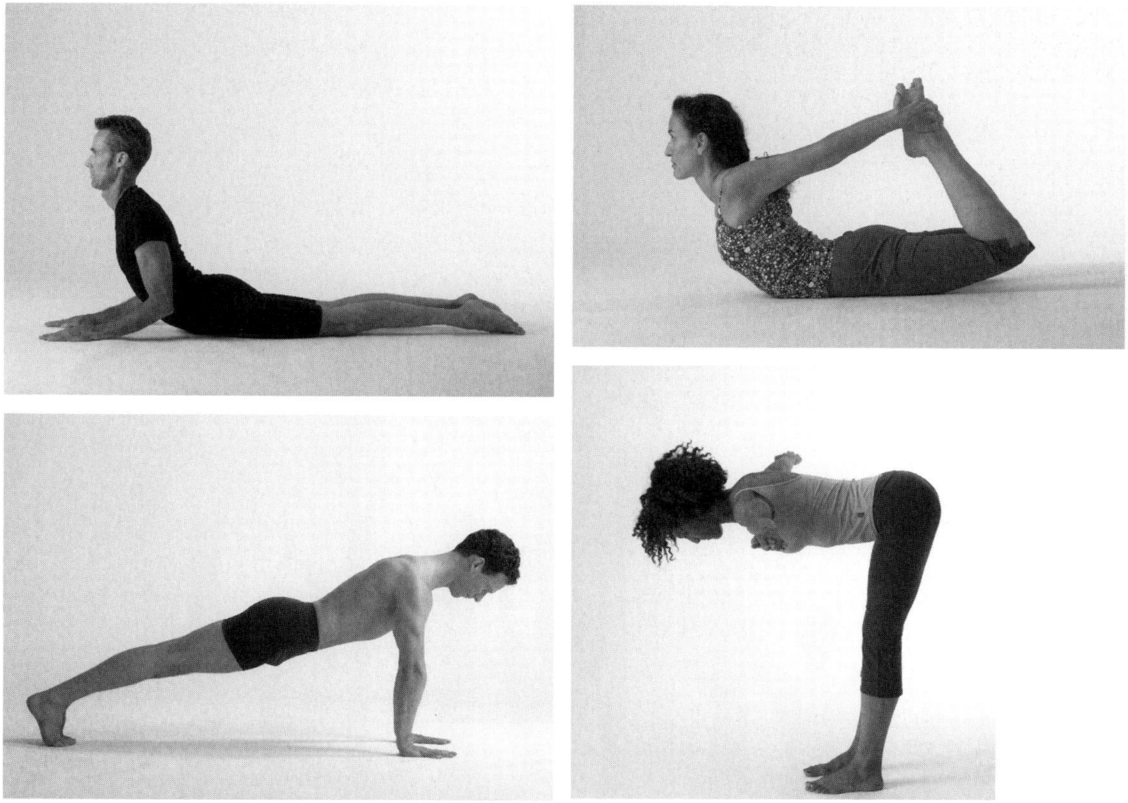

In Kripalu Yoga, the neck remains elongated and aligned with the rest of the spine during postures.

EXPERIENCE: POSITIONING THE SHOULDERS

This experience leads you into several overhead arm positions used in yoga postures. Explore how these positions support, or don't support, your shoulder alignment.

1. Stand with the feet parallel, hip-width apart, arms at your sides. Stabilize the core and elongate the spine. Press the sternum forward to open the chest.

2. Allow the tops of the shoulders to relax down, away from the ears. Roll the shoulders back and down, drawing the wing points together and letting the shoulder blades drop deep in the shoulder girdle. Press the fingertips toward the floor to enhance the downward movements of the shoulders and shoulder blades.

3. Inhale and raise the arms overhead into a broad V. As you exhale, press the sternum forward and once again allow the tops of the shoulders to relax down and away from the ears. Keep the wing points drawn together and shoulder blades deep in the shoulder girdle, even while pressing through the fingertips to lengthen the arms. Let your breath flow freely as you feel your way into proper shoulder alignment.

4. Inhale and bring the arms straight overhead, shoulder-width apart and palms facing. As you exhale, once again allow the tops of the shoulders to relax down while keeping the arms straight. Notice if your wing points want to spread apart, causing the shoulder blades to lift and shoulders to round forward. Keep the wing points drawn together and shoulder blades deep in the shoulder girdle.

5. Inhale and bring the palms together. Interlacing fingers and thumbs, extend the index fingers. This hand position is called *Steeple Position.*

6. Press the index fingers toward the ceiling to lengthen the arms, and notice if you are able to keep the top of the shoulders relaxed and away from the ears, wing points drawn together and shoulder blades pressed back and down.

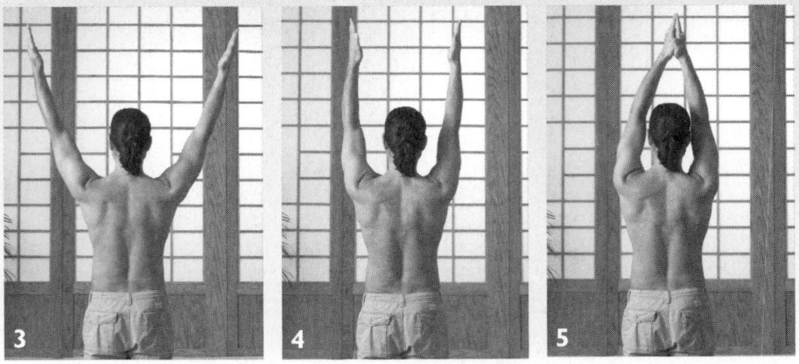

7. Take a deep breath in, and slowly release the arms back to your sides on an exhalation. Feel any sensations of warmth, tingling, or energy flowing in your shoulders and arms. Remember how proper shoulder position felt, and what instructions and movements helped you get there.

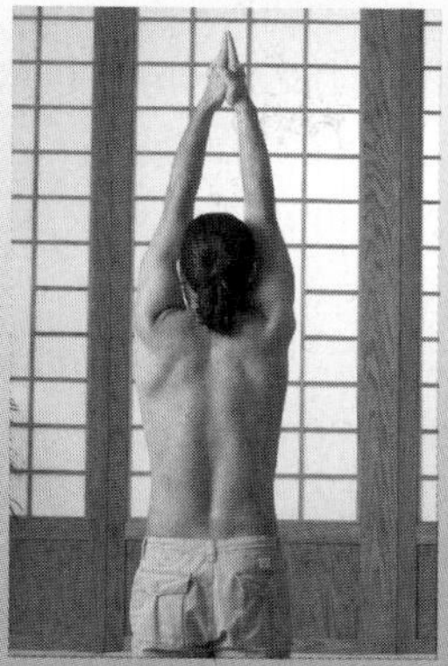

Avoid lifting the shoulders to the ears, which collapses the chest and pulls the shoulder blades up and out of their optimal position in the shoulder girdle.

Sitting postures and twists: *Press the sitz bones into the floor. Lift out of the waist. Lift the sternum without arching back. Tuck the chin slightly and extend through the crown of the head.*

• Open the Chest, Position the Shoulders

Many of us stand with the tops of the shoulders rolled forward, which collapses the chest and pulls the shoulder blades up and out of the shoulder girdle. To return the chest to its natural open position, press the sternum forward without puffing the chest out military style. Then two movements make it easy to position the shoulders.

The first is to *allow the tops of the shoulders to relax down, away from the ears.* When anxious, we are all prone to the *startle response,* an unconscious tendency to lift our shoulders toward our ears. This positioning of the shoulders can become chronic and a source of considerable upper body tension. The second is to *draw the wing points together, letting the shoulder blades drop deep into the shoulder girdle.* This provides maximum support for the arms. Once these movements are taught, the actual posture instructions are simplified to *roll the shoulders back and down.* To get a feel for shoulder alignment, try the experience on page 60.

• Keep the Neck an Extension of the Spine

Imagine a bowling ball attached to a short length of chain and you will gain greater respect for the work performed by the neck each and every day. Your head weighs about ten pounds, a considerable weight for the delicate cervical vertebrae and neck muscles to support, especially as you move through a series of yoga postures. As you articulate the spine and major joints of the body, *keep the neck an extension of the spine.* This means the neck remains aligned with the rest of the spine, bending smoothly forward in forward bends, and bending smoothly back in backbends, but never collapsing forward or back. In some schools of yoga, the head is dropped back in certain backbending postures. In Kripalu Yoga, however, the chin is kept slightly tucked and the crown of the head extended in backbends. This greatly reduces the risk of injury to the cervical vertebrae and associated nerves.

• Position the Limbs

Many who come to yoga for relief from back pain or other structural problems strain to get their arms and legs in the right position, while compromising the alignment of the spine. As a result, they only aggravate their condition. As you come into the posture with the body grounded and spine elongated, you are supported from the core and able to position the limbs to accomplish the desired stretch. In a number of postures, the limbs can be used to generate significant leverage. Leverage should assist the natural movement of the spine and joints; it should never be used to force the body beyond healthy limits.

• Hold and Release with Awareness

When you come into the posture consciously and find your best alignment, there is a sense of kinesthetic and neurological "rightness," as if the posture helps you remember the right relationship between its various parts. Hold there for several flowing breaths.

Keep the principles of alignment in mind as you slowly and smoothly release the posture. The majority of postures are released by engaging the same press points that brought you into the posture, returning you to the starting position. All postures contain clear instructions on how to release. Avoid quick or sudden movements, which can lead to strain or injury. Don't forget to take a moment to drink in all the delicious sensations associated with coming out of a good stretch.

THE SOUL OF YOGA

What is the soul of yoga?
Follow your heart into the
center of the pose and find
in the midst of detail and
precision, in breath, alignment,
balance, bliss, fear and sadness—
at the very core of all of this
is love.

CHAPTER SIX

REJUVENATION THROUGH RELAXATION

When you are relaxed, all that is highest and best comes to you as grace.

—YOGI AMRIT DESAI

For thousands of years, yoga practitioners have used relaxation techniques to access a state called *Yoga Nidra* meaning *yogic sleep*. Yoga Nidra is a kind of twilight state between waking and sleep, a state of profound rest that quickly renews body and mind. Contemporary practitioners generally use the term *deep relaxation,* and often find that as little as ten to fifteen minutes of Yoga Nidra can leave them feeling as refreshed as a full night's sleep.

For those seeking healing, learning how to consistently access a state of deep relaxation is essential. When relaxed, your nervous system works at peak efficiency, monitoring any deviation from the delicate balance that is wellness and acting to restore harmony. Your endocrine system is finely tuned, sending the precise amount and mix of hormones to regulate organ function. Your immune response is strong, boosting your capacity to heal. All these things happen spontaneously, and happen best, when you are relaxed. When stress inhibits these or other functions, relaxation is the natural antidote.

Beyond its health benefits, yoga teaches that learning how to relax is the first step on the path of meditation. The ability to relax the body while the mind remains present and aware is what makes deeper states of consciousness accessible. For all these reasons, the Sun and Moon Series conclude with deep relaxation.

Being led into deep relaxation by a skilled instructor at the end of a yoga class can feel so natural that it is easy to overlook what actually happens. If you want to practice on your own, it is important to understand the relaxation process. Deep relaxation is actually a combination of several different techniques, which are taught in sequence below. The first is the posture called *Shavasana* meaning *Corpse Pose.*

Relaxing in Corpse Pose

Although it looks easy, Corpse Pose is actually a challenging yoga posture. The difficulty involved is learning how to surrender the full weight of your body into the support of the floor, which requires the capacity to relax all the voluntary skeletal muscles. As you come into Corpse Pose, it is common to first become acutely aware of all the places that are not relaxed. If you can breathe into the sensations and simply feel them, muscular tension gradually lets go.

All postures, including Corpse Pose, require proper alignment. The guiding principle in Corpse is to keep the body symmetrical, which supports an even flow of energy through the nervous system. The classic position is with the arms palms up near the sides and feet splayed out about hip-width apart. Along with symmetry, comfort is important. Some people like to rest their hands on the belly or on the chest, or position the feet a little closer or wider apart.

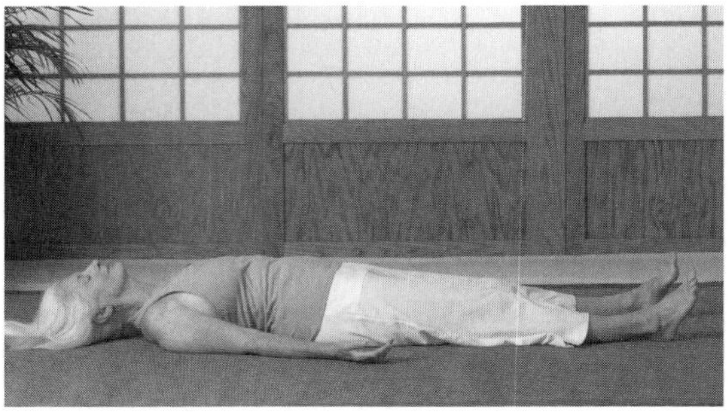

It is not uncommon to find it difficult to relax on your back. Try placing a pillow beneath the knees, which releases the hamstring muscles and relieves low back tension. Alternatively, draw the feet up close to the buttocks and let the

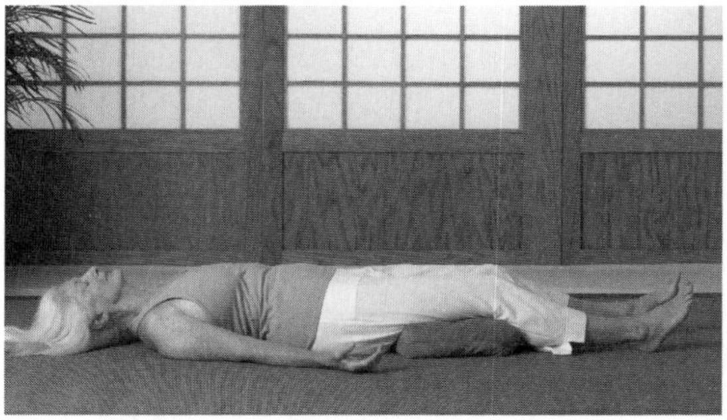

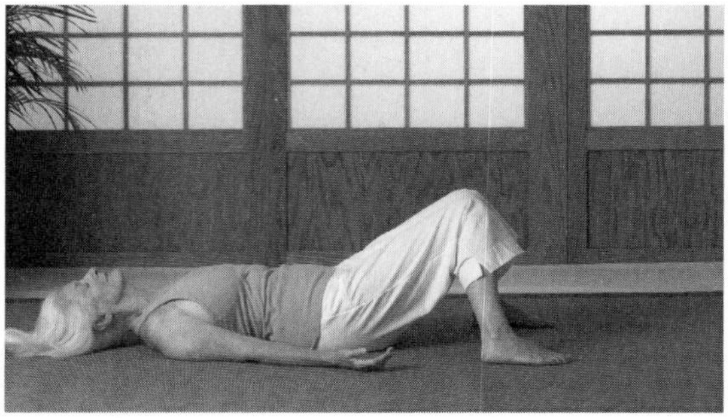

MORE RELAXATION TIPS

- If you wear eyeglasses, take them off. Some people like to cover their eyes with an eye pillow designed to block light and apply a light pressure to keep the eyelids closed. You can also use a folded washcloth for this purpose.

- As your body relaxes, its surface temperature tends to drop precipitously. Putting on an extra layer of clothing or covering up with a blanket is a big aid to entering the state of Yoga Nidra. If you don't cover up, you may not feel cold. You may just find yourself unable to let go into deep relaxation for no apparent reason.

- As you follow the instructions to progressively relax the body, make sure you are actually feeling each part of the body. Avoid the tendency to just vaguely think about relaxing. Let your awareness actually drop from your head into your body, feeling all the sensations present in each part. Invite it to relax completely, and move on to the next part.

- If a part of your body holds on to tension despite your invitation to relax, rest your awareness there for a minute or two. Give up any effort to make it go away and fully feel whatever is there. Open to receive any message your body may be trying to send you. If the tension remains, allow it to be there and relax all around it. Then continue with the steps of the relaxation process.

- During relaxation, you will undoubtedly fall asleep from time to time. This is to be expected. Just keep practicing with the intention to learn how to relax completely while remaining lucid and aware of what is happening. Conscious relaxation enables you to access and release subtle layers of physical, emotional, and mental tension that are normally unconscious. This is what distinguishes Yoga Nidra from a catnap.

knees fall together, so that they support the weight of the legs. If your head tilts back uncomfortably, place a folded blanket or thin pillow beneath it to bring the neck into alignment. Don't use a large pillow, which crimps the neck and obstructs the free flow of breath.

> *In my first experience of deep relaxation, I had a vision of the night sky and a feeling of being suspended in awe and knowing. I still access this same vision each time I go into Corpse Pose. It calms me in times of stress and allows me to see that I carry peace with me at all times. I can always go to that place of universal knowing.*
>
> —Julie Garland

Relaxing Breath

Relaxing Breath is the simplest and most powerful of all relaxation techniques. Come into Corpse Pose and give the body a minute or two to gradually sink into the support of the floor. Then let the breath begin to flow freely, gradually lengthening out your exhalations. The inhale happens naturally, and the exhale just rolls out long, slow, and smooth. After a few minutes of focused breathing in this way, the abdominal muscles relax and exhalations grow to about twice as long as inhalations. This means if you were inhaling to a count of three, you would exhale to a count of about six.

This is Relaxing Breath, and it has a stunning number of benefits:

- Decreases heart rate
- Lowers blood pressure
- Reduces stress chemicals in bloodstream
- Boosts immune response
- Internalizes awareness
- Enhances self-awareness and empathy
- Increases creativity

Relaxing Breath has all these benefits because it induces the *relaxation response,* a physiological state associated with a marked increase in the activity of the parasympathetic nervous system. After a yoga session, the body is primed for relaxation and a few minutes of Relaxing Breath will accomplish this crucial shift in physiology. Then gently release any conscious control of the breath, letting it flow naturally in and out, and continue with the relaxation technique.

Progressive Relaxation

Progressive relaxation is the technique of relaxing the entire body, part by part. Beyond being a highly effective way to release tension, the act of directing awareness from one part of the body to another helps you remain awake and aware during the relaxation process.

Most forms of progressive relaxation begin with the feet and work up the body, relaxing the major muscles and joints. The technique in the experience on pages 68 and 69 is more comprehensive, guiding you to focus not only on muscles and joints, but also on your organs, glands, and nervous system; your mind and heart; and the free flow of energy and awareness through your being.

To deliver its message of relaxation, progressive relaxation always employs some form of another technique: *suggestion*.

Suggestion and Affirmations

Suggestion is the delivery of a message or instruction to a deeply relaxed mind. Suggestion bypasses the mind's normal tendency to examine, criticize, and block input, allowing the message of relaxation to be delivered to the psyche in a way that avoids normal shields and defenses. *Auto-suggestion* is when you deliver the message to yourself, versus having a therapist, yoga teacher, or relaxation tape give it to you.

In the experience that follows, you are guided to *invite each part of the body to completely relax*. This wording conveys an important principle. You don't have to consciously learn how to relax. Your body already knows how; you are just inviting it to do something that is natural and innate. To support the body, the mind provides a clear mental suggestion. For example, when guided to focus on the feet you mentally affirm: *I am relaxing my feet. I am relaxing my feet. My feet are completely relaxed.* Although this phrasing is recommended, the same suggestion can be delivered in many ways. You can use phrasing that engages your kinesthetic sense of feeling: *My feet feel heavy and completely relaxed.* Or you can include the element of visualization: *My feet are surrounded by radiant light and completely relaxed.*

Other suggestions used in the experience include *invite the mind to relax* and *release any worries or concerns* and *allow mental and emotional defenses to fall away,* and ultimately *let go into deep relaxation*. Regardless of form or phrasing, it is important to voice the suggestion clearly in your mind and to listen to it attentively. Begin with the technique as given. As you become familiar with the relaxation process, feel free to experiment and discover what forms of suggestion work best for you.

Many relaxation techniques also include the use of *affirmations,* positive statements repeated silently and internally to engender a positive state of mind. As practice deepens, some practitioners find that deep relaxation provides an opportunity to reprogram the subconscious mind, countering the negative messages that undermine happiness, health, and effectiveness in life.

Affirming a Different Truth

Delivered at a surface level of consciousness, affirmations tend to be deflected by the mind's defenses. Even when repeated often, spoken aloud, or written, they can fail to effect real change or modify behavior. Affirmations delivered to a mind that is deeply relaxed, highly

EXPERIENCE: PROGRESSIVE RELAXATION IN CORPSE POSE *(Yoga Nidra in Shavasana)*

This experience combines all of the techniques described above. Before beginning, put on an extra layer of clothes or better yet cover yourself with a blanket. If it is uncomfortable for you to lie flat on the floor, make yourself comfortable by modifying Corpse Pose in any of the ways suggested on page 64.

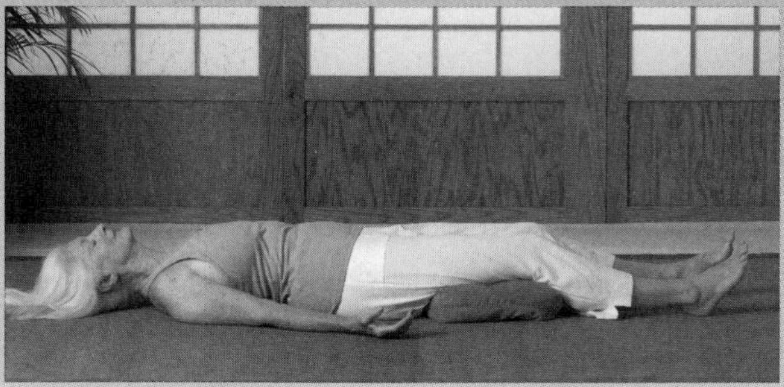

1. Lie on your back with the legs extended. Adjust the feet so they are a comfortable distance apart, and let the toes fall out to the sides. Bring the arms a comfortable distance from the sides, palms up and fingers naturally curled. Rock the head gently from side to side a time or two to release the muscles of the neck. Then bring the head back to center, and elongate the neck by slightly tucking the chin. Then release the chin tuck and allow the back of the head to rest solidly on the floor.

2. Close the eyes to facilitate feeling. Let the whole body sink into the floor, especially the backs of the legs, sacrum, shoulder blades, and back of the head.

3. Focus your attention on the flow of breath. Allow the breath to flow freely for a minute or two, smoothing out the shifts between in-breaths and out-breaths, just watching and feeling the process of breathing. Then gradually move into Relaxing Breath by lengthening your exhalations. Do this without any strain, letting the inhale happen naturally, and then letting the exhale just roll out of you long, slow, and smooth. Then draw in another breath and repeat.

4. Continue Relaxing Breath for several minutes, feeling the belly and the whole body deeply relaxing. Then release any conscious control of the breath, letting it flow naturally in and out.

5. Bring your awareness down to your feet. Starting with the feet and slowly coming up the body, consciously invite each part of the body to completely relax. Give a clear mental suggestion, such as: *I am relaxing my feet. I am relaxing my feet. My feet are completely relaxed.* Relax the feet, ankles, calves, knees, thighs, hips, abdomen, low back, chest, shoulders, upper back,

arms, hands, and fingers. Continue relaxing the throat, back of the neck, head, and scalp. Then relax the muscles of your face, letting any facial expression fall away. Release the jaw, letting the teeth separate slightly. Allow any tension held in the cheeks, muscles around the eyes, forehead, temples, and sides of the head to melt away. Then scan the whole body, inviting any subtle muscle tension that remains to let go.

6. Once again drop your awareness deep inside the body and down to the bowl of the pelvis. Consciously invite energy to freely circulate through the organ and glandular system, harmonizing and balancing its function. Give a clear mental suggestion, such as: *Energy flows freely and easily through my organs and glands.* Focus on the organs and glands in the following order: organs of reproduction and elimination; all the abdominal organs; kidneys and adrenals, which are located in the low and mid-back; thymus, heart, and lungs; thyroid and parathyroid; and brain. Let the entire nervous system gradually calm and grow quiet.

7. Allow the heart to open to full feeling. Invite the mind to relax, surrendering any control over the flow of emotion or thought. Release any worries or concerns. Allow mental and emotional defenses to fall away. Let go into deep relaxation. You may want to consciously affirm: *Energy flows freely through every level of my being.*

8. Stay in this state as long as you wish. When your consciousness begins to surface, come out of relaxation gently. Gradually deepen the breath. Wiggle your fingers and toes to bring awareness back to the body. Take a few minutes to stretch in ways that feel good. Roll over onto one side and slowly come back to sitting, taking care to bring relaxation with you.

9. For a minute or two, just be, noticing the quality of body and mind. If you wish, you may choose to sit for a time in meditation. When you feel complete, draw your practice to a close with a sense of gratitude. Return to whatever is next in your life with a renewed sense of focus and calm.

As you become familiar with the relaxation process, you can shorten the instructions to the following:

- Come into Corpse Pose
- Engage Relaxing Breath
- Relax the body from the feet to the head
- Rebalance the organs and glands from the pelvis to the brain
- Allow worries, concerns, and defenses to fall away
- Let go into deep relaxation
- Come back gently

A CD or audiotape that skillfully guides you into relaxation can be a helpful learning tool. Even after learning, some people prefer the ease of having an external voice provide the suggestions. See the Resource List for recommendations.

aware, and free of defenses tend to have a very different effect. Even a single affirmation can be life changing.

Some approaches teach that the way an affirmation is worded is very important. They recommend using the first person, the present tense, and short, clear statements that don't allow for mixed messages. Other approaches emphasize the importance of one's intention and the feeling state in which the affirmation is uttered. All agree that only a small number of affirmations should be used at any one time, and that they must be repeated consistently to alter the conditioning of the subconscious mind.

Here is a short list of affirmations to get you started:

- I am enough, just as I am.
- My heart is open to feeling.
- I am free of limiting beliefs.
- I am happy, healthy, and deeply at peace.
- Energy flows freely through every level of my being.
- I rest in the presence of Spirit.

The best affirmations emerge from your own practice and life experience. Once you identify a repetitive and limiting pattern of thought, you can choose to affirm a different truth.

> *It's a paradox that relaxation requires a kind of effort. Letting go isn't easy. It means stepping into unknown territory, relinquishing the familiar shape of my being. Relaxation also requires attention. Untying grosser knots of tension, I discover more subtle, deeper knots. Each one I untie liberates more energy and brings me to a more inclusive state of health. When I practice deep relaxation, I emerge peaceful, clear, and refreshed.*
>
> —Charles Eisenstein

When to Practice

When practiced at the end of a yoga session, deep relaxation comes naturally and is extremely rejuvenating. Resist the tendency to view yoga as just exercise, a belief that will make you want to end your practice after finishing postures. It's the *combination* of postures and deep relaxation that frees the body and mind of tension, returning you to a balanced state of health. Even if you have to shorten some other part of your session, try to allow at least ten minutes for deep relaxation.

Other good times to practice Yoga Nidra include before lunch as a midday break, after work as a way to let go of the day's events, or after getting into bed as a way to relax the body prior to sleep. If you work out, ending with some cooldown stretches and a few minutes of deep relaxation will multiply its benefits. Complementing a morning posture practice with deep relaxation before dinner is a nice way to bookend your day with yoga.

Relaxation Experiences

People report a variety of experiences in deep relaxation. Some of this can be understood through the shifts in brain wave activity that take place. Beta brain waves are dominant when the mind is engaged in normal activity. As you relax, slower alpha brain waves increase and you may notice a heightened sense of feeling and flow. Thoughts seem to slow and creative ideas often slip into consciousness.

As you relax more deeply, even slower theta brain waves increase and you may have the experience of being profoundly at rest while quite awake and aware. In the theta state, your sense of time and space is altered. Minutes often pass by like seconds. Sometimes a few minutes can seem like hours. You may be aware of sounds and the space that surrounds you but lose all sense of your physical body. Or you may have the feeling that your body is heavy as iron, or that it is weightless and floating freely a few inches above the floor, or has expanded to fill the room. Since most people only experience the theta state during sleep, these experiences can at first be disorienting. Knowing that these experiences are the result of natural and beneficial states of consciousness can help you relax into them. Over time these experiences occur almost universally as positive and deeply nurturing.

> *I have found practicing relaxation to be an art. The unstringing of muscles never comes immediately. It takes time. Layers have to be peeled off to reach real relaxation. The first layers disappear as I release each posture. Then, in Corpse Pose, I listen to my heartbeat gradually slow—who said yoga isn't aerobic? I feel the little knots in the surface muscles let go the same way I used to hear the wooden floors of my old apartment settle down for the night. They'd give over to gravity one creak at a time.*
>
> *The tingle of relaxation spreads from the sacrum upward, moves laterally between my shoulder blades, then radiates down my back muscles along the ribs. Just when I start to think that deeper wave of relaxation isn't going to come, I feel the final release spreading through me like liquid mercury. The feeling is bright, smooth, heavy, drawn by gravity to gather at the points touching the earth. I'm always surprised when it happens. That last release into the depth of relaxation dawns like an orchestra sneaking up on a key change. It breaks through and opens into a major chord.*
>
> —Kim Coleman Healy

Using Visualization to Relax

Relaxation techniques that use *visualization* or *imagery* are based on the principle that thoughts and images have the capacity to shift your brain activity and state of being. By harnessing the power of imagination, visualization

EXPERIENCE: LIQUID LIGHT VISUALIZATION

1. Come into Corpse Pose.

2. Take a few deep breaths and let the body sink into the floor.

3. Let your awareness flow down to your feet. Visualize and feel a warm, luminous, liquid light flowing into the soles of your feet. Allow this liquid light to gradually fill your feet. Then watch and feel as the liquid light slowly but steadily fills the legs, pelvic area, abdomen, chest, throat, and head. See and feel the whole body filled with this warm, luminous, liquid light.

4. When the body has filled, visualize and feel this liquid light streaming through the arteries, veins, and nerves in flowing currents. Feel this flow renewing and recharging your being on every level.

5. As you are bathed in this energy, see your body surrounded by a radiant glow. Let the glow increase in intensity until you are powerfully radiating light in all directions.

6. Let go of any mental effort and allow yourself to rest in deep relaxation.

creates thoughts and images that temporarily take the place of external sensory input. The idea is to create scenes and situations that are safe, relaxing, and otherwise desirable. The body responds to these imagined scenes as if they were real, which is why positive images can dispel stress and encourage feelings of well-being. The more vivid the images, the greater the effect on the mind and body.

An especially popular visualization is imagining yourself in a place where you are completely comfortable and at peace. Some people see themselves lying in the sun on a sandy beach, listening to the ocean waves. Others sit on mountaintops, stroll through quiet gardens, or visit a childhood haven. Bring all of your senses into play, feeling the sun on your face, hearing the sounds of birds, smelling the fragrance of flowers in bloom, and tasting the cool water.

> *When we moved into final relaxation, it felt as though the floor actually softened and cradled my body. I felt very heavy and then profoundly light, expansive, and without boundaries, above and beyond it all, and also part of everything, all at the same time. When the teacher called us back, I found for the first time I could remember that there was joy in my body. I knew there was something more, something bigger, and I was a part of it.*
>
> —Jennifer Cann

CHAPTER SEVEN

THE ART OF PRACTICE

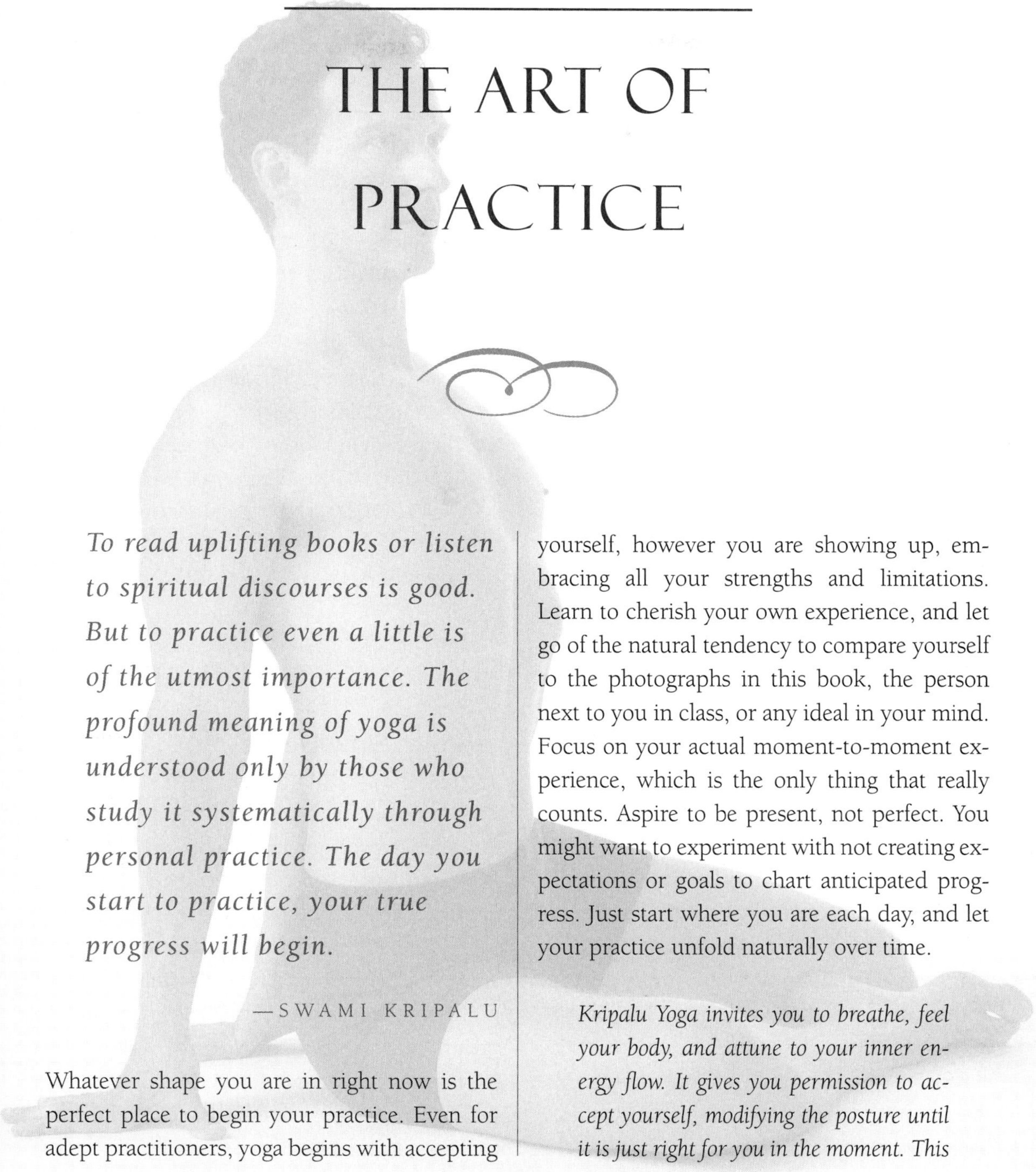

To read uplifting books or listen to spiritual discourses is good. But to practice even a little is of the utmost importance. The profound meaning of yoga is understood only by those who study it systematically through personal practice. The day you start to practice, your true progress will begin.

—SWAMI KRIPALU

Whatever shape you are in right now is the perfect place to begin your practice. Even for adept practitioners, yoga begins with accepting yourself, however you are showing up, embracing all your strengths and limitations. Learn to cherish your own experience, and let go of the natural tendency to compare yourself to the photographs in this book, the person next to you in class, or any ideal in your mind. Focus on your actual moment-to-moment experience, which is the only thing that really counts. Aspire to be present, not perfect. You might want to experiment with not creating expectations or goals to chart anticipated progress. Just start where you are each day, and let your practice unfold naturally over time.

Kripalu Yoga invites you to breathe, feel your body, and attune to your inner energy flow. It gives you permission to accept yourself, modifying the posture until it is just right for you in the moment. This approach allows you to come home to your body and yourself. Regular practice helps you access and live from a stronger connection to who and what you really are. The hidden power of Kripalu Yoga is that it uses postures as a tool to discover your authentic self.

—Lawrence Noyes

Create Sacred Space

Your outer environment will either support your practice or present frequent opportunities for distraction. Kripalu Yoga describes the optimal environment as *safe and sacred space,* and learning how to create short periods of sanctuary in your life is essential to sustaining a practice. You need enough floor space to stretch out in all directions. A setting that is clean and comfortable helps foster a sense of order that facilitates focus and relaxation. The ability to adjust the temperature, flow of fresh air, and lighting is a nice amenity. Traditional texts recommend that you avoid either direct sun or cool drafts. Having what you need close at hand, perhaps a yoga mat for firm footing, a pillow for sitting on the floor, and a blanket for relaxation, makes things simple.

Psychological safety is also important. Set aside a block of time where you can be free from distractions. If possible, create privacy by closing the door behind you and turning off the phone. Many people find that soothing background music is a big help in calming the mind and opening to deeper feeling. To foster a sense of the sacred, you may want to decorate an altar with candles, flowers, meaningful symbols, or photographs. Lighting candles, hearing familiar music, or just putting on sweats and getting out the mat becomes a ritual, a symbolic act that sends a powerful message to your body and mind that this is a time for self-nurturance.

I created my own sacred space to do yoga in my daughter's room—she's away at college. I have candles and a window to see the sunrise. No one interrupts me there because I'm the first one up and everyone else is still asleep. I tend to be high-strung and have found that when I start my day this way, I don't get rattled so easily.

—Gail Barraco

Learn to Slow Down

For the majority of people living active lives, the mind moves quickly all day long, shifting back and forth from one thing to the next, often recollecting the past or imagining the future. The body moves at a much slower pace, always in the here and now, flowing with the pulse of the heartbeat, the rise and fall of breath, and the natural cycles of various life processes. In order to bring body and mind together, you must learn to slow the mind down to the pace of the body.

Be prepared for the mind to put up a fight. At the beginning of a session, it often feels like the mind simply won't let go, and that the effort to breathe, relax, and feel is a futile exercise. Resistance arises and the mind loudly cries out in protest. Then something shifts. As the body softens and the mind comes to focus, what seemed impossible a few moments ago happens effortlessly. The same posture that felt like drudgery now feels blissful. As the movement from posture to posture smooths into flow, the satisfaction that comes from being deeply present in your body occurs as an epiphany. In the face of resistance, it is easy to forget that you simply need to stay with it. As your practice matures, you are likely to become so accustomed to this experience of shifting gears that it hardly registers. In the initial stages of practice, it can pose a significant barrier.

> *One of my favorite aspects of Kripalu Yoga is the pause between postures. This wasn't always the case. When I first started yoga classes, I was impatient to get to the next posture, the next level of practice, and then on to the next activity. Even though I loved the class, I watched the clock. I always left before the relaxation because I couldn't bear to lie still and do nothing for ten minutes.*
>
> *Over and over, my yoga teacher invited me to pause, breathe, and feel. At first, I felt nothing. Then one day after holding the boat posture for what felt like forever, I welcomed the rest. I enjoyed feeling my body slowly melt back onto the floor. As I relaxed, a marvelous thing happened. I felt my body release on deeper and more subtle levels. It felt that every single cell, right down to my bone marrow, had let go with a huge sigh of relief. I could have stayed there in stillness enjoying the sensations for a very long time, but of course my teacher interrupted my peace with an invitation to move on to the next posture. I was able to enjoy the irony of the moment.*
>
> *Now I love the pause between things. I have also integrated this wisdom into how I schedule my days. I used to pack my days so full I never had a moment to spare. Whenever possible, I now give myself time to receive the richness of each experience before dashing off to the next. And when I need to, I can voluntarily repeat that experience of deep release.*
>
> —Rebecca Johanna Stephans

Respect the Body's Need to Warm Up

Warm-ups stimulate respiration and increase pulse rate, lubricate the joints with synovial fluid, raise the temperature of muscles and connective tissues that may be cold and tight, and awaken the mind and nervous system to greater body sensitivity. Taking the time to warm up honors your body's need to move gradually into movement and deeper stretching.

If you don't begin your yoga practice slowly, gradually increasing the intensity of your stretches, you not only risk injuring yourself, but your practice will remain superficial. An unprepared body will resist the mind's efforts to force it into challenging postures before it is ready.

> *For two years after my divorce, I was unable to quiet my mind. I pushed away the things I most wanted to do—paint, write, and listen to music—and held my body in a constant state of tightness. I tried to calm my mind through meditation but was unsuccessful. Then I spent a weekend doing Kripalu Yoga and breathing and my mind became still. Since then, I've found it easy to slip into a meditative state. When I notice that I'm not breathing, I make a conscious effort to deepen and then follow my breath. When my body feels tight, I've been able to let it go and feel myself relax. I'm listening to music and painting again.*
>
> —Noreen Owens

Come Back to the Breath

So much of yoga comes naturally if you can just remember to breathe. Again and again during your practice, bring your attention back to the breath, letting it flow freely. After releasing a posture, take a deep breath in and let out an audible sigh to release tension. Integrate the beneficial effects with a few three-part breaths. Then breathe your way into the next posture. As you become more attuned to the breath you see that yoga practice—and life—unfolds one breath at a time.

Let the Postures Evoke Feeling

Practicing at the edge assures that you will encounter a broad range of sensations and emotions. Kripalu Yoga postures are intended to evoke a depth of feeling, as this provides an opportunity for the deeper work of regaining emotional sensitivity and balance. Resist the tendency to go "into your head" and try to understand or fix your feelings. Simply breathe, relax, and feel, letting sensation and emotion flow through you. Over time, areas of numbness wake up. Buried and banished feelings surface to be felt, and emotional armoring melts away. Celebrate this process of opening to feeling as the pathway to greater vitality and full aliveness.

> *What I experience in Kripalu Yoga is the luxury of getting to know myself. I see the pockets of memory that cause me to hold back my love because I feel unlovable. Postures give me the ability to release these memories and return to my natural state of being. When I get back in touch with that, I always find comfort, peace, and connection with my higher self.*
>
> —Paula Linda Reed

Listen to Self-Talk

Practice generates an inner focus that allows your mental dialogue to be heard and examined. Psychologists call this *self-talk* and consider it a normal and healthy phenomenon. Although some level of inner dialogue is going on almost all the time, it tends to be less audible when you are engaged in external activities. When engaging in a contemplative practice like yoga, it can seem like your self-talk is greatly intensified. What is actually happening is that you are hearing more of the things you are saying to yourself all the time.

Kripalu Yoga presents a rare opportunity to closely watch the flow of thought and listen attentively to the inner workings of your mind. You do not have to control or change your thinking in any way, or once and for all win the argument with your inner critic. Simply watch objectively, and listen with compassion to what is being said. As you grow comfortable watching thoughts that range from the ridiculous to the sublime, you may notice that the inner space around your thinking has expanded, and find that what you think carries less of an emotional charge.

Attune to Energy

As your practice deepens, you may begin to experience that sensations, emotions, and thoughts are all aspects of a single intelligence, the energetic source of body and mind.

Attuning to this source energy can lead to moments when you go beyond accustomed ways of experiencing yourself. The yoga tradition is replete with stories of people whose practice led them to encounter a wide spectrum of what are commonly called *peak experiences*. These may be as simple as becoming deeply absorbed in the flow of breath and sensation, having powerful insights, or feeling your body in new ways. They can be as powerful as experiencing a deeper or higher level of reality. Peak experiences cannot be forced. All you can do is stay present to your experience, attune to energy, and let the wisdom of your own body express.

> *One day I drove home after yoga class and the day was brilliant. There was newly fallen snow. The roadside sparkled, and light shined as though from the heavens. I felt pure joy.*
>
> —Sheila deMagalhaes

The Practice Session

It is not the deep breathing, or the active stretching, or the balanced strengthening, or the moments of relaxed calm that make yoga so effective. It is all of them together. As a review and final step toward practice, here is a basic template for a Kripalu Yoga session:

The Yoga of Conscious Awareness

BY SENIOR TEACHER RUDY PEIRCE

When I joined the Kripalu Center staff in 1982, everything from dawn to dusk was about awareness. In all our activities, we were guided to look within and notice "what's going on inside." At times, it felt like being under a microscope. I took this guidance into my yoga practice and became able to pick up more and more subtle sensations in my body. Cultivating this type of self-awareness gradually became part of my lifestyle. I learned to honor my inner workings, and even my inner grumblings. As a yoga teacher, I now see how this awareness permeates my classes. Each moment on the mat is an opportunity to notice what's happening and deepen your awareness of it. In the midst of doing postures, I find myself asking students to inquire:

Where do you feel the stretch?
Where is the breath flowing, where is it blocked?
Notice if any subtle changes accompany the exhalation.
Bring awareness to your belly, what's happening there?
What is your body asking for right now?
What is your heart saying?
Where is your mind's attention?

I teach this way, because this is how yoga became a spiritual practice for me. Just by looking within, I discovered a connection to spirit that had become covered over with the busyness of my life. When I ask myself: "What does the soft voice of spirit have to say to me right now?" the answer is often: "Let go. You can relax now. There is nothing that you need to do in this moment. Simply be. Simply be."

• Bring Yourself Present

Come into a sitting or standing position and bring yourself present by going through the steps of breathe, relax, feel, watch, and allow. As the breath begins to flow, let your awareness drop from the head into the body, permeating each and every cell. Inwardly affirm an intention to remain present to the sensations, emotions, and thoughts that arise during practice. Setting a clear intention to remain present helps you to stay mentally engaged, avoids the tendency to become habitual and unconscious in your movements, and allows you to draw on body wisdom.

• Engage the Breath

Relax your abdomen and come into Ocean Sounding Breath, letting your breath flow freely in and out. Invite the breath to gradually deepen into Three-Part Breathing, and breathe deeply for several minutes as you oxygenate the blood and charge the system with energy. Come back into a relaxed and rhythmic Ocean Sounding Breath. You will sustain this flowing breath throughout the entire practice session, breathing as deeply as comfortable given the movement or posture you are doing. Whenever your mind wanders and your breath stops flowing smoothly, just reengage the breath.

• Take Time to Warm Up

Taking the time to warm up produces a more enjoyable, safe, and beneficial yoga experience. Warm-ups can be done either on the floor or from standing, but take care to gently work the whole body with repetitive movements that do not require either a lot of exertion or stretching to your full range of motion.

• Perform a Balanced Sequence of Postures

Kripalu Yoga enlivens the entire body through a balanced routine of postures performed in synchronization with the breath. After warm-ups, both the Sun and Moon Series begin with standing postures and end with floor postures. Standing postures provide many structural benefits, stretching and strengthening the major muscle groups to produce a balanced muscle tone supportive of good posture and proper body alignment. Floor postures provide many deeper health benefits. Done in the proper order, they systematically revitalize the organs and glands.

• End with Deep Relaxation

Postures release excess muscle tension and prepare you for the rejuvenating experience of deep relaxation. If a yoga session were likened to a sumptuous meal, relaxation would be a wholesome dessert worth saving time to savor fully. Try to allow at least ten minutes for final relaxation to allow the body to integrate and rebalance.

Coming to Completion

Come out of relaxation slowly. A nice way to bring your awareness back to your physical body is to wiggle your fingers and toes. Roll over to one side and rest for a minute or two in a fetal position, and then stretch in any way that feels good. Gradually work your way back up into a sitting position. Close your eyes and be present—breathe, relax, feel, watch, and allow. If you wish, sit for a few moments in meditation. Return to whatever is next in your life with a renewed sense of focus and calm.

2. THE PRACTICE SESSIONS

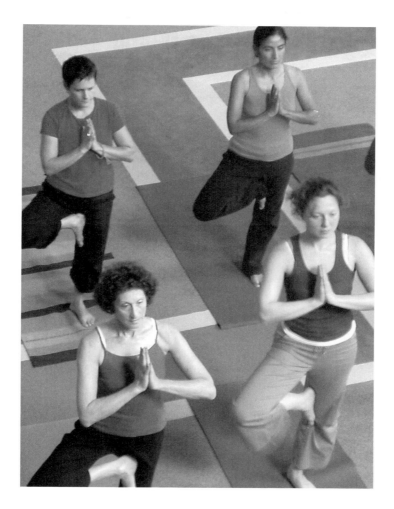

BASIC TIPS FOR YOGA PRACTICE

- Consult a physician before beginning a practice if you have health conditions, are pregnant, or had a recent surgery or medical procedure. If you are taking a yoga class, let the teacher know about any injuries or health challenges you are facing so they can fine-tune and modify your practice.
- Allow time to digest after eating, generally an hour after a snack, two hours after a light meal, and three to four hours after a heavy meal.
- Wear clothing that lets the body move freely and the pores breathe. Some prefer loose-fitting sweats, others tights. Try practicing barefoot, which gves you better footing and stimulates the many nerve endings in the feet.
- Traditional yoga advises women not to practice during menstruation. Contemporary approaches differ, but many teachers recommend rest during the first three days of flow and the avoidance of inversions and vigorous breathing exercises for the full period.
- Good times to practice are first thing in the morning, late afternoon after work, and late evening before bedtime. Depending on your lifestyle and work schedule, you may need to practice at other times. More important than the time of practice is consistency. The best time to practice is when you can make room in your schedule to practice regularly.
- Morning stiffness is partially the result of dehydrated connective tissues. Drinking a glass of water before beginning practice helps.
- Move slowly and smoothly and keep the breath flowing, which increases the benefits of practice and minimizes the risk of injury.
- Always heed pain, which is a clear message from the body that you are exceeding healthy limits. Learning to distinguish between pain and discomfort is a key component of a safe and effective yoga practice. (See chapter 4.)
- Supplement a regular home practice with a weekly yoga class, which allows a certified yoga teacher to oversee your progress and puts you in touch with other people interested in and practicing yoga. For a Kripalu Yoga teacher near you, log on to www.kripalu.org or call (413) 448-3202.

SUN FLOW

Warm-Ups

Mountain Pose and Centering
Standing Twists
Monkey Stretch
Forward Fold
Sun Salutation
Breath of Joy

Standing Postures

Warrior
Triangle
Standing Angle
Crane

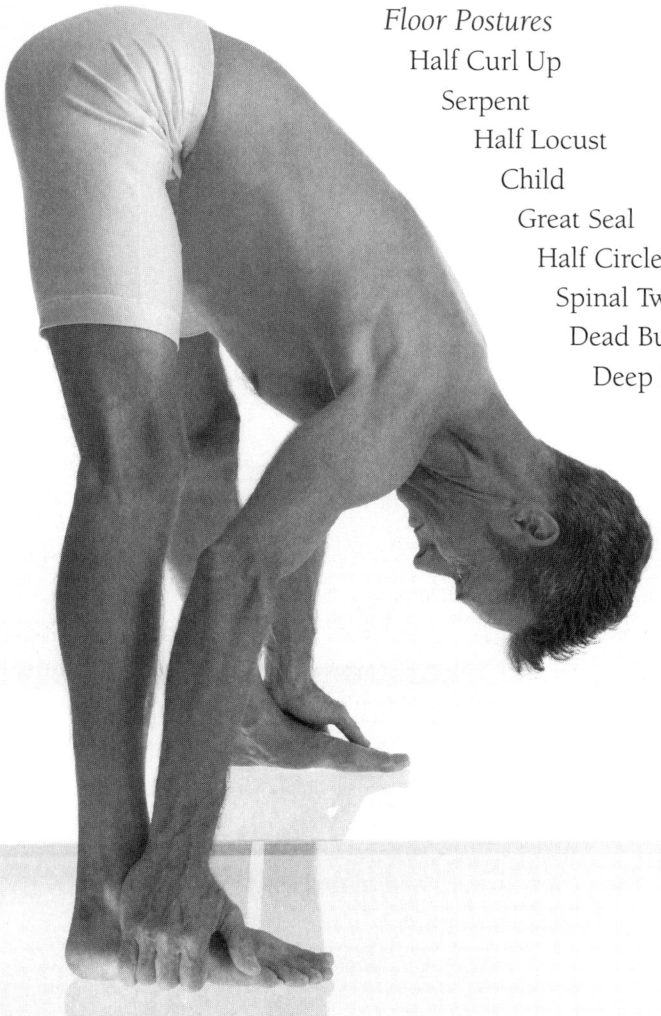

Floor Postures

Half Curl Up
Serpent
Half Locust
Child
Great Seal
Half Circle
Spinal Twist
Dead Bug
Deep Relaxation in Corpse

MOUNTAIN POSE AND CENTERING

(Ujjayi Pranayama in Tadasana)

1. Stand with your feet parallel, hip-width apart, and arms at the sides.

2. Lift the toes, spread them wide, and place them back on the floor. Press down evenly into all four corners of the feet, engaging the muscles of the legs without locking the knees. Balance your body weight between the heels and toes, and between the right and left legs.

3. Stabilize the core of your body by pressing the tailbone down and pubic bone forward to level the pelvis, and gently contracting and lifting the muscles of the pelvic floor. Elongate the spine by lifting out of the waist.

4. Press the sternum forward without arching the spine back or puffing the chest out military style. Allow the tops of the shoulders to relax down, away from the ears. Draw the wing points together, pressing the shoulder blades down. With the chin parallel to the floor, extend through the crown of the head to elongate the neck.

5. Lift the hands into Prayer Position and gently press the palms together. Bring yourself present: breathe, relax, feel, watch, and allow. Affirm the intention to remain present in your body as you practice.

6. Come into Ocean Sounding Breath, allowing the friction of the breath against the back of the throat to make a sound like the rise and fall of waves at the beach. Use the sound of the breath to help you smooth out its flow, letting in-breaths and out-breaths flow smoothly one into the next. You will sustain Ocean Sounding Breath for the duration of your practice. Whenever the mind wanders, just come back to the breath.

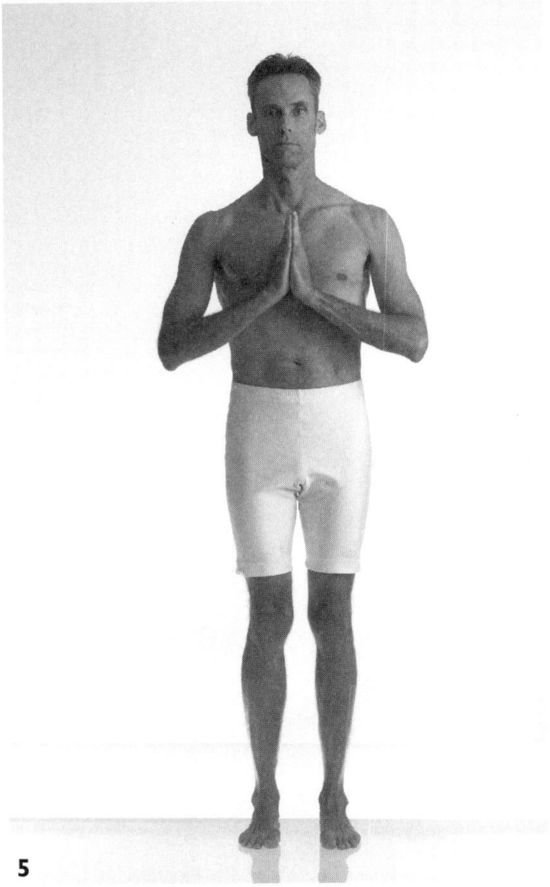

5

Be Aware:

Practiced as a centering, Mountain Pose is a tangible reminder of the importance of alignment principles. At the beginning of practice,

Ocean Sounding Breath is an invitation to breathe deeply, and you are likely to find yourself moving naturally into Three-Part Breathing. Let that happen, returning to a flowing breath for warm-ups and sustaining Ocean Sounding Breath for the duration of your practice session. Whenever the mind wanders, just come back to the breath.

STANDING TWISTS

1. Stand with the feet parallel, a little wider than hip-width apart, arms near your sides.

2. Begin to rotate the hips and shoulders from side to side. Allow the relaxed arms to flap against the sides like empty coat sleeves, with the hands gently striking the body down by the hip bones. Let the head join in the motion, turning to look over one shoulder, and then the other. Coordinate breath and motion, exhaling as you twist and inhaling back to center.

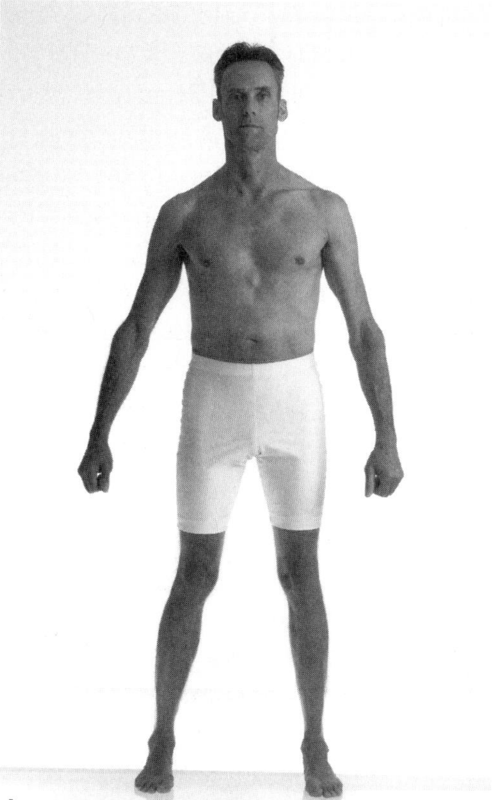

1

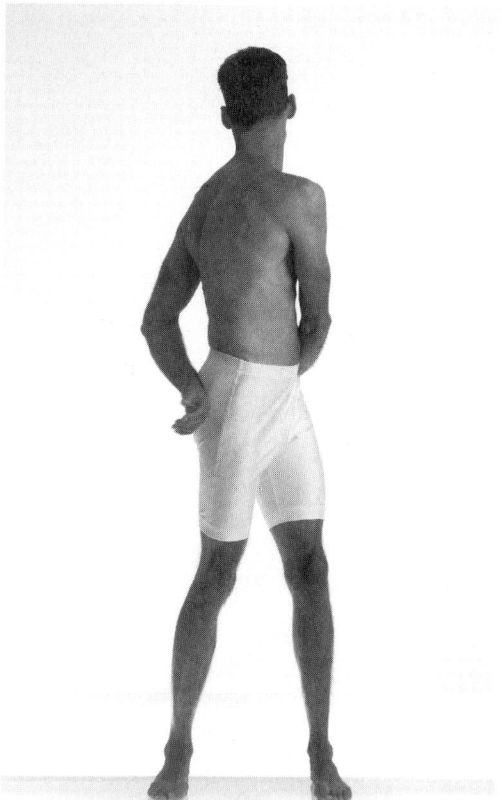

2

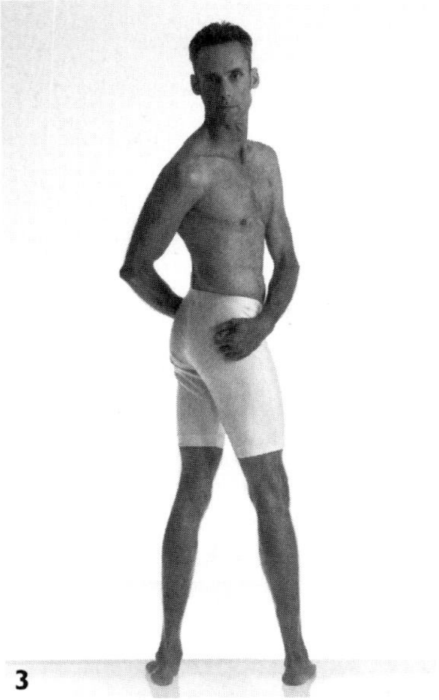

3

3. Keep the spine erect and the hips and shoulders rotating as if in a barrel—versus swaying—from side to side.

4. As you twist from side to side, let the hands gradually lift to belly button height, then chest height, then shoulder height, moving the stretch progressively up the spine. As the hips, shoulders, and arms swing to the right, let the left heel lift slightly to allow the hips a greater range of movement and avoid straining the left knee.

5. Lower the hands the way they came up, returning to the arms flapping against the sides like empty coat sleeves. Let the twisting slow down and then come into stillness. Take a deep breath in and let it out with an audible sigh.

Be Aware:
Gently twisting one way, then the other is a great way to begin warming up the body. Another variation is called Stirring the Pot. Stand as above but with the feet slightly splayed out to the sides. Soften the knees and bring the hands in front of you to grasp an imaginary kettle spoon. Begin to move as if you were stirring a huge kettle of oatmeal, shifting the weight from one foot to the other. Pause and reverse, stirring in the opposite direction.

MONKEY STRETCH

1. Stand with the feet a little wider than hip-width apart, arms at the sides, loose fists resting lightly on the outside of the upper thighs.

2. Take a deep breath in. Slowly exhale as you bend the torso to the right. Slide the right hand down the outside of the leg and draw the left hand up into the armpit. Keep the hips and shoulders facing forward, emphasizing the lateral stretch of the spine and avoiding the tendency to twist.

3. Inhale back to center, bringing both hands back to the thighs, and repeat on the opposite side.

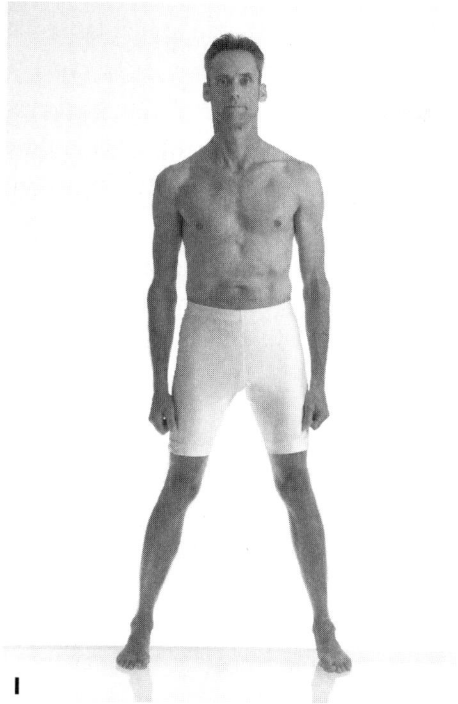

1

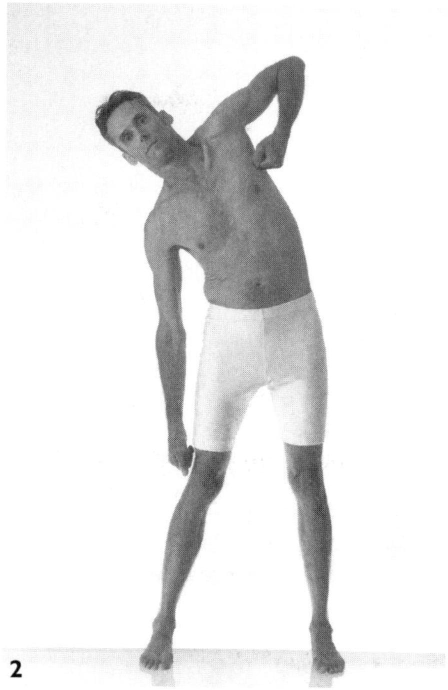

2

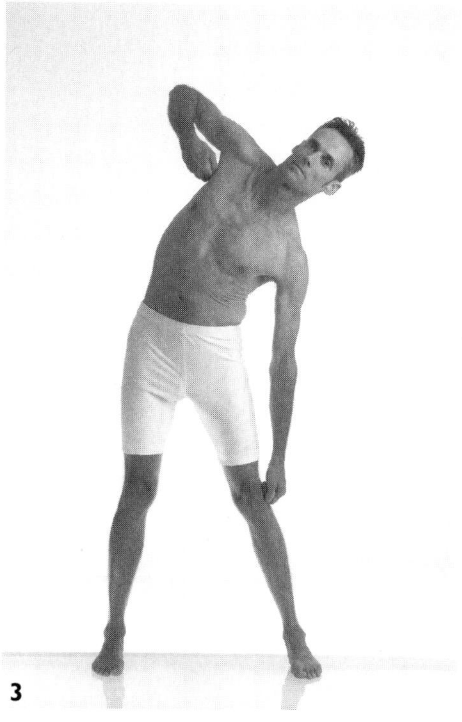

3

4. Repeat this movement several times on each side, coordinating breath and movement.

5. On the last stretch to each side, hold the stretch for a deep breath in and out.

Be Aware:

This warm-up is called Monkey Stretch because the way the hand is pulled into the armpit resembles a child's imitation of a monkey. It can be done slowly and gently, emphasizing a deep breath. You can also make it faster and more vigorous, emphasizing an active breath. Or combine both by starting slow and gradually picking up the pace. You can also substitute Quarter Moon. Either way, you are preparing the body for deeper side stretches later in the session.

FORWARD FOLD

(Pada Hastasana)

1. Stand with the feet hip-width apart. Reach the arms behind you and interlace the fingers. Squeeze the palms together, pressing the knuckles down and back to straighten the arms and draw the shoulder blades together. Press the sternum forward to open the chest. Breathe deeply as you hold.

2. Release the interlaced fingers and rest the hands on the thighs.

3. Take a deep breath in. As you exhale, lift the tailbone and begin to hinge at the hip joints, folding forward with a straight spine. Slide the hands down the legs, using the arms to support the weight of the torso. Bend the knees as needed to avoid strain. Let the breath flow freely as the body adjusts to this mild inversion.

4. If you want more stretch, grasp one elbow, and then the other, with the opposite hands. Relax and let gravity gently elongate the spine and neck. Breathe deeply as you hold.

5. To release, bring the hands back to the legs and bend the knees deeply. Inhale and press into the feet, sliding the hands back up to the thighs. Hinge at the hips, coming up with a straight spine and using the hands for needed support.

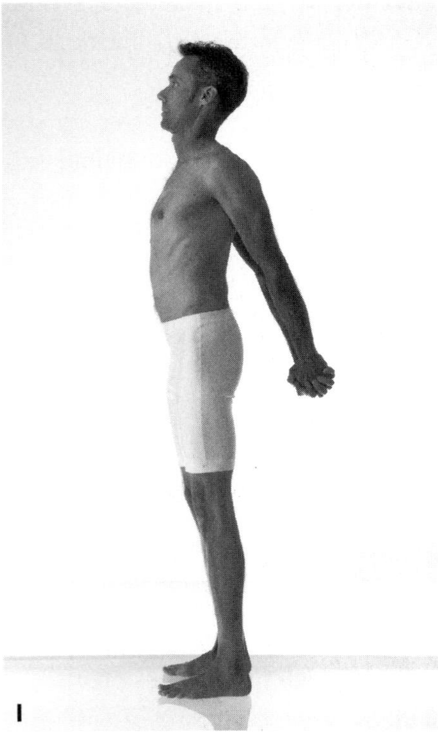

1

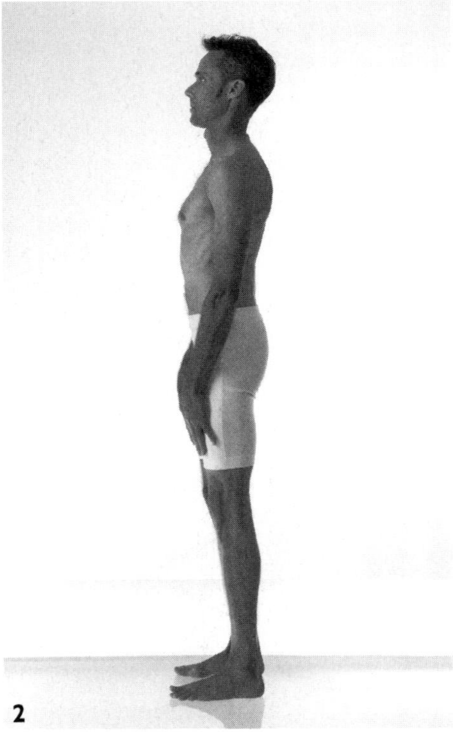

2

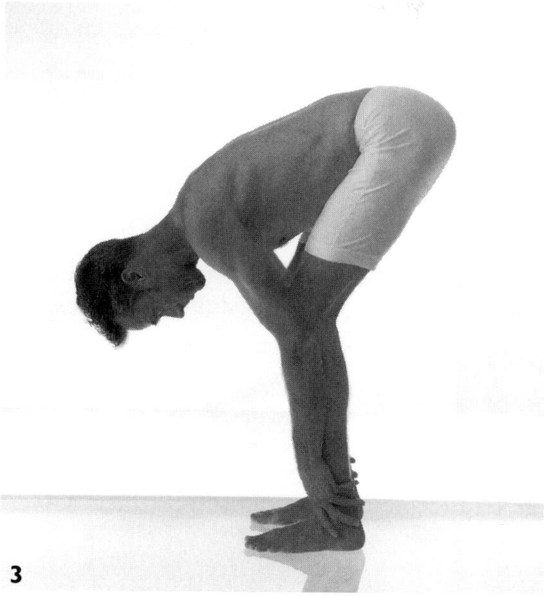

3

Be Aware:

Pada Hastasana means ***hands to feet pose*** and describes a number of standing forward bends. Forward bending can be challenging if your low back is sensitive. Done properly, forward bending preserves the mobility of the hip joints needed to resist the tendency to round forward from the lumbar spine.

If you want less challenge, do steps 1 to 3. Allow the knees to bend deeply to avoid strain, and use the hands to help support the weight of the torso. If you want more challenge, come to step 4. Press the feet into the floor to straighten the legs and press the elbows toward the floor to elongate the spine.

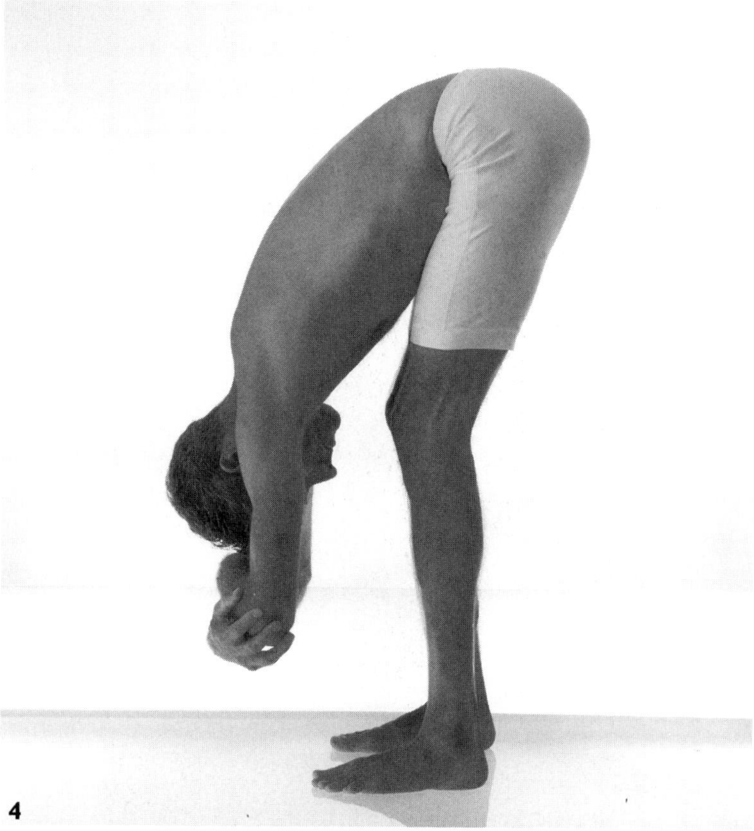

4

SUN SALUTATION

(Surya Namaskar)

1. Stand erect with your feet hip-width apart. Inhale and bring your hands into prayer position. Exhale as you gently press the hands together and slightly bow the head.

2. Inhaling, reach the hands forward and then sweep them overhead. Press the pubic bone slightly forward, lift the sternum, and press the fingertips up and back. Keep the neck elongated, allowing the upper spine to gently arch. Do not overstretch the low back or drop the head back.

3. Exhale and lift the tailbone, hinging forward from the hips. Sweep the arms out to the side like a swan dive. Let the knees be soft to avoid any strain to the low back.

4. Keep the spine long and neck extended as you come forward. Bend the knees as needed to rest the hands on either side of your feet.

5. Inhale and step the right foot back into Lunge Pose, keeping the hands on the floor on either side of the front foot. Position the left knee directly over the left ankle, and press the right heel back to straighten the right leg. Press both hips down, the sternum forward, tuck the chin slightly, and extend through the crown. You may want to come onto the fingertips in what is called Teepee Position. Take several breaths in Lunge.

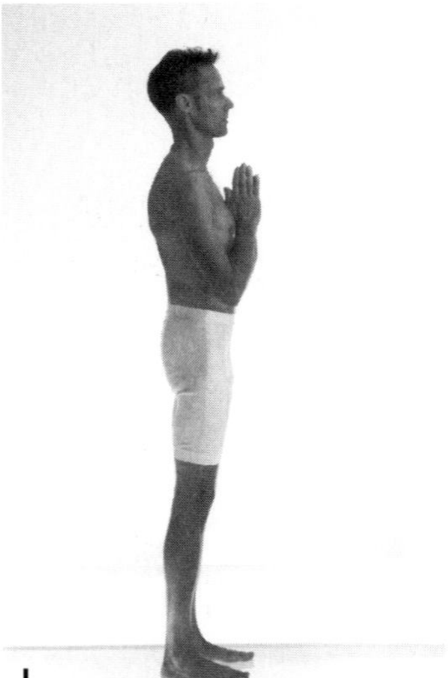

1

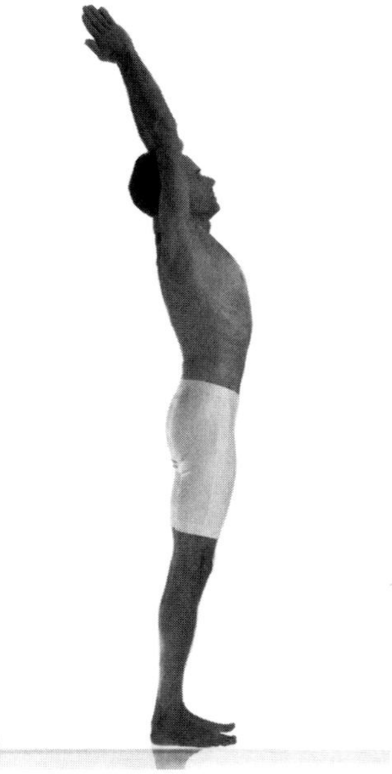

2

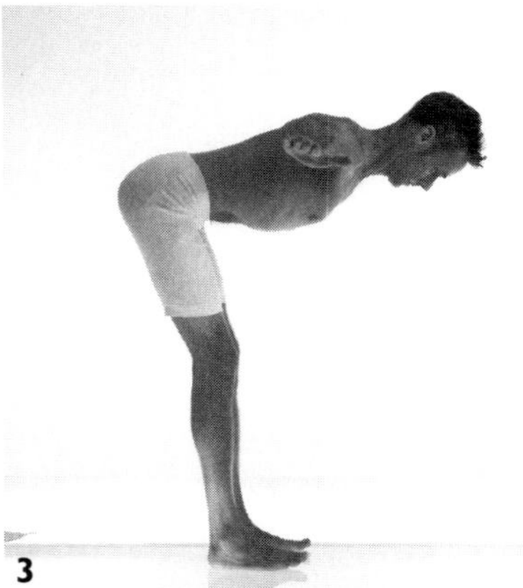

3

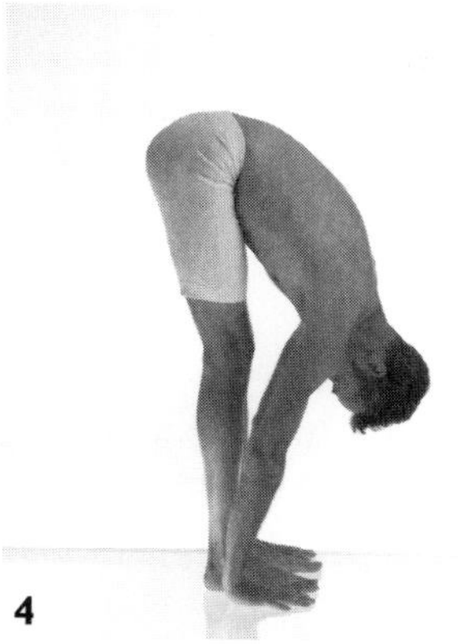
4

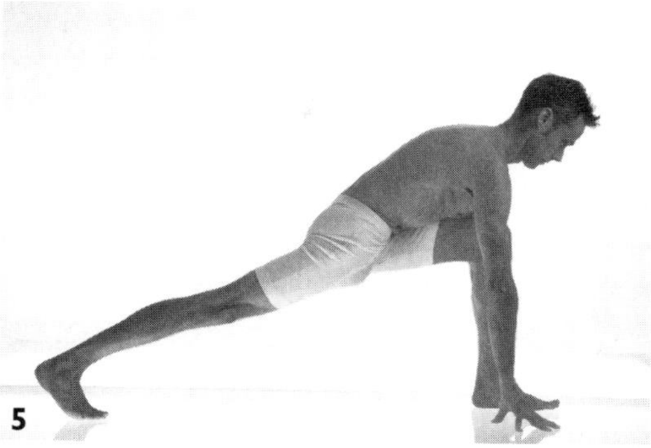
5

6. Drop the right knee down to the floor, and bring the left knee back to meet it, coming into Table Pose, curling the toes under. Take a deep breath in.

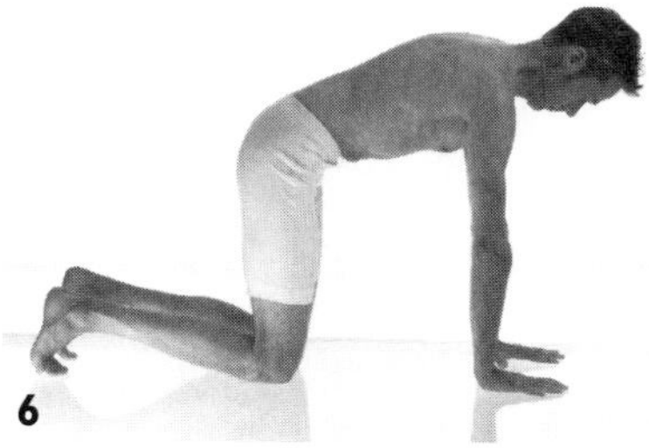
6

7. Exhale and press into the hands and lift the hips high, coming into Downward Dog. Lift the tailbone into a dog tilt. Press the buttocks back and the hands into the floor to elongate the spine, extending through the crown. Hold for several breaths.

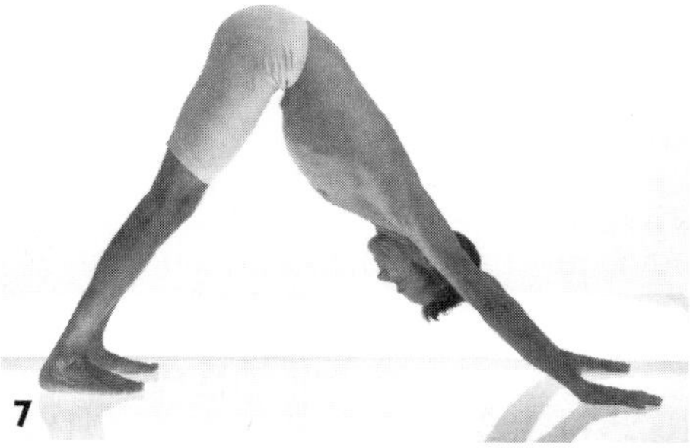
7

8. Inhale and step the right foot forward into Lunge Pose as detailed in step 5. Take several breaths in this position.

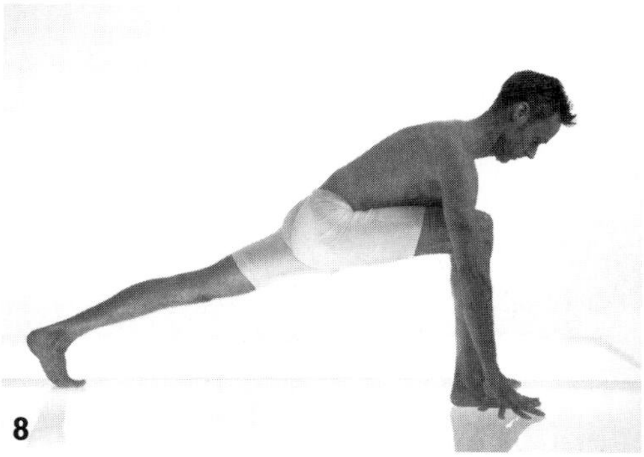
8

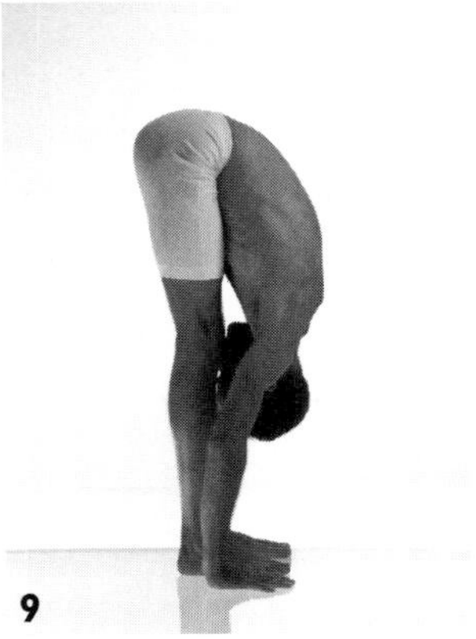

9

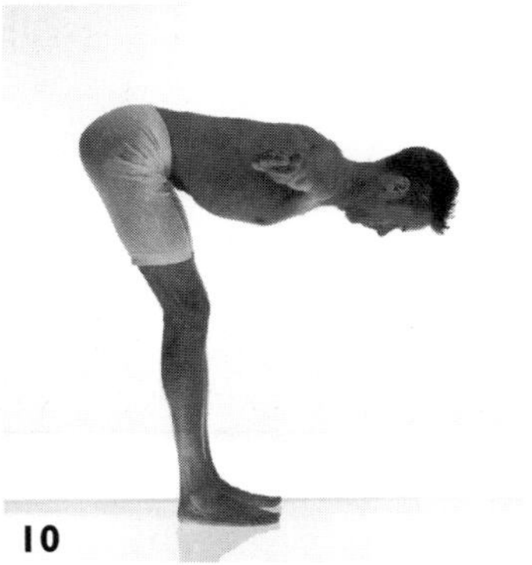

10

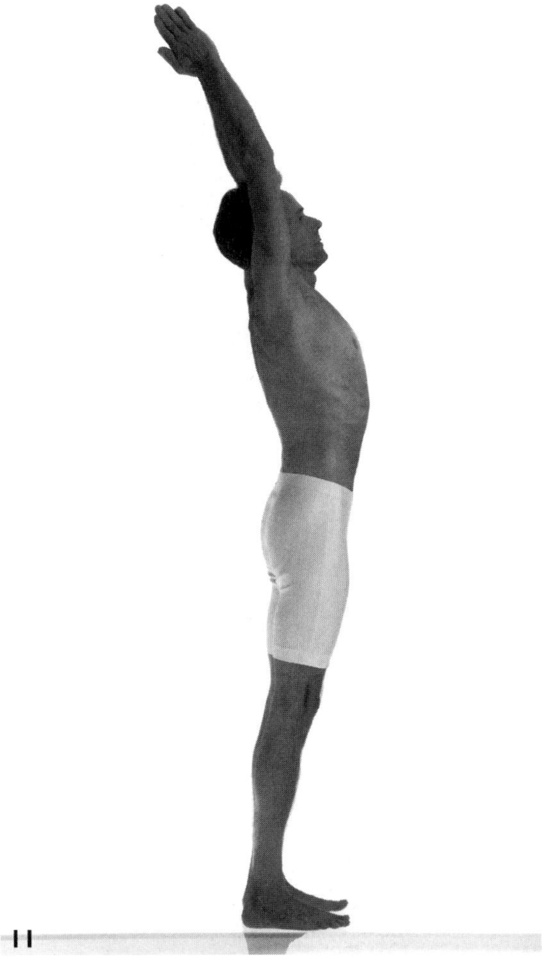

11

9. Exhale and step the left foot forward and even with the right foot. Bend the knees as needed to rest the hands on the floor on either side of your feet. Press into the feet to straighten the legs as much as possible without strain, and bring the belly and forehead toward the legs. Let the breath flow freely in and out as you hold.

10. Inhale as you hinge at the hips and come up with a straight spine, arms reaching out to the sides in a reverse swan dive. Bend the knees as needed to avoid strain.

11. As you complete the inhalation, reach the arms overhead. Press the pubic bone slightly forward, lift the sternum, and press the fingertips up and back. Keeping the neck elongated, allow the upper spine to gently arch.

12. Exhale as you return the hands to Prayer Position.

13. Repeat the sequence, initiating the movement into Lunge by stepping the left foot back.

Be Aware:
The Sun Salutation is a classic yoga exercise and there are many ways to incorporate it into a yoga sequence. In this series, the Sun Salutation is used to warm up the body before standing postures. Two repetitions is sufficient for this purpose. In some approaches, Sun Salutation is the core practice and different variations are repeated numerous times. A sequence of forward and backward bends, Sun Salutation is complemented by the side stretches and twists of the Moon Salute.

BREATH OF JOY

1. Stand with your feet hip-width apart and knees slightly flexed. This exercise combines deep breathing with fluid motion, and the knees remain soft throughout to protect the low back.

2. Exhale. As you begin to inhale, raise your arms in front of you to shoulder height with the hands palms down. Let your knees flex slightly with the movement.

3. As you continue to inhale, sweep the arms a little down and then out to the sides to shoulder height, again letting the knees flex slightly.

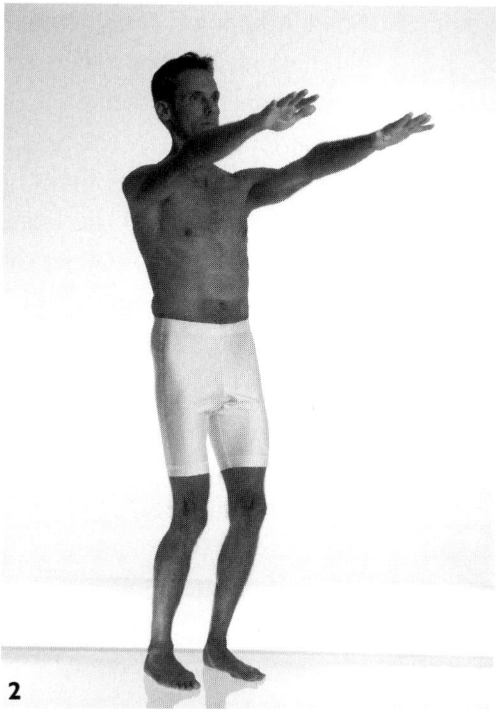
2

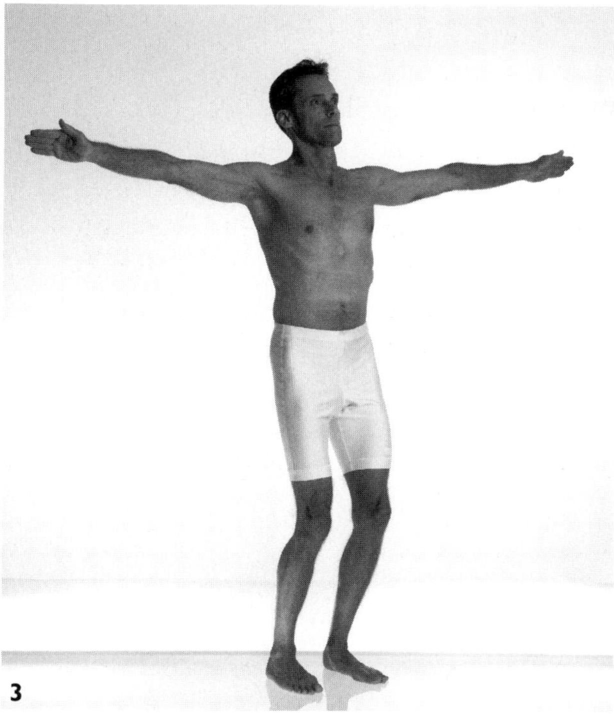
3

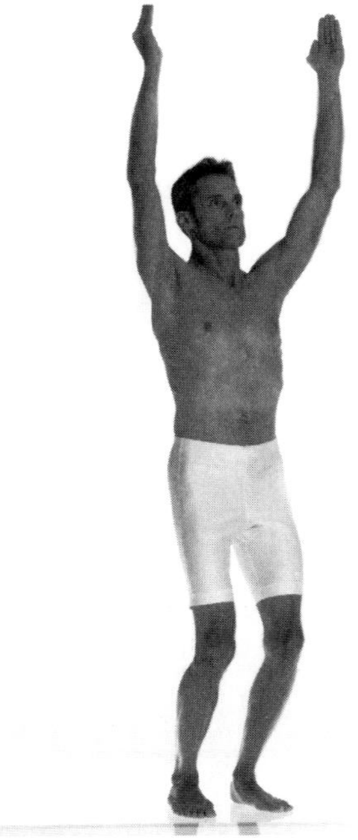

4

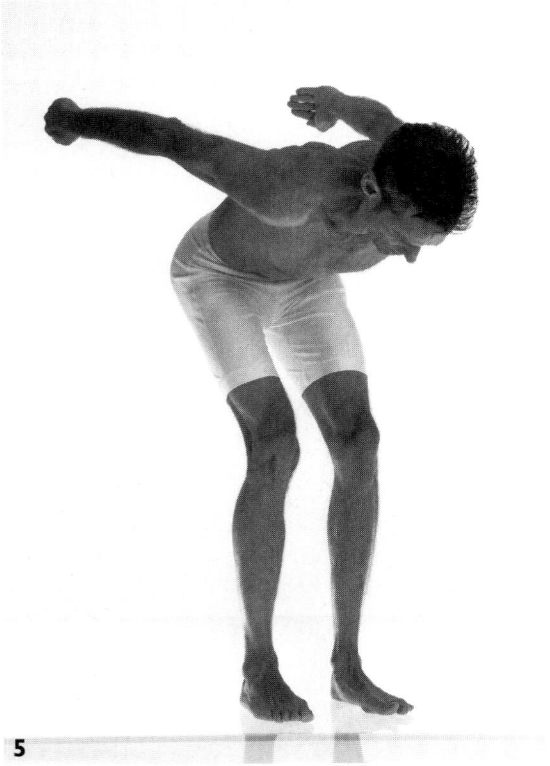

5

4. Complete your inhalation as you raise the arms overhead, palms facing.

5. Swing the arms toward the ground, exhaling with a breathy "ha" sound. Bend forward from the hips and let the momentum of the movement carry the arms behind you. Emphasize the breath, letting the motion be fluid and unforced.

6. Inhale as you bring the torso up and lift your arms in front of you, moving directly into a second repetition. Sweep the arms out to the sides, and then raise them overhead, once again exhaling with a "ha" sound. Repeat ten times.

Be Aware:

This energizing warm-up uses a rhythmic body motion to facilitate deep breathing. The arm motion helps fill the lower, middle, then upper lungs. By charging the body with energy, Breath of Joy enhances the beneficial effects of postures that follow. Allow the breath to guide the movement, letting the motion be fluid and unforced. The flexing of the knees creates a slight bounce that helps protect the low back. If your low back is sensitive, try doing the exercise with a minimum of torso movement.

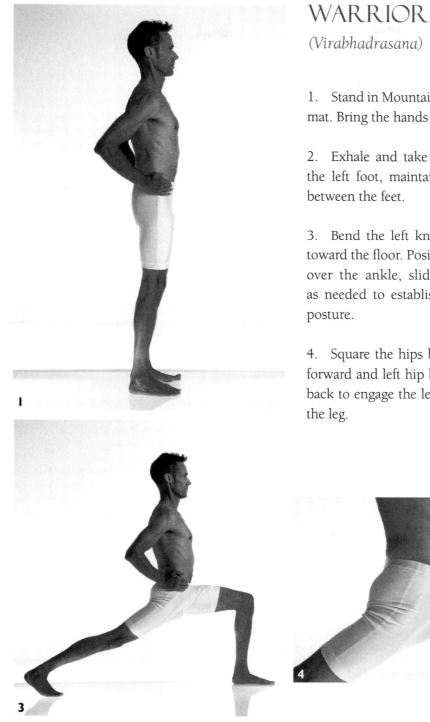

WARRIOR

(Virabhadrasana)

1

1. Stand in Mountain Pose at the back of your mat. Bring the hands onto the hips.

2. Exhale and take a big step forward with the left foot, maintaining hip-width distance between the feet.

3. Bend the left knee and let the hips sink toward the floor. Position the left knee directly over the ankle, sliding the right foot back as needed to establish a strong base for the posture.

4. Square the hips by bringing the right hip forward and left hip back. Press the right heel back to engage the leg muscles and straighten the leg.

3

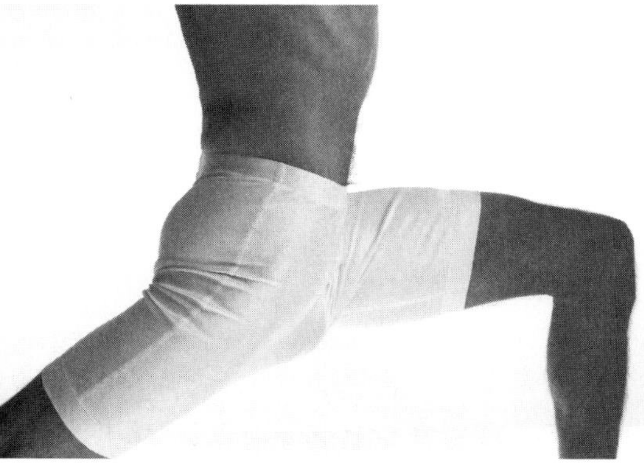

4

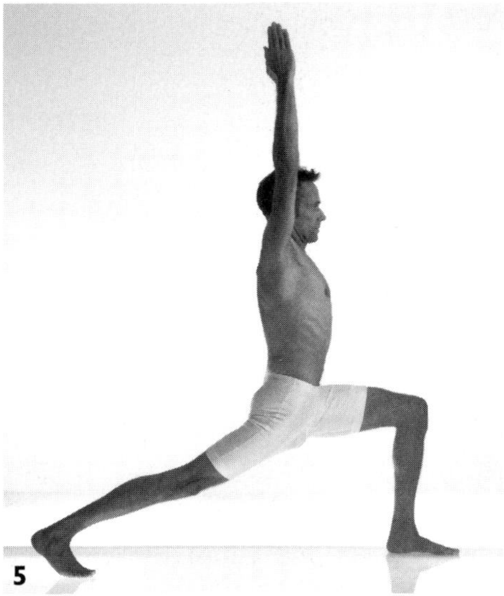
5

5. If your posture feels steady and balanced, inhale and sweep the arms out to the sides and overhead, shoulder-width apart and palms facing. Elongate the spine by letting the hips sink toward the floor while extending through the crown, and pressing the fingertips toward the ceiling. The eyes look straight ahead.

6. Release by bringing the hands down to the thigh just above the front knee. Press the hands into the knee to support your weight as you step the back foot forward and return to Mountain Pose.

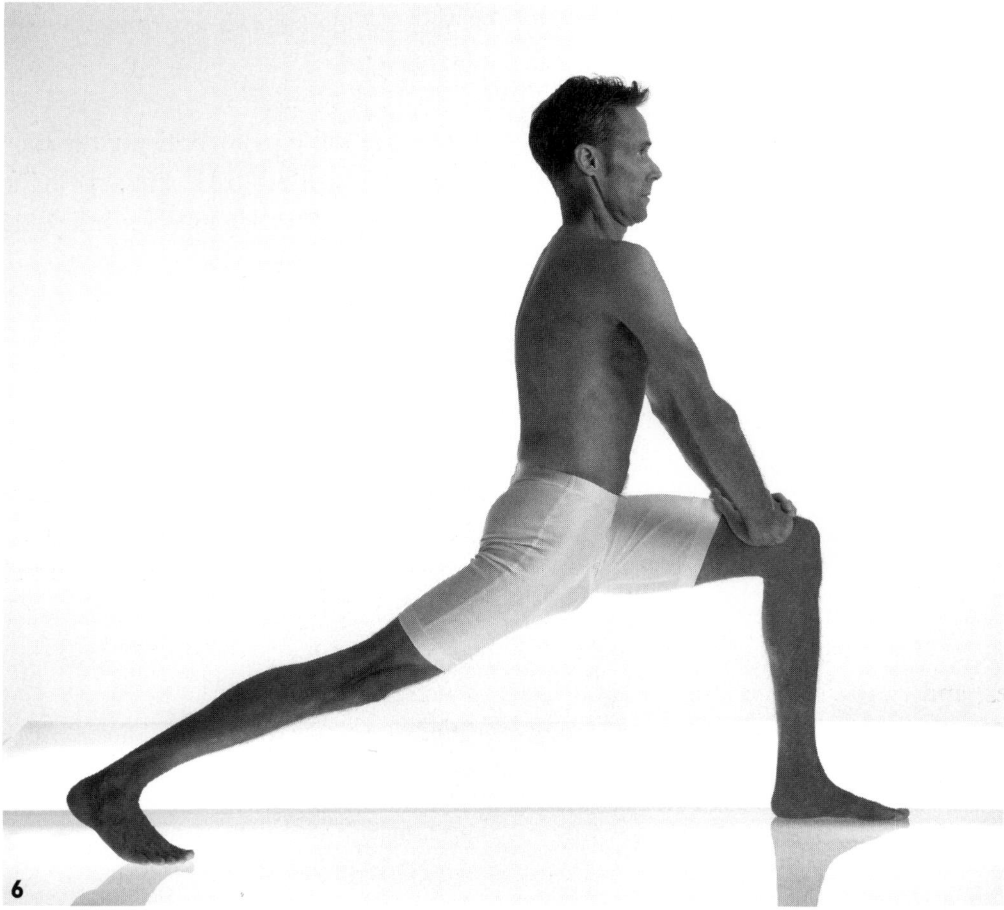
6

7. Come to the back of your mat and repeat on the opposite side.

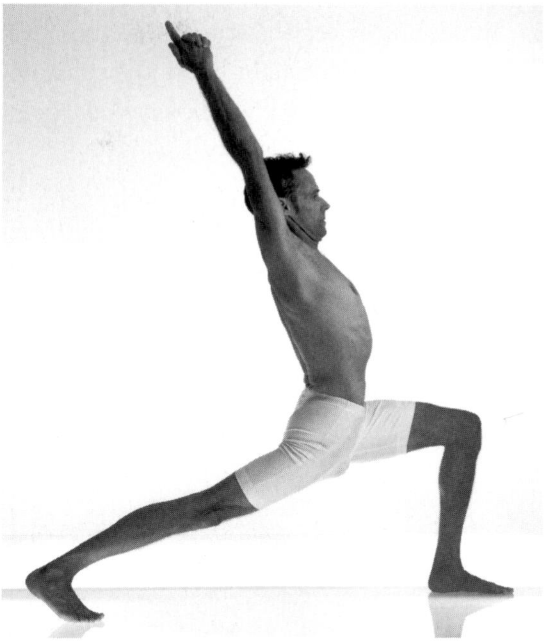

Be Aware:

Warrior Pose stretches and strengthens the legs, hips, shoulders, arms, and chest. If you have knee problems, proceed carefully and make sure the front knee is aligned directly over the ankle. If the front knee extends beyond the ankle, slide the rear foot farther back.

Warrior is a good posture to hold, although its intensity makes prolonged holding challenging. If you want less challenge, hold with the hands on the knee as in step 6. Over time you will build the strength required to raise the arms overhead. You can also lower the back knee to rest on the floor in a variation called Supported Warrior, which reduces the effort required to hold the posture and makes it easier to balance.

If you want more challenge, sweep the arms overhead and interlace the fingers, extending the index fingers in Steeple Position. Let the hips sink as you arch back and press the fingers skyward.

TRIANGLE

(Trikonasana)

1. Step the feet as wide apart as your legs are long. Turn the left foot out a full turn of ninety degrees, and turn the right foot in a quarter turn. Align the left knee to point directly over the left foot.

2. Press into the feet to engage the muscles of the legs. Stabilize the core by pressing the tailbone down and pubic bone forward to level the pelvis, gently contracting the muscles of the pelvic floor. Elongate the spine by lifting out of the waist and extending through the crown of the head.

3. Inhale and sweep the arms out to the sides and up to shoulder height. Press the sternum forward, roll the shoulders down and back, and extend through the fingertips.

4. Exhale as you slide the arms and shoulders to the right, extending the torso and coming into a lateral stretch of the spine. Keep both hips and shoulders facing forward, resisting the tendency to twist. Let the left hip bone drop slightly, and the right hip bone lift slightly.

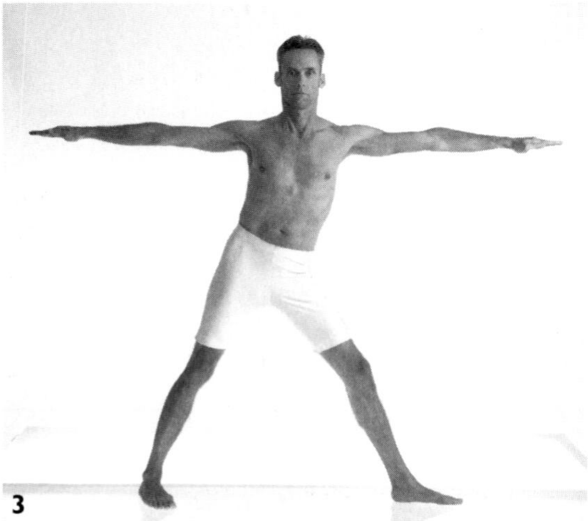
3

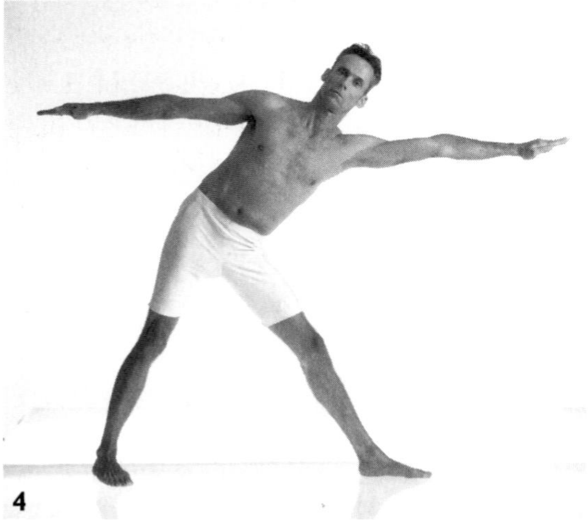
4

5. Breathe deeply as you continue to reach left, relaxing into a deep stretch across the hips and shoulders. Allow the left knee to bend slightly if necessary to avoid strain, while pressing firmly into the front foot, which presses the back hip away. Extend through the crown to keep the spine long.

6. On an exhalation, rotate the left arm down and right arm up. The left hand rests lightly on the left leg and the right hand reaches up toward the ceiling. Keep the body in one plane, as if you were doing the posture with your back against a wall. If your balance is steady, slowly turn the head to look at the

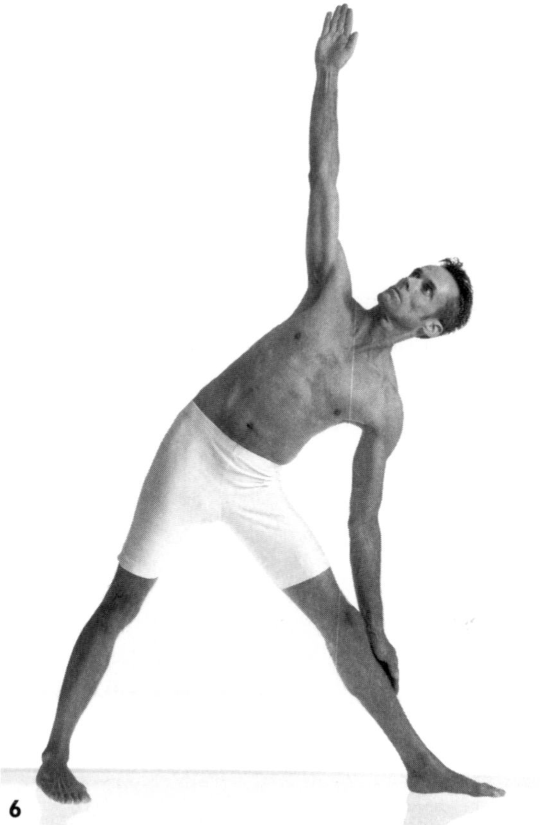
6

upturned right hand, keeping the back of the neck long. Breathe deeply as you hold.

7. To release, inhale as you press into the feet and up through the right hand, returning to standing.

8. Exhale and lower the arms to the sides. Rotate the right foot out a full turn of ninety degrees, turn the left foot in a quarter turn, and repeat on the other side.

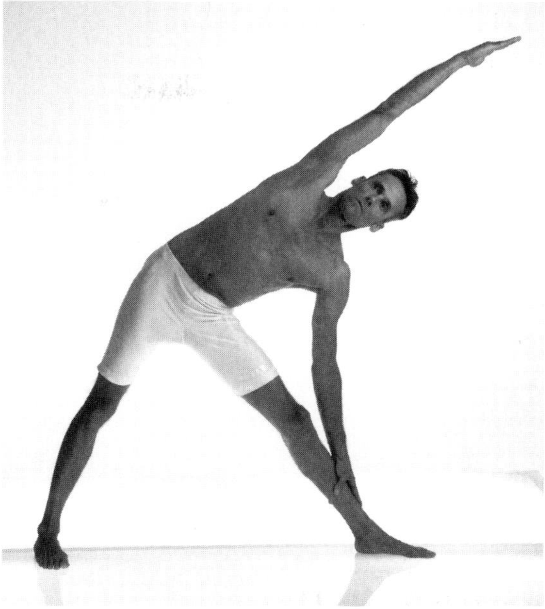

Be Aware:

Triangle builds a balance of strength and flexibility in the upper and lower body. To reap its benefits, you must be willing to not compromise alignment. As you begin practice, your full expression of Triangle is likely to be a side stretch. Steps 4 and 5 teach you how to involve more of your body. This movement of the hips and shoulders is sometimes described as *slide and glide.* The shoulders slide to one side, and the hip joints glide so one slightly lifts and the other slightly lowers.

In working to keep the hips and shoulders square, do not compromise the alignment of the front knee. Make sure the knee continues to point in the same direction as the foot throughout the posture. If the knee is pulled out of alignment, bend it slightly to avoid any torque to the knee joint.

Resist the tendency to use the lower hand to bear the weight of your torso. Rest the hand lightly on the leg, or even keep it just off the leg, to build core strength. If you are unable to comfortably rotate the neck to gaze at the upturned hand, look to the horizon. If you want more challenge, bring the top arm in line with the side. Press out through the fingertips to deepen the side stretch.

The Triangle is a good posture to hold. Come into the posture a first time on both sides to warm up. On the second time, come into the posture slowly, staying with the deep stretch across the hips and shoulders for several breaths before rotating the arms into the full expression of the posture. Hold for several flowing breaths.

STANDING ANGLE

(Dandayamana Konasana)

1. Step the feet as wide apart as your legs are long. Bring the hands to the hips. Press into the feet to engage the muscles of the legs. Stabilize the core by pressing the tailbone down and pubic bone forward to level the pelvis, gently contracting the muscles of the pelvic floor. Elongate the spine by lifting out of the waist, pressing the sternum forward, and extending through the crown.

2. Take a deep breath in. As you exhale, lift the tailbone and begin to hinge at the hips, coming forward with a straight spine. Feel the movement of the hip joints with the hands. Let the knees bend as needed to ease any feeling of strain in the low back. As the torso approaches parallel, slide the hands slowly down the legs. Extend through the crown to keep the spine and neck elongated. Let the breath flow freely as your body adjusts to having the head below the heart.

3. Bring the palms onto the floor directly beneath the shoulders, elbows bent and fingertips in line with the big toes. Rock your weight forward onto the balls of the feet and press the buttocks back. With the knees bent as needed to protect the low back, press into the feet to straighten the legs while continuing to extend through the crown. Then press gently into the palms to enhance the forward hinging of the hips. Breathe deeply as you hold.

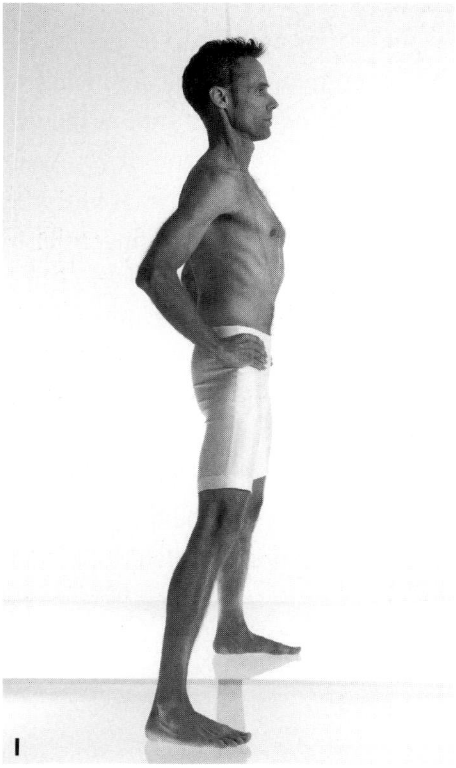

1

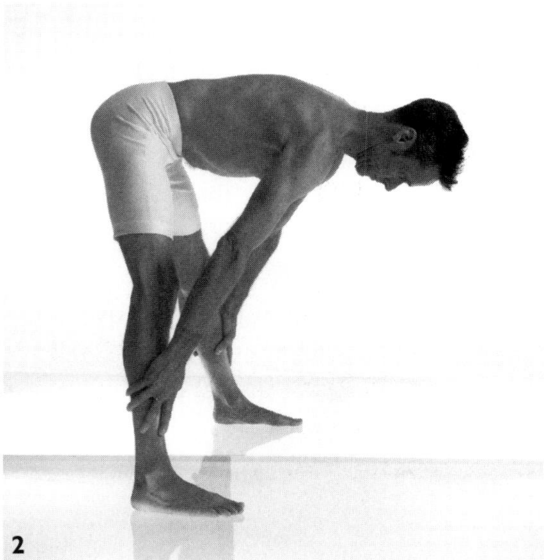

2

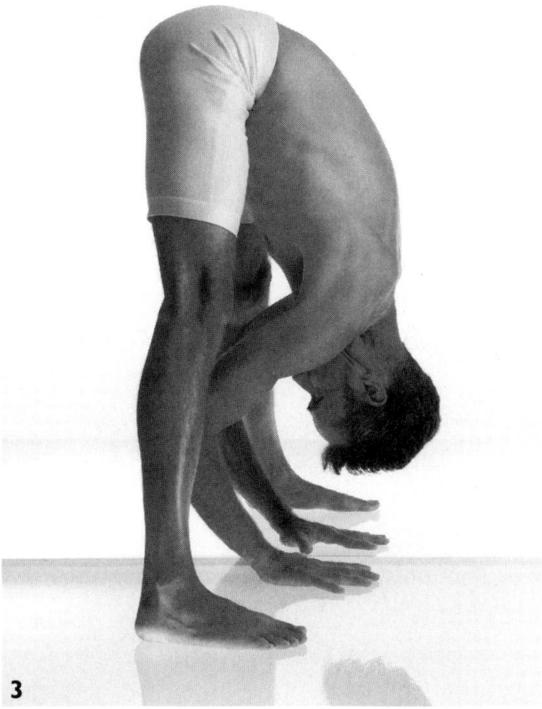

3

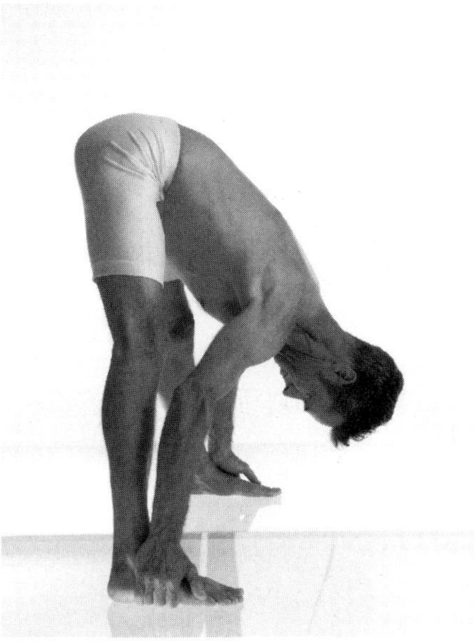

4. To release, bring the hands back to the feet or legs. Inhale as you press into the feet to engage the hips and come up with a straight spine, sliding the hands up the legs.

5. Step the feet together. Pause to receive the posture, drinking in all its benefits.

Be Aware:

This posture brings the head below the heart and should not be practiced if you have unmedicated high blood pressure, glaucoma, detached retina, or other eye problems.

If you want less challenge, keep the knees noticeably bent and use the hands to support your movement down and up. Relax into the holding, letting gravity do all the work. Experiment rocking the hips ever so slightly from side to side to enhance the hip stretch.

If you want more challenge, grasp the outside of the feet by bringing the fingers under the arch. Use your arm strength to hinge forward from the hips and draw the head toward the floor, keeping the spine straight.

CRANE

1. Stand in Mountain Pose. Focus your gaze at a point on the wall in front of you.

2. Transfer the weight onto the left foot, pressing it firmly into the floor.

3. Inhale as you lift the left knee and sweep the arms out to the sides and into a T position with the palms down.

4. Keep the hips level and right foot pressed into the floor to fully engage the thigh muscles of the standing leg. Lift the left knee as high as possible.

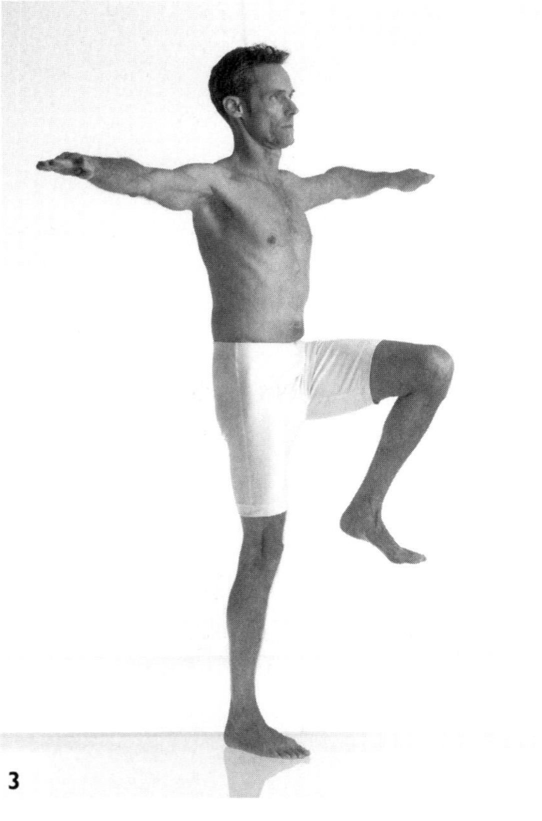

3

5. Press out through the fingertips to open the chest. Lift the sternum and extend through the crown to elongate the spine. Relax the left foot, even as you keep the left knee lifted.

6. To release, exhale and lower the arms to the sides and the left foot back to the floor.

7. Inhale and press the left foot firmly into the floor, moving directly into the posture on the opposite side.

Be Aware:

Crane brings body and mind into balance. As you hold the posture, let the body be still and the mind peaceful.

This posture uses the technique of standing on one leg to build lower body strength. Work to keep the standing leg straight by fully engaging the thigh muscles. By raising one

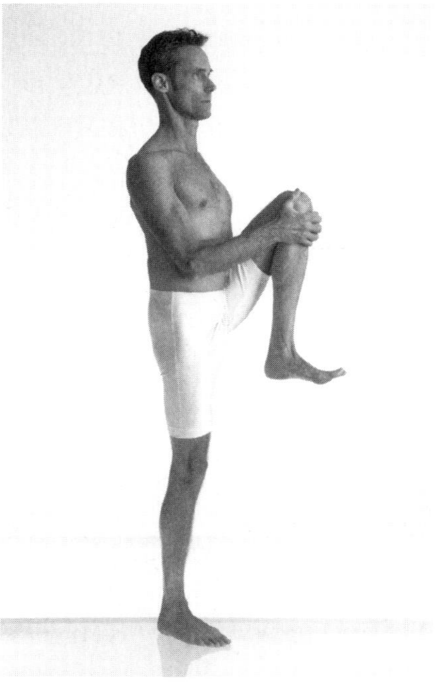

knee while the other leg is fully engaged, hip flexibility is increased.

If you want more challenge, flow into Standing Wind Relieving pose by interlacing the fingers around the knee. Keep the standing leg engaged by pressing the foot strongly into the floor as you draw the opposite knee into the chest.

HALF CURL UP

1. Lie on your back with the legs extended. Reach the arms overhead on the floor, palms up. Wriggle from side to side, stretching the arms overhead and walking the shoulder blades up to elongate the spine, shoulders, and arms. Then flex both feet and press away one heel, and then the other, moving from side to side and lengthening the sacrum, hips, and legs. Stretch your body to its full length using the support of the floor.

2. Interlace the fingers and rest the hands on the lower belly. Bend the left knee, bringing the left foot close to the buttocks.

3. Take a deep breath in. As you exhale, press the left foot gently into the floor and contract the abdominal muscles to "curl up" the torso.

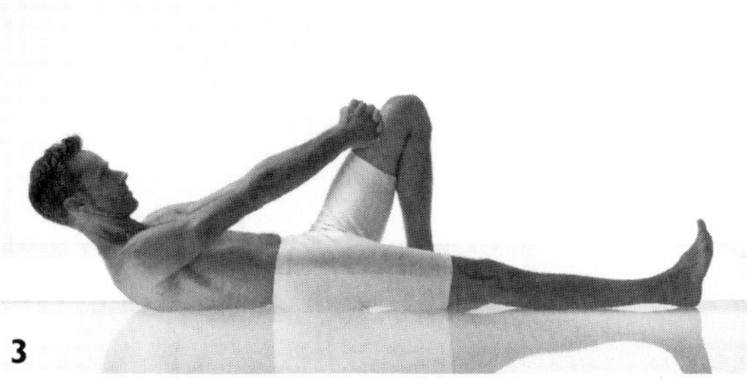

3

Press the knuckles away to straighten the arms. Tuck the chin slightly to protect the neck from any strain.

4. Let the breath flow freely as you hold, feeling the core strengthening taking place.

5. To release, take a deep breath in. As you exhale, slowly lower to the starting position. Before moving on to the second side, rest for a moment and feel any sensation of warmth, enhanced blood circulation, or energy flow in the belly.

6. Interlace the fingers the other way, and repeat on the opposite side.

Be Aware:

Half Curl Up is a particularly safe and effective abdominal strengthener. Resist the tendency to hold the breath, and you will be able to hold the posture longer and obtain better results. Most of us have a dominant grip. Alternating the way you interlace the fingers is a nice way to explore your nondominant way of doing things.

SERPENT

(Sarpasana)

1. Lie on your belly with the forehead on the floor. Reach the arms in front of you, palms down. Wriggle slightly from side to side, stretching the arms overhead and walking the rib cage forward to elongate the spine. Then lift one leg and then the other, pressing the toes away to lengthen the legs and open the sacrum and hip joints. Stretch your body to its full length using the support of the floor.

2. Bring the arms down to your sides palms up. Adjust the legs so they are hip-width apart, tops of the feet flat on the floor. Exhale fully.

3. Inhale and press the pubic bone, hip bones, and lower abdomen into the floor to stabilize the core of the body. Use the press as a firm base to lift the head and torso by engaging the back muscles. Keep the neck elongated by gazing at the floor and extending through the crown. The backward bend of the spine is a smooth curve, without any sharp bend in the low back or neck. Pause in this position for several breaths, feeling the strengthening of the back muscles that is taking place.

4. Bring the hands behind your back and interlace the fingers. Press the knuckles back and the sternum forward to open the chest. Let the breath flow freely in and out.

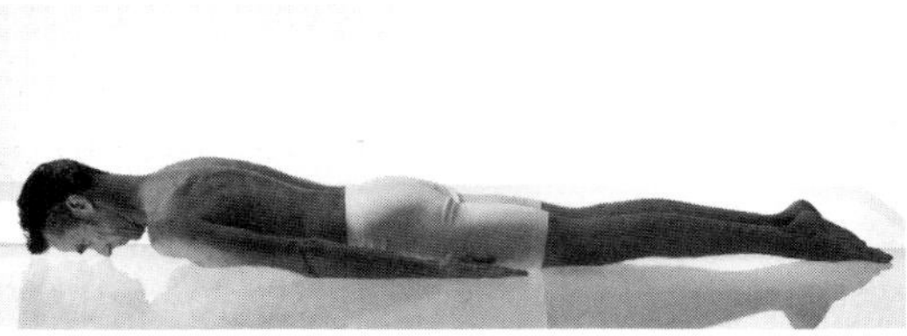

2

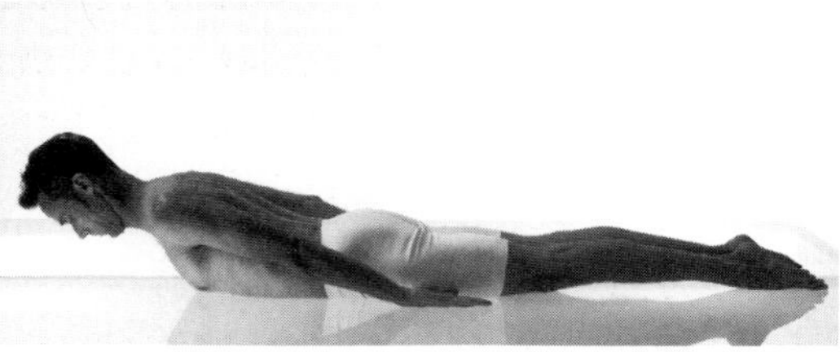

3

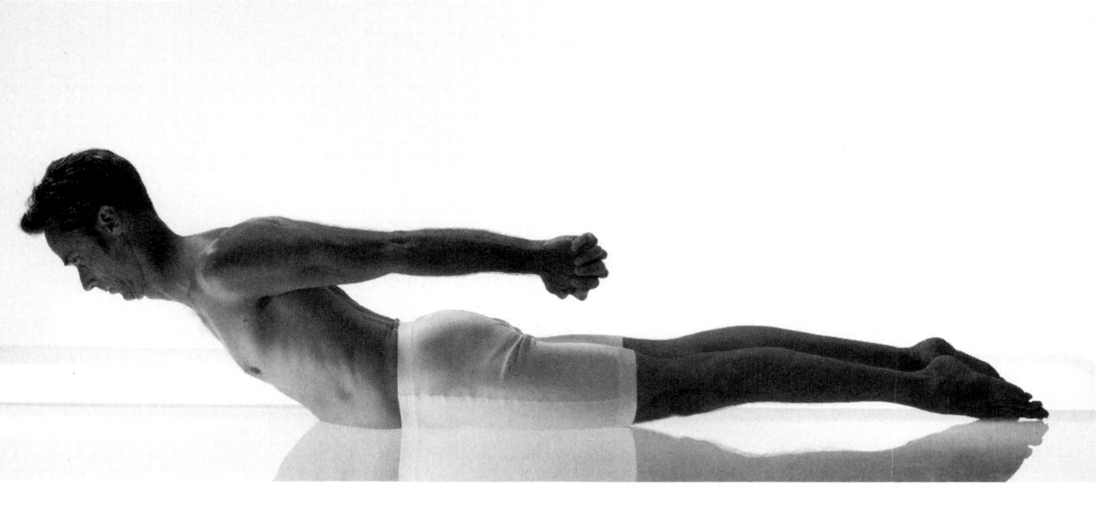

4

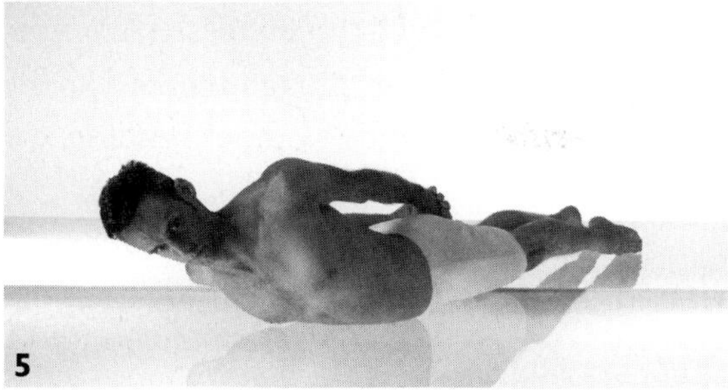

5

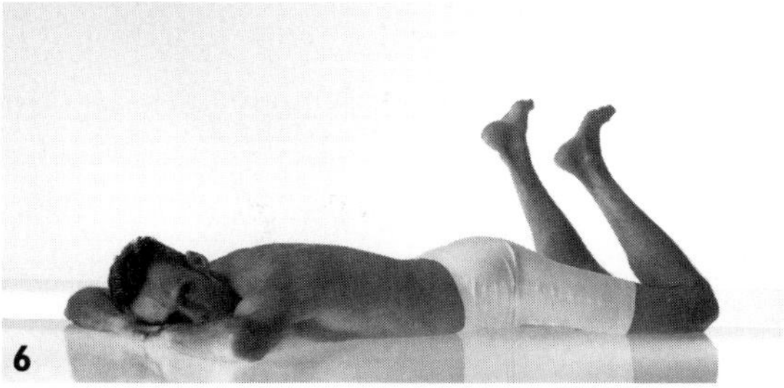

6

5. Take a deep breath in, and as you exhale roll the head and shoulders slowly to one side, and then the other. Roll from side to side several times, feeling the back muscles working and the stretch of chest, shoulders, and neck.

6. To release, come back to center and take a deep breath in. As you exhale, lower the forehead to the floor and release the hands. Turn your head to one side and overlap the fingers to form a small pillow under the temple. Bend the legs at the knees and bring the heels toward the buttocks. Release any low back tension that may have built up by waving the feet gently from side to side like windshield wipers, feeling the sensation of release in the sacrum and low back.

Be Aware:

Elongating the spine prior to backward bending makes it safe and beneficial. The movements in step 1 open the vertebrae, sacrum, and hips to create space for unobstructed movement. Don't skip this step.

The press of the pubic bone, hip bones, and lower belly is the foundation of Serpent and all forms of Cobra. It provides the solid base needed to safely lift the torso off the floor. The backward bend emphasized in Serpent is to the middle and upper back, not the lower back or neck. If you feel any low back tension after Serpent, wave the lower legs side to side to release it.

If you want less challenge, do steps 1–3 to build the strength needed in the abdominal and back muscles to go further. If you want more challenge, explore Diagonal Stretch and Cobra.

HALF LOCUST

(Ardha Salabhasana)

1. Lie on the belly with the arms by your sides, hands palms down. Stretch your chin forward, resting the bottom of the chin on the floor to open the throat. If this neck position is uncomfortable, you can keep the forehead or mouth on the floor.

2. Adjust the feet so they are hip-width apart. Bring the elbows in to touch the sides. Focus your attention on the right leg.

3. On an exhalation, press into both hip bones and slowly lift the left leg off the floor. Keeping both hips pressed equally into the floor, press out through the left toes to lengthen the leg. Then press up through the heel to lift the leg as high as possible without bending.

4. Allow the right side of the body to remain relaxed. Isolate the work in the muscles of the left buttock, hip, and leg. Breathe deeply as you hold.

5. To release, exhale and slowly lower the left leg to the floor.

6. Repeat on the opposite side.

7. Turn your head to one side and overlap the fingers to form a small pillow under the temple. Bend the legs at the knees and bring the heels toward the buttocks. Release any tension that may have built up by circling the heels, noticing any sensation of release in the sacrum and low back.

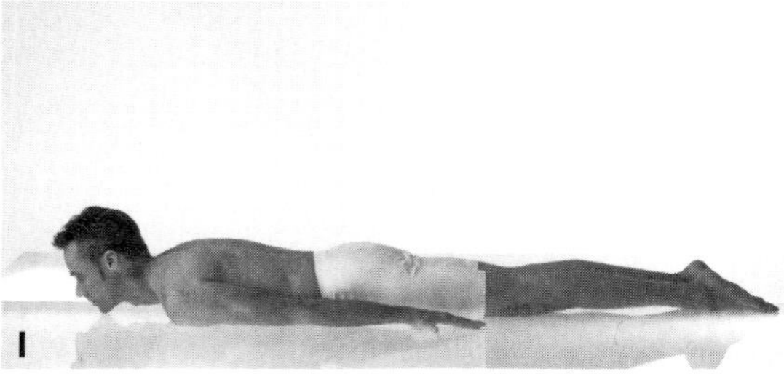

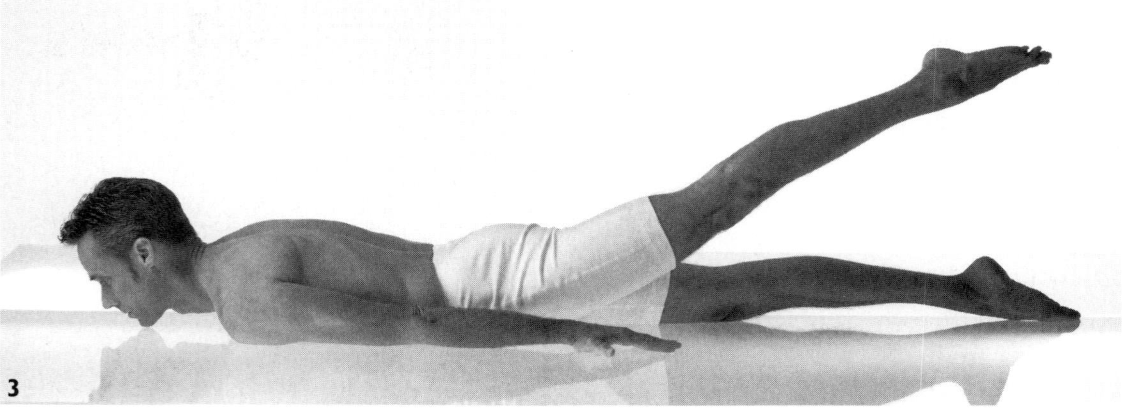

Be Aware:
Half Locust teaches you the paradox of effort and relaxation. While fully engaging the muscles of one leg, the rest of the body remains relaxed. It also stretches the hip; strengthens the muscles of the lower back, buttocks, pelvis, and legs; and massages the abdominal organs. Stretching the chin forward on the floor is intended to increase circulation to the thyroid and parathyroid glands located in the throat. After Half Locust, it is not uncommon to feel some tension in the low back. Turn your head to the opposite side from Serpent—the previous posture—and circle the heels to release it.

If you want less challenge, try lifting and lowering the right then left leg in a slow scissors-like movement versus holding them up.

If you want more challenge, you can explore a simple version of Full Locust. Bring your mouth onto the floor. Take a deep breath in. As you exhale, press firmly down on the pubic bone, hip bones, and lower belly to lift both legs off the floor. Keep the legs straight and feet hip-width apart. Press out through the toes to lengthen the legs and up on the heels to lift the feet. After releasing, rest for a few moments before moving on to the next posture. Don't do Full Locust if you have high blood pressure or a heart condition.

CHILD

(Garbhasana)

1. Come onto your hands and knees. Place the hands under the shoulders, palms down with the fingers spread wide. Position the knees under the hips. The torso, back, and neck form a straight line. This is Table Pose. Take a deep breath in.

2. As you exhale, slide the hips and buttocks back toward the heels. The palms remain on the floor and the arms overhead.

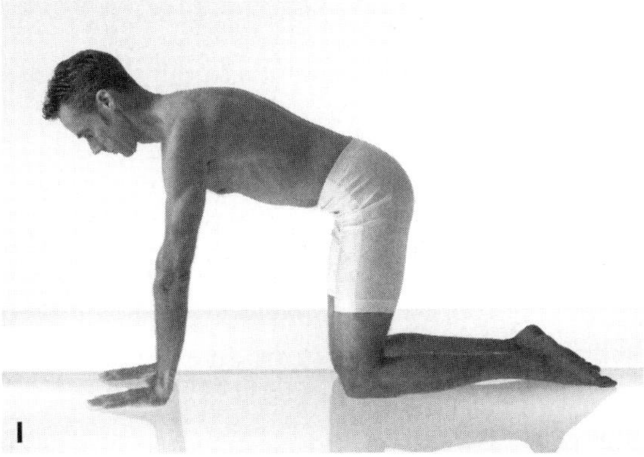

1

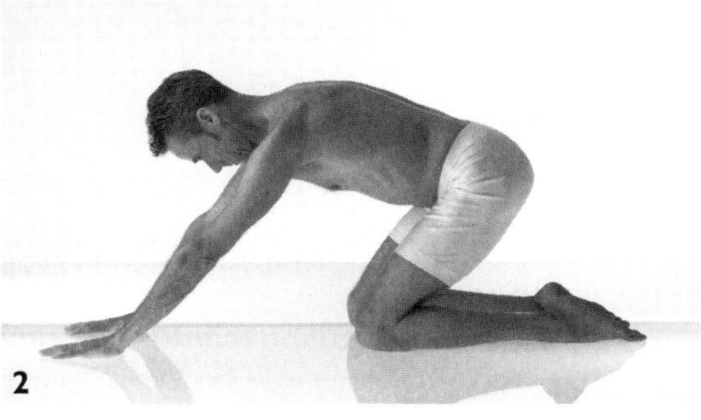

2

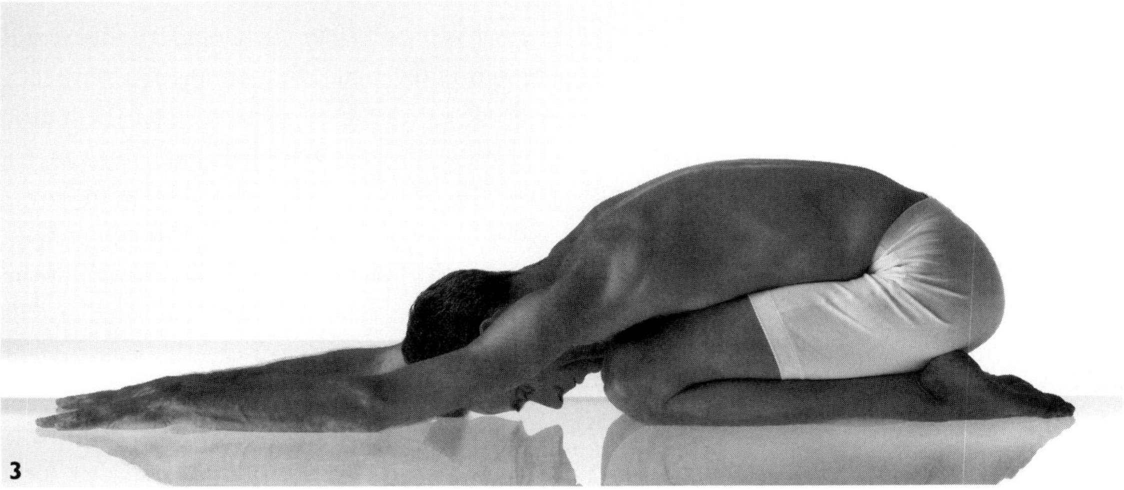
3

3. Let the torso extend over the thighs, the buttocks sit on the heels, and the forehead rest on the floor.

4. Relax and let the breath flow freely as you hold for a minute or more.

5. To release, bring the hands under the shoulders and press up into Table.

Be Aware:

Child is a resting pose and a nice complementary stretch for all backbends and especially belly down postures like Cobra and Locust. It relaxes the muscles of the low back and encourages blood flow to the abdominal organs, kidneys, and adrenal glands. Remain in Child Pose for a minute or more to drink in its benefits.

It is important to find a way for your body to be comfortable. Child Pose can also be done with the arms by the sides, hands palm up. If you cannot easily bring the forehead onto the floor, stack one fist on the other. You can also place a cushion between the buttocks and heels, or between the chest and thighs. Make room for your belly by touching the big toes together and spreading the knees apart.

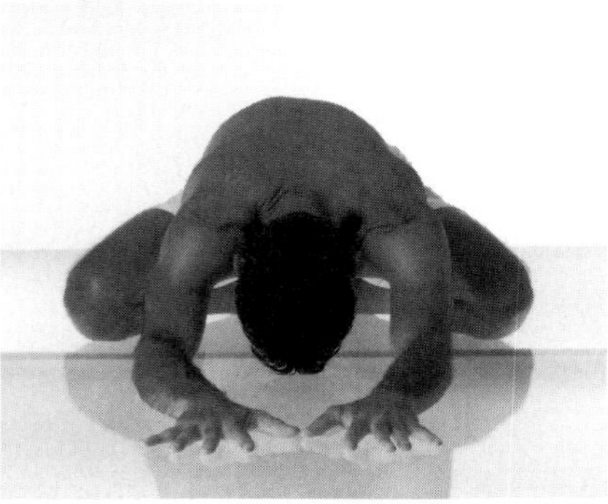

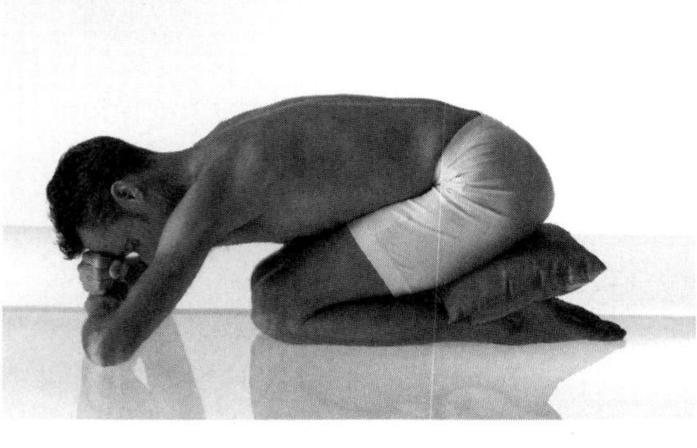

GREAT SEAL

(Maha Mudra)

1. Sit with the legs extended. Draw the sole of your left foot against the right thigh, bringing the left heel as close to the pubic bone as you can while keeping the left knee on the floor. Square the hips so they both face forward. Rest the hands on the floor in front of you.

2. Press both sitz bones into the floor. Flex the right foot to engage the muscles of the right leg. Gently contract the muscles of the pelvic floor. Elongate the spine by lifting out of the waist and extending through the crown.

3. Inhale as you sweep the arms out to the sides and overhead, palms facing. Extend through the fingertips to further elongate the spine. Exhale and relax the top of the shoulders down away from the ears.

4. Take a deep breath in. As you exhale, lift the tailbone and tip the pelvis forward. Slowly hinge forward with the spine elongated, rotating the hip joints rather than rounding from the lumbar spine. You should feel the stretch in the back of the right leg and hamstring versus the low back.

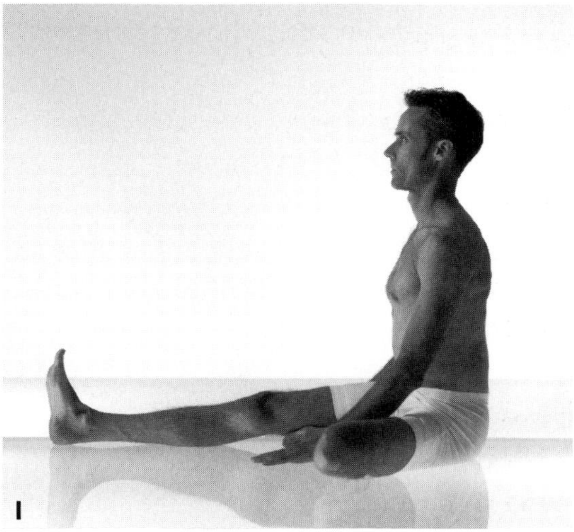

1

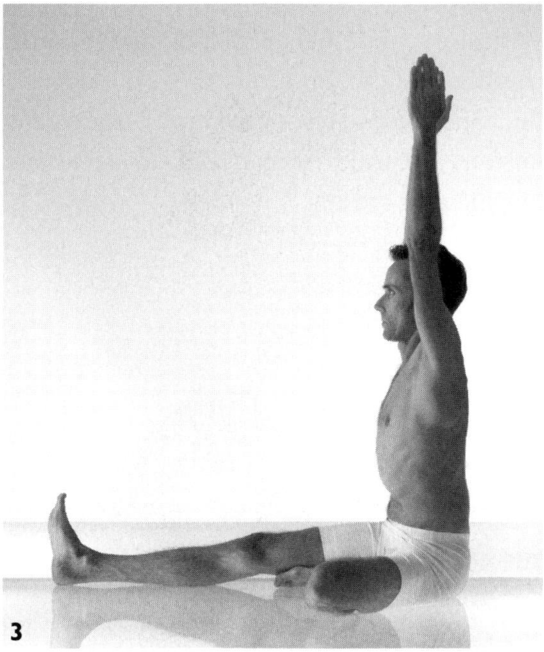

3

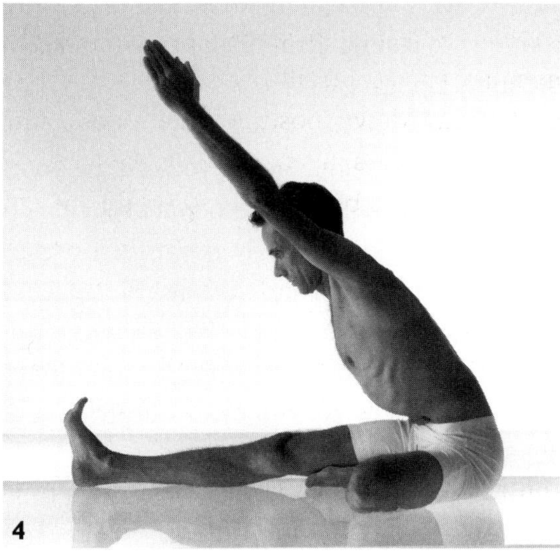

4

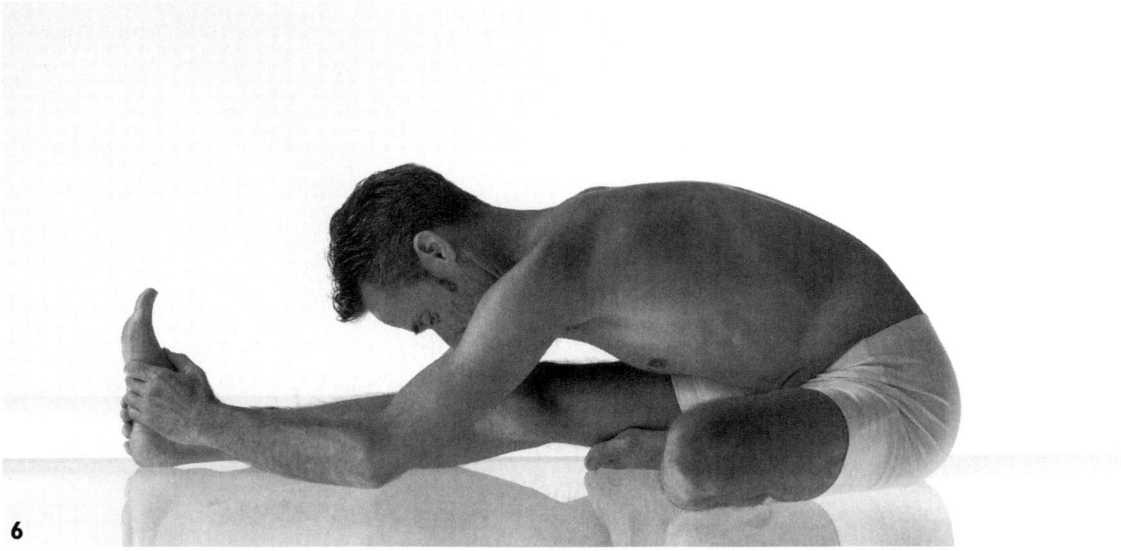

6

5. Come to your full forward extension with a straight spine. If your hamstrings or hips are tight, you may not come very far forward. Pause for a moment to let the breath flow and feel the leg stretch.

6. Allow the upper spine and neck to gently round and the hands to rest on the shins, ankles, or feet. Relax the back of the neck, but continue to extend through the crown to keep the spine elongated.

7. If you want more stretch, you can use your hands to gently enhance the forward rotation of the hips, bringing the belly toward the upper thigh, the sternum toward the knee, and extend the crown toward the toes. Do not use excessive hand strength to round the spine forward from the waist and low back. Breathe deeply as you hold, emphasizing a long exhalation in which residual air is actively squeezed out of the lungs by a gentle contraction of the abdominal muscles.

8. To release, bring the hands to rest palms down on either side of the extended leg. Rotate the hip joints to bring the torso back to vertical. As you come up, do not raise the arms overhead. Allow the hands to slide along the floor and come to rest by the hips. Integrate the posture, feeling the effects and taking several long flowing breaths.

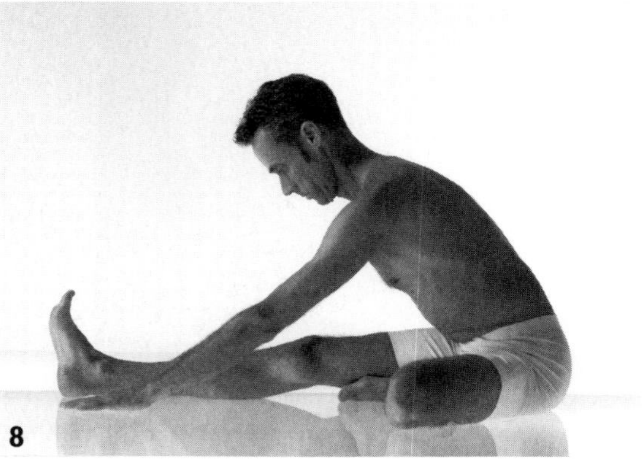

8

9. Instead of repeating Great Seal with the left leg extended, flow directly into Half Circle, the next posture in the Sun Series. Then repeat both postures on the opposite side.

Be Aware:

Forward bends foster an attitude of surrender. The flexibility required in the hamstrings, pelvis, and hips to fold forward cannot be forced. If you push your body beyond its edge, you are likely to experience low back pain from muscle strain or spinal misalignment. Emphasize the forward rotation of the hip joints, coupled with an attitude of self-acceptance, and you will gradually gain hip mobility and hamstring flexibility.

If coming down with the arms overhead is a strain, try this modification. Lift the arms as described in step 3 to elongate the spine to its maximum length. Then lower the hands palms down to either side of the extended leg. Exhale as you lift the tailbone, tipping the pelvis forward and hinging from the hips. Gently slide the palms along the floor as you come forward with a straight spine. Continue with steps 5–9 as described above.

If you want more challenge, you can reengage the arms after holding and come out of the posture the same way you came into it. Reach the arms forward, pressing out through the fingertips to straighten the arms. Then rotate the hips to lift the torso and return the arms overhead. Press up through the fingertips to elongate the spine a final time, and sweep the arms back down to the sides.

The Great Seal is an excellent posture for holding. Come into the posture and hold for an extended period of time by relaxing and letting gravity do the work of stretching the body forward. Emphasize a long exhalation and notice how simply breathing in this way brings you more deeply into the posture. Release in slow motion, taking delight in the movement up and into Half Circle.

HALF CIRCLE

(Ardha Mandalasana)

1. From the Great Seal ending position, bring the heel of the left hand onto the floor a few inches behind the left hip. Spread the fingers of the hand wide, and press the rim of the palm firmly into the floor.

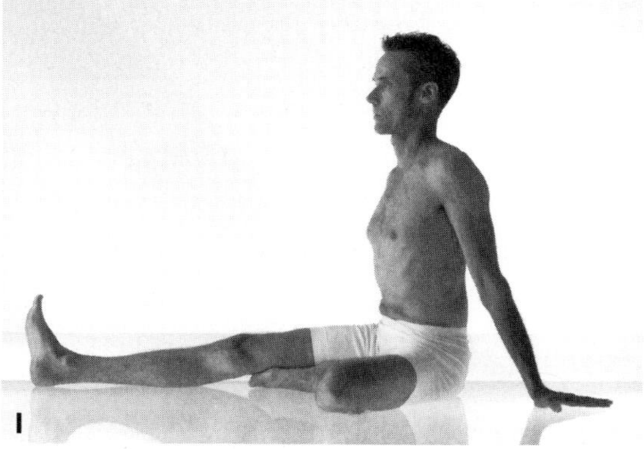

1

2. Inhaling, turn to look over your left shoulder and sweep the right hand up and across the body to the left, pressing down into the left hand and left knee to lift the hips and right leg up.

3. Press the hip bones forward and right foot into the floor. Lengthen the whole right side of the body by pressing the fingertips of the right hand away from the toes. Breathe deeply as you hold, fully feeling all the sensations.

4. To release, take a deep breath in. Exhale as you lower the hips to the floor and bring the right arm down, returning to the starting position.

5. Repeat the Great Seal and Half Circle on the opposite side.

Be Aware:

Half Circle is a side stretch that complements Great Seal. It opens the belly and chest, stretching and strengthening the arms, shoulders, chest, and abdomen. If you want less challenge, you can come into the posture without lifting the hips off the ground, emphasizing the arm and shoulder stretch. If you want more challenge, hold the posture with a flowing breath.

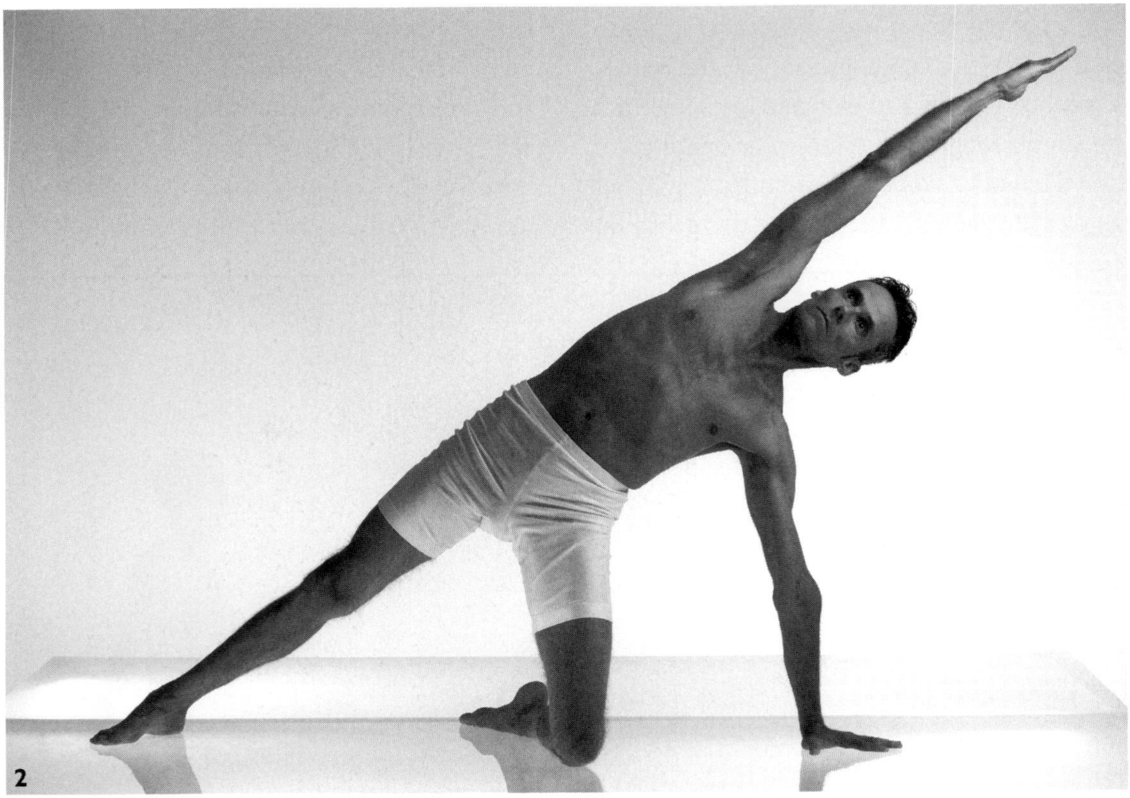
2

SPINAL TWIST

(Matsyendrasana)

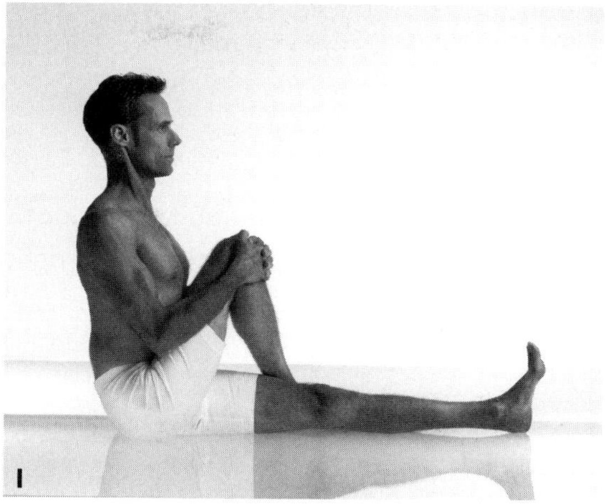

1

1. Sit with the legs extended, feet together, and hands resting on the floor at the sides. Bend the right knee, sliding the right heel close to the buttocks and interlacing the fingers around the knee. Cross the right foot over the left leg, placing the sole of the right foot on the ground by the left knee or thigh. Press the right sitz bone into the floor, allowing the weight to rest evenly on both sitz bones.

2. Elongate the spine by using your hand strength to pull the knee toward the sternum, lifting out of the waist and extending through the crown. Flex the left foot to lengthen the left leg.

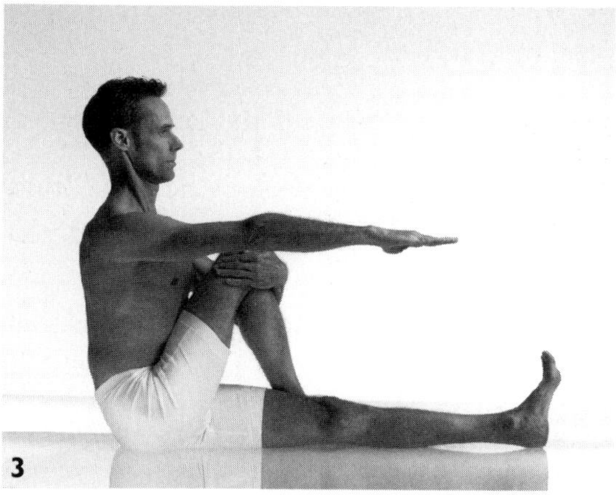

3

3. Hold the right knee with the left hand. Raise the right arm up to shoulder height and extend through the fingers.

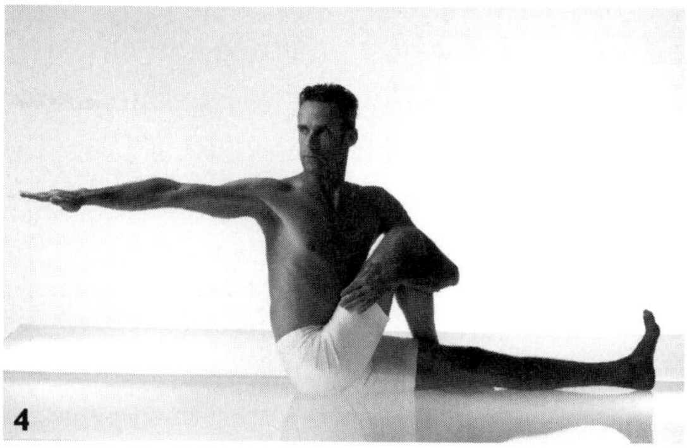

4

4. Take a deep breath in. As you exhale, begin to rotate the spine and sweep the right arm around the body to the right, following the movement of the hand with your gaze. As you twist, it becomes easy to wrap the arm around the knee, or hold the knee in the crook of the arm.

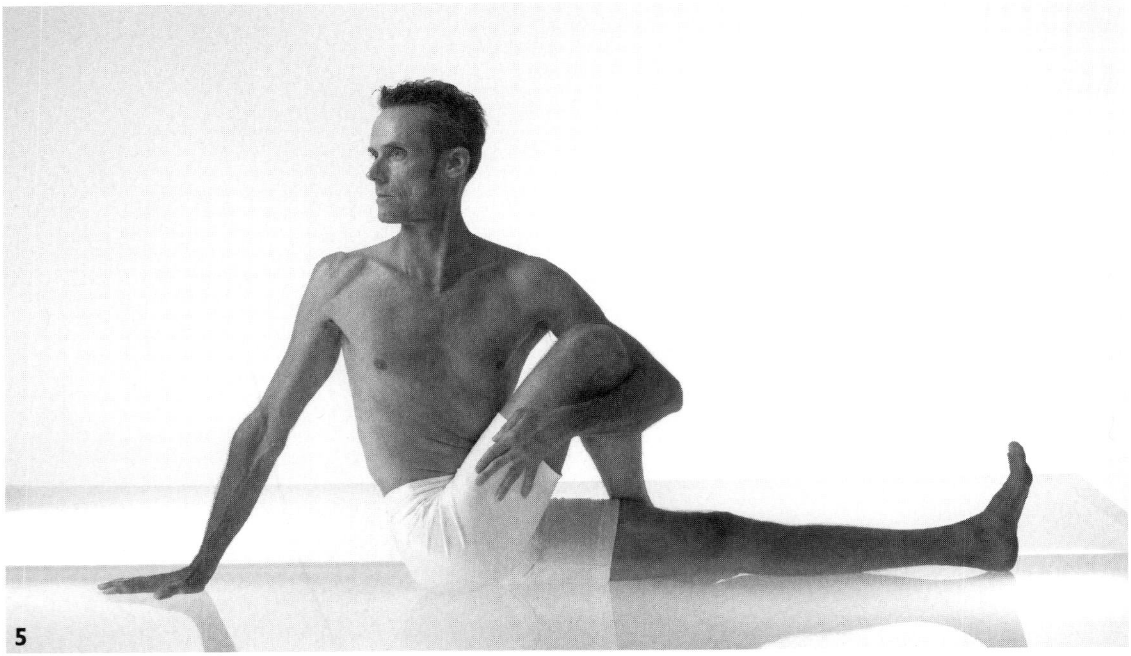
5

5. When you have rotated the spine fully, lower the right palm to the floor behind you. Press into the right palm to help keep the spine long. If your arms are short, or your wrists are sensitive, you can make a fist with the right hand, and press the fist into the floor.

6. With each inhalation, press down on the sitz bones and extend through the crown to lengthen the spine. With each exhalation, draw the belly in, twisting from the base of the spine to the back of the head, allowing the abdomen, rib cage, shoulders, and chin to twist to the right. Keep the chin level, looking as far to the right and behind you as possible. Breath deeply as you hold.

7. To release, lift the right arm back to shoulder height. Inhale and sweep the right hand around to center, following the movement of the hand with the eyes as you rotate the torso back to center. Lower the right hand to the ground, and straighten both legs.

8. Repeat on the opposite side.

Be Aware:
To twist safely, the spine must be kept elongated to avoid putting pressure on the delicate spinal nerves. Follow the instructions closely in step 2 to use the knee position and your arm strength to elongate the spine.

The Spinal Twist is an excellent posture to hold. At first, use the breath and instructions in step 6 to twist deeply. Once you have come into a deep twist, relax the muscles completely and breathe deeply.

If you want less challenge, try Supine

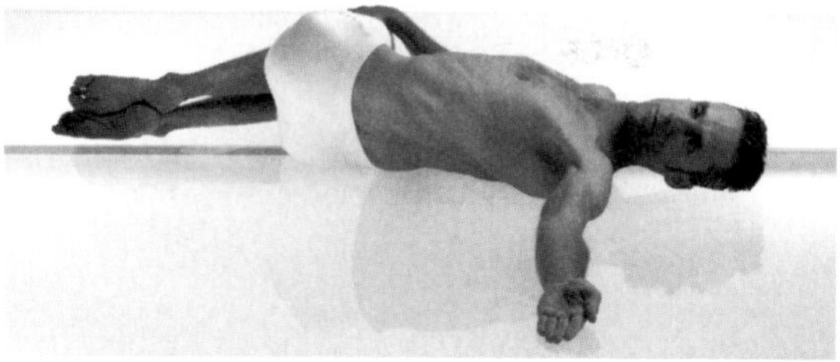

Twist. Come onto your back and bring both knees into the chest. Let the arms come out to the sides in a T, palms up. Take a deep breath in, and as you exhale let both knees rock over to the right. Turn your head to look left and hold the left knee with the right hand. Many people find this position soothing to the low back.

DEAD BUG

(Urdhva Prasarita Padasana)

1. Lie on your back with the feet close to the buttocks and arms at the sides.

2. Bring both knees into the chest. Let the sacrum and low back rest solidly on the floor. Rock the head side to side a time or two. Bring the head back to center and tuck the chin slightly to elongate the back of the neck.

3. Exhale. As you inhale, lift the legs and arms until they are vertical.

4. Let the breath flow freely. Explore micro-movements of the feet and hands, letting the ankles, toes, wrists, hands, and fingers move as you hold for several minutes.

5. To release, take a deep breath in. Exhale and lower the knees into the chest, arms to the sides. Extend the legs into Corpse Pose.

6. Close the eyes and see if you can feel an increase in blood circulation and energy flow from holding this inversion.

Be Aware:
Simply lifting the limbs and holding with a flowing breath is a surprisingly effective inversion. Work up to holding Dead Bug for

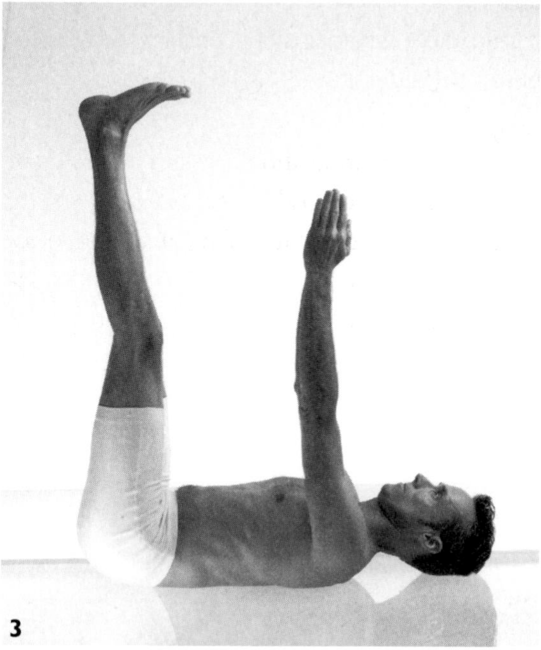

3

three minutes or more, using the breath and micromovements of the hands and feet to keep the body relaxed. When an inversion is held, the whole body is stimulated by its need to adjust to a new relationship with gravity and a different pattern of blood flow. When the inversion is released, the whole body rebalances as gravity and circulation return to normal. Moving from Dead Bug to Corpse, close the eyes and experience this for yourself.

Because the weight of the body rests on the back and floor, the Dead Bug is a particularly safe inversion and especially appropriate for heavier individuals. Since the hips are not raised above the rest of the torso, the Dead Bug is an inversion that can be practiced during menstruation.

DEEP RELAXATION IN CORPSE

(Yoga Nidra in Shavasana)

1. Lie on your back with the legs extended. Bring the arms by the sides, palms up and fingers gently curled. Adjust the feet so they are a comfortable distance apart, and let the toes fall out to the sides.

2. Close the eyes to facilitate feeling. Let the whole body relax and sink into the floor.

3. Focus your attention on the flow of breath, simply watching and feeling the breath rebalance after postures.

4. Gradually move into Relaxing Breath. Inhale naturally and let the exhalation roll out long, slow, and smooth. Over time, the exhalation will grow approximately twice as long as

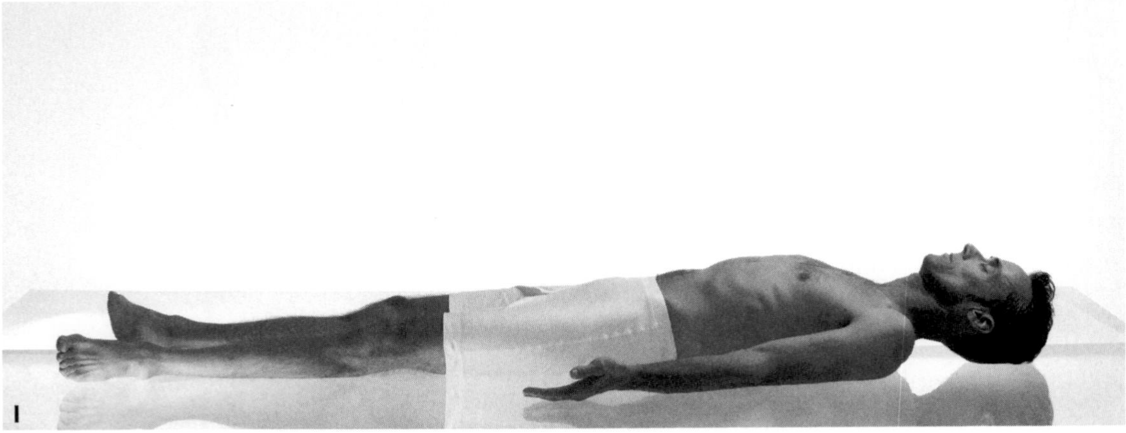

1

the inhalation. Stay with Relaxing Breath for three minutes or more. Feel the heartbeat grow slow and steady. Notice the state of introversion that naturally arises from breathing in this way.

5. Release any conscious control of the breath and begin any of the relaxation techniques detailed in chapter 6.

6. Let go into deep relaxation, allowing worries, concerns, and defenses to fall away.

Be Aware:
As your body relaxes, its surface temperature tends to drop, so put on an extra layer of clothing or cover yourself with a blanket prior to entering Corpse. If it is uncomfortable to lie flat on the floor, a pillow beneath the knees helps relieve low back tension. If your neck is uncomfortable, try placing a folded towel or blanket under your head. Don't use a large pillow, which will cramp the neck and obstruct the free flow of breath. For more relaxation tips, see page 65.

MOON FLOW

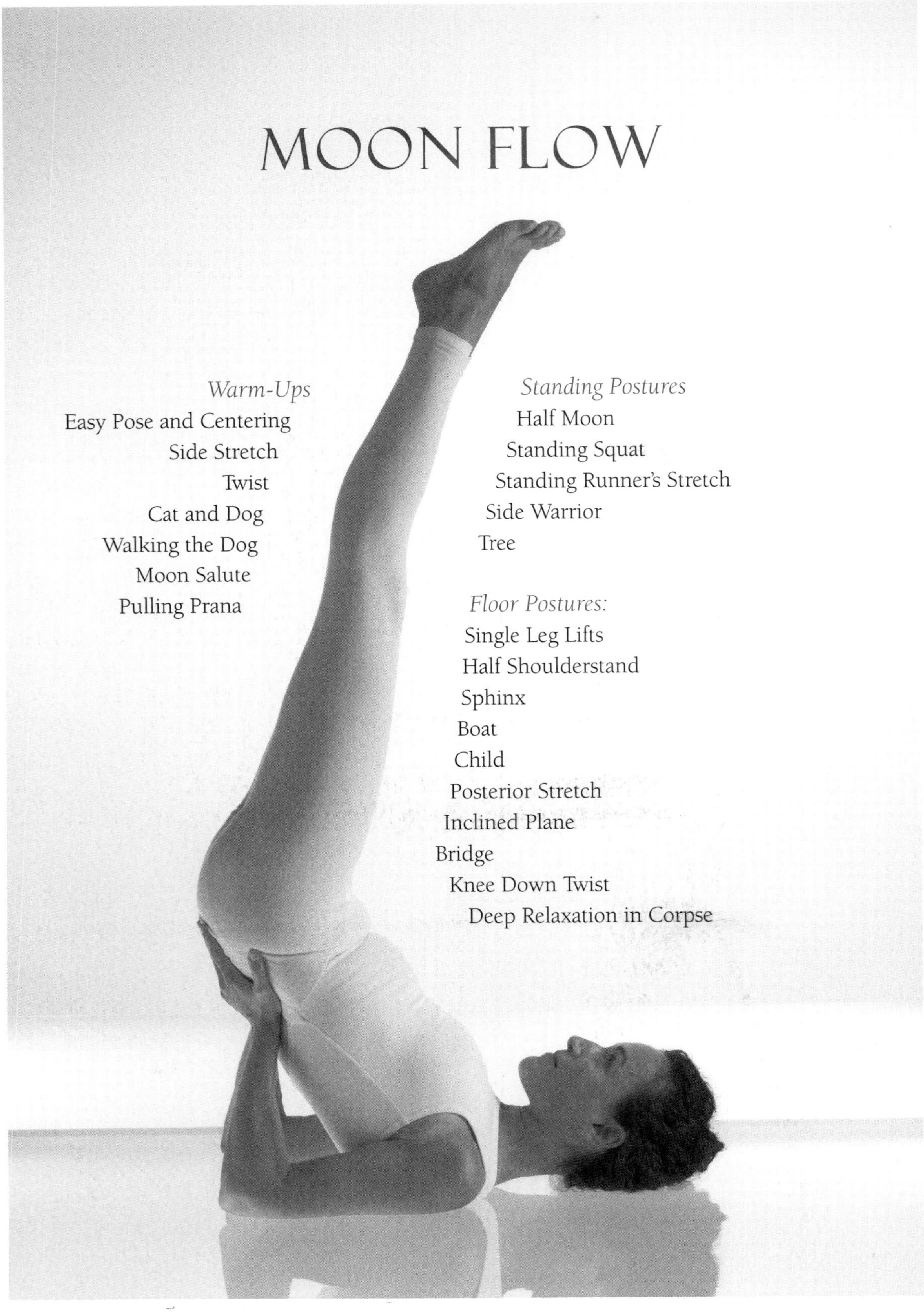

Warm-Ups

Easy Pose and Centering
Side Stretch
Twist
Cat and Dog
Walking the Dog
Moon Salute
Pulling Prana

Standing Postures

Half Moon
Standing Squat
Standing Runner's Stretch
Side Warrior
Tree

Floor Postures:

Single Leg Lifts
Half Shoulderstand
Sphinx
Boat
Child
Posterior Stretch
Inclined Plane
Bridge
Knee Down Twist
Deep Relaxation in Corpse

EASY POSE AND CENTERING

(Ujjayi Pranayama in Sukhasana)

1. Sit near the front edge of a cushion with the legs extended. Bend the knees and slide the feet toward the body until the feet rest comfortably on the floor. Place the hands on the knees, palms up or down.

2. Press the sitz bones into the floor to provide a stable base for your sitting posture. Elongate the spine by lifting out of the waist, tucking the chin slightly and extending through the crown. Open the chest by pressing the sternum forward and rolling the shoulders back and down.

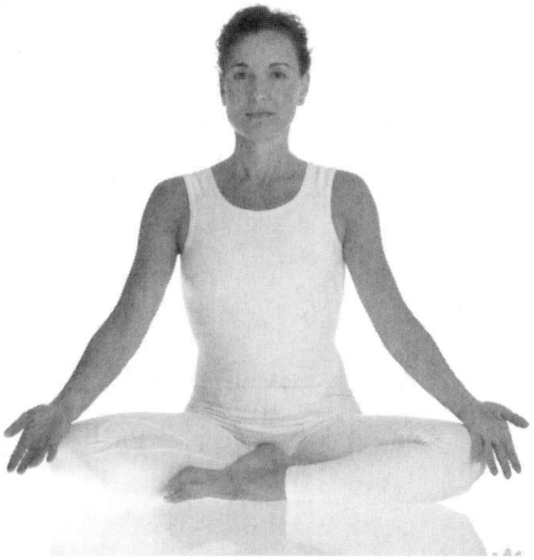

2

3. Bring yourself present: breathe, relax, feel, watch, and allow. Affirm the intention to remain present in your body as you practice.

4. Close your eyes and focus the attention on the flow of the breath. Come into Ocean Sounding Breath, allowing the friction of the breath against the glottis to make a sound like the rise and fall of waves at the beach. Use the sound of the breath to help you smooth out its flow, letting in-breaths and out-breaths flow smoothly one into the next with a sense of ease and timelessness.

Be Aware:

This simple cross-legged sitting position is one you can use for breathing exercises and meditation. Sitting toward the front edge of the cushion encourages the pelvis to roll slightly forward, inhibiting the tendency to round the low back. It is much easier to sit with a straight spine when the hips are higher off the ground than the knees. To raise the hips, most people need to sit on one or more cushions.

Even sitting on a cushion, you may find your knees remain off the ground. In this position, the weight of the legs can torque the knee joints and cause pain. Placing a cushion under each knee provides needed support. With practice, you will probably need less hip lift and knee support. If floor sitting just doesn't work for you, use a chair.

At the beginning of practice, Ocean Sounding Breath is an invitation to breathe deeply and you are likely to find yourself moving naturally into Three-Part Breathing. Let that happen, returning to flowing breath to begin warm-ups and sustaining Ocean Sounding Breath for the duration of your practice session.

SIDE STRETCH

1. From Easy Pose, bring the right palm to rest on the floor a comfortable distance from the right hip. Exhale.

2. Inhale as you sweep the left arm out to the side and overhead. Feel the stretch along the left side of the torso, creating space between the hip and rib cage, stretching the muscles between each rib, and opening the armpit.

3. Exhale as you lower the left arm, resting the left palm on the floor a comfortable distance from the left hip.

4. Inhale and sweep the right arm out to the side and overhead, repeating on the opposite side.

5. Repeat this side-to-side movement several times, moving with the breath to stretch out one side, and then the other.

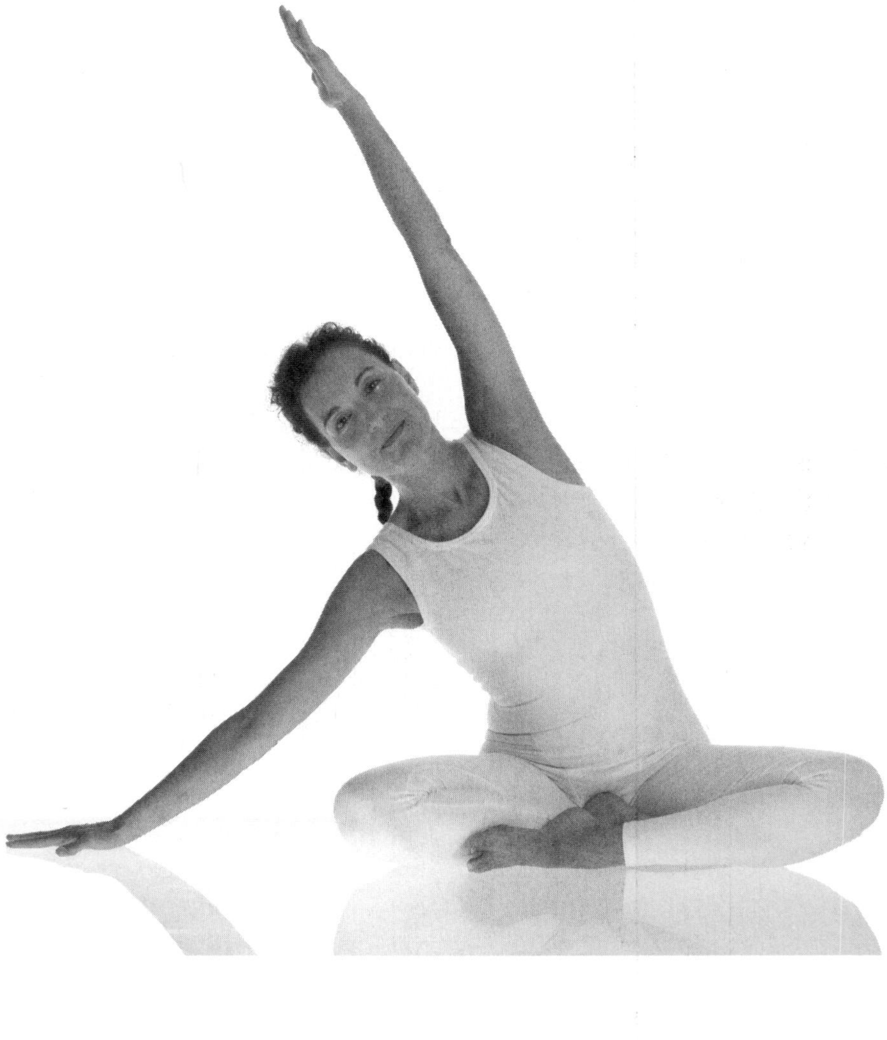

2

6. On the final repetition, inhale the left arm up and hold the stretch for a few flowing breaths in and out. Press both sitz bones and the left hand into the floor. Extend through the crown and fingertips of the left hand. Stay present in your body as you hold, feeling all the sensations. Take a deep breath in, and let out an audible sigh. Take another deep breath, and release on the exhalation. Repeat on the opposite side.

Be Aware:

This warm-up combines a side and shoulder stretch with a gentle lateral bend of the spine. Keep both sitz bones pressed down and the sternum lifted to avoid any tendency to twist the hips or shoulders. You can enhance the stretch by bending the elbow of the lower arm or sliding the hand a little farther away from the hip.

TWIST

1. Sit in Easy Pose. Press both sitz bones down, stabilizing the core and elongating the spine. Exhale.

2. Inhale the arms out to the sides and overhead in a wide V. Press the fingertips away and extend through the crown to further elongate the spine.

3. Exhale and twist to the right as you lower the right hand to the floor behind your right hip and the left hand onto the right knee. Turn the head to look over the right shoulder.

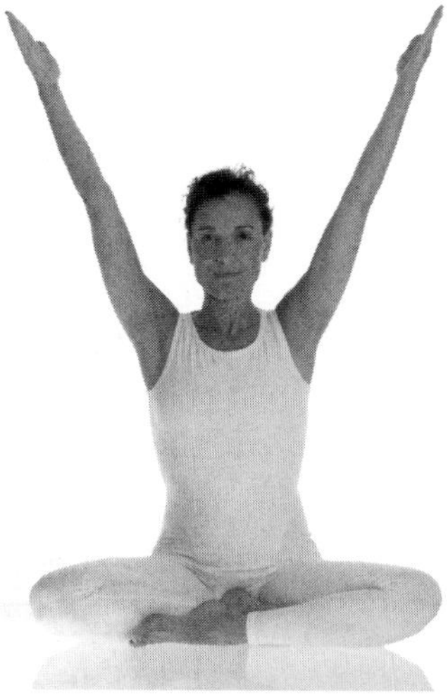

2

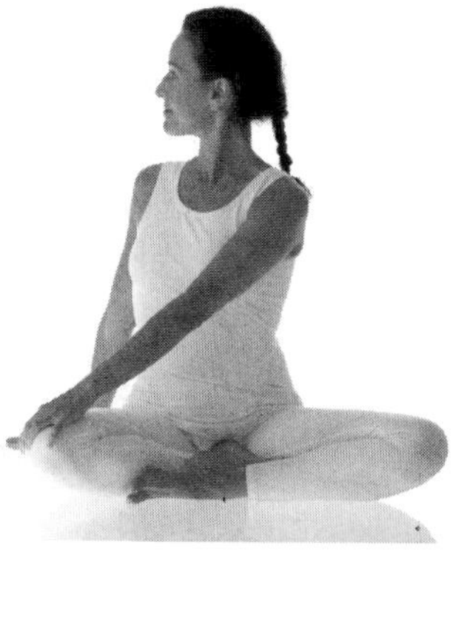

3

4. Inhale the arms back up into a wide V. Exhale and twist to the opposite side.

5. Repeat this twisting motion several times, inhaling the arms up to stretch the spine long, and exhaling as you lower the arms and twist. Let the exercise become a flow of breath and movement.

6. On the final repetition, hold the twist to the right for several flowing breaths. Press into both sitz bones and the right palm to keep the spine elongated. Apply gentle pressure with the left hand, level the chin, and look to the right to enhance the twist. Inhale the arms back up, and hold the twist for several flowing breaths on the opposite side.

7. Inhale the arms up into a wide V a final time. Take a few breaths in this position, pressing the sitz bones down and extending through the crown and fingertips. Inhale deeply, then

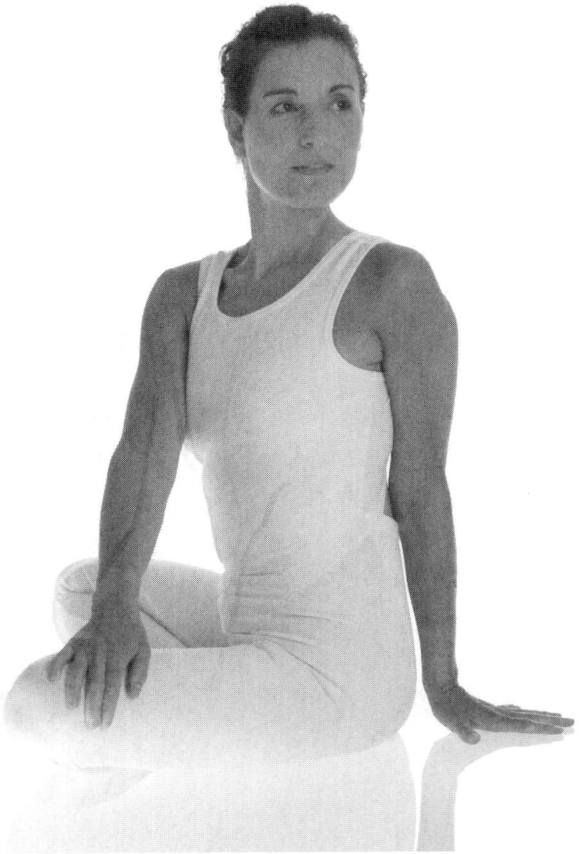

4

slowly lower the hands to the knees on the exhale. Close the eyes and feel your spine from bottom to top.

Be Aware:

To twist safely, the spine must be elongated to create ample space for the vertebrae to rotate without putting pressure on the delicate spinal nerves. In this exercise, the movement of the arms keeps the spine long as you twist from side to side. Because twisting compresses alternative sides of the abdomen and chest, it is impossible to breathe deeply while twisting. While holding, let the breath flow as freely as possible without strain.

CAT AND DOG

1. Come onto your hands and knees. Place the hands under the shoulders, palms down with the fingers spread wide. Place the knees under the hips. The torso, back, and neck form a straight line. This is Table Pose.

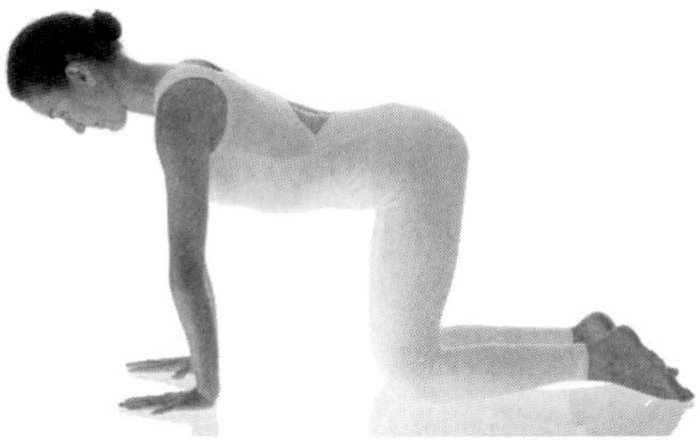

1

2. Inhale into Dog Tilt by lifting the tailbone high, letting the belly and mid-spine fall toward the floor, and looking upward.

3. Exhale into Cat Stretch by tucking the tailbone under, arching the mid-back up like an angry cat, and tucking the chin into the chest.

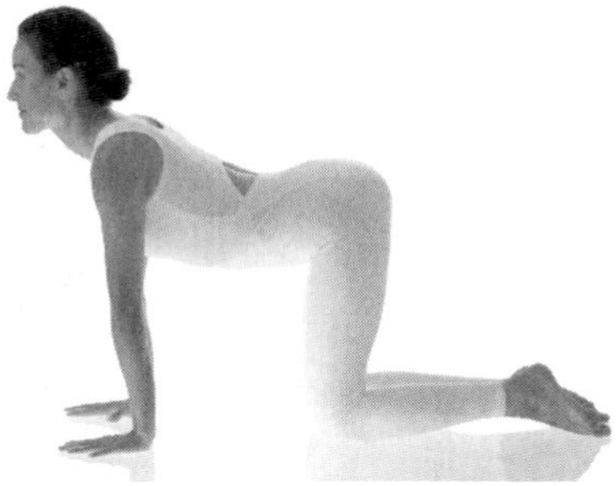

2

4. Coordinating breath and motion, begin to flow smoothly from Cat to Dog. Initiate the movement with the tailbone and let it ripple through the spine, neck, and head to create a fluid and undulating movement of the spine.

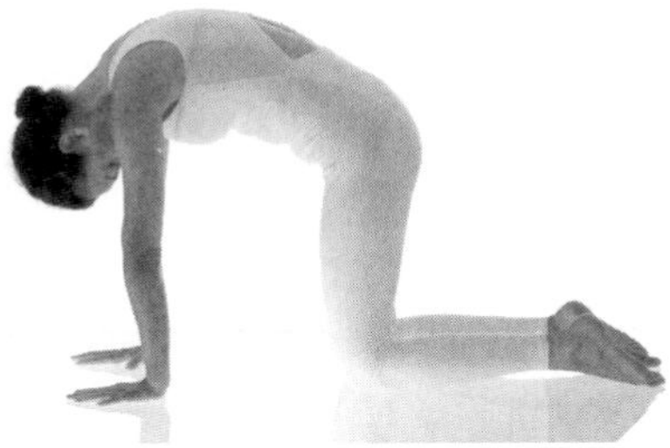

3

5. Repeat several times, noticing where the spine flexes easily and where it doesn't move so easily.

Be Aware:

These two simple stretches emphasize the root movement of the spine that underlies all forward and backward bends. Use them to become acquainted with the lifting and tucking of the tailbone, instructions used in many postures that may be unfamiliar to you.

Holding the Cat Stretch releases tension from the upper back and neck. Breathing deeply, press the hands into the floor, tuck the tailbone under, and press the chin into the chest. As you hold, press the mid-back up toward the ceiling, letting out any sighs or sounds that release tension.

The last three warm-ups stretched your spine side to side, twisted it right then left, and flexed it forward and back. These are the six primary movements required to maintain the flexibility of the spinal column.

WALKING THE DOG

(Adho Mukha Svanasana)

1. From Table Pose, spread the fingers wide apart and curl the toes under.

2. Take a deep breath in. Exhale as you press into the hands and balls of the feet to lift the hips up. Keep the knees bent, the spine straight, and the neck long. Let the breath flow, giving your body a moment to adjust to this position.

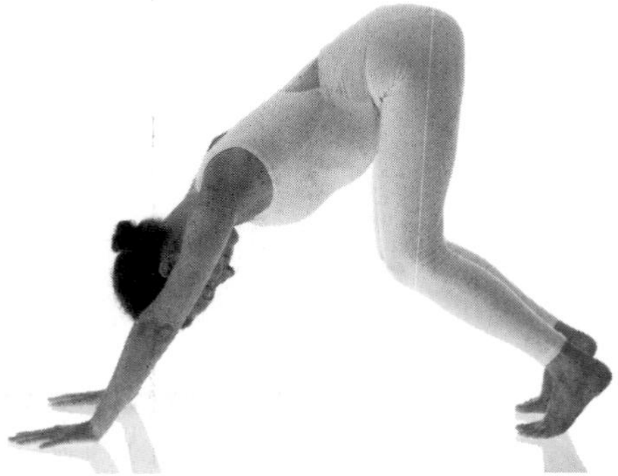

2

3. Bend the left knee and press the right heel toward the floor, feeling the stretch to the back of the right leg. Then bend the right knee and press the left heel toward the floor, feeling the stretch to the back of the left leg. Move smoothly side to side, letting the hips swivel as

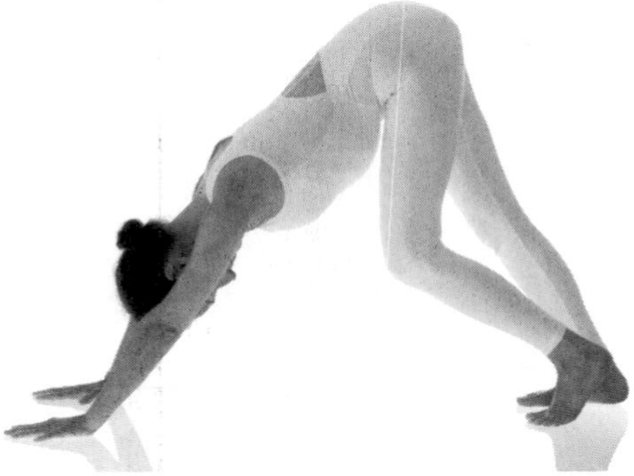

3

you stretch out the legs. This is called "walking the dog."

4. Come back to center with both knees comfortably bent. Lift the tailbone toward the ceiling, coming into a Dog Tilt. Inhale and lift the hips as high off the floor as possible. As you exhale, press the buttocks back toward the wall behind you, bringing the heels toward the floor.

5. Press the rims of the palms into the floor, engaging the muscles of the arms and shoulders. Allow the shoulder blades to move down and back, dropping deep into the shoulder girdle. Gently engage the abdominals to help keep the spine long. Extend the crown of the head away from the lifted tailbone, letting the head and neck be framed by straight upper arms. Feel the spine being pulled in opposite directions and lengthened by this combination of movements. This is Downward Facing Dog Pose.

6. To release, bend the knees and gradually walk the hands toward the feet until all of your weight rests on the feet.

7. Bend the knees deeply enough that the torso rests on the thighs. Lift the head slightly to lengthen the neck. Bring the hands to the knees for support and slowly press up to standing in the most supportive way for your body.

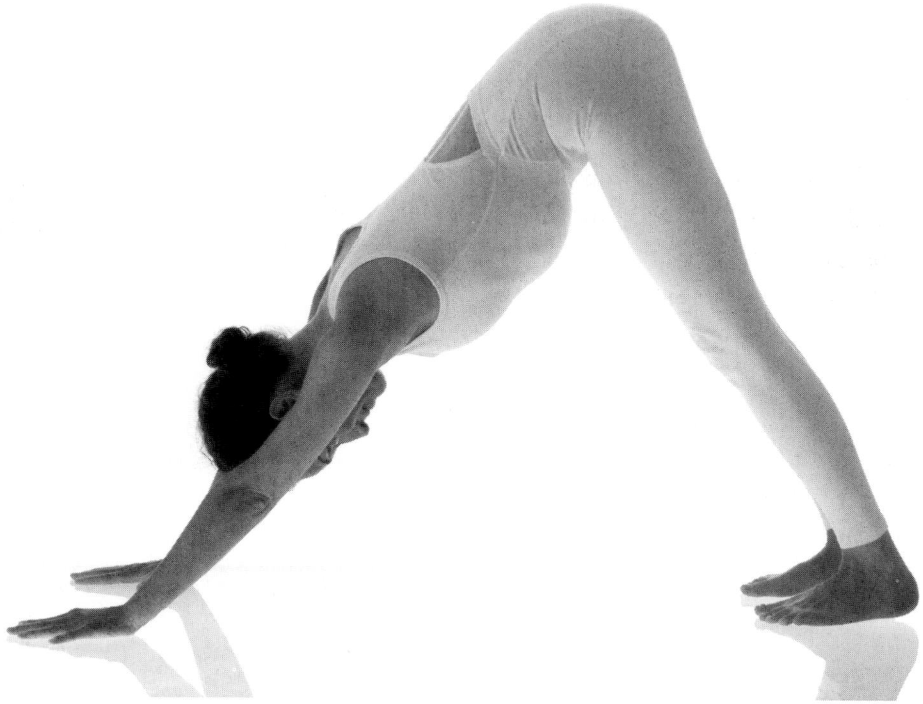

5

Be Aware:
Downward Facing Dog has many benefits, elongating the spine and stretching the muscles of the arms, legs, and back. Along with being a good upper body strengthener, it is also a mild inversion. Do not practice if you have unmedicated high blood pressure, glaucoma, detached retina, or other eye problems.

If you want less challenge, don't straighten the legs. Walk the Dog and release back into Table Pose. To build endurance, come in and out several times, resting in Table Pose in-between. Over time, your flexibility and strength will increase. If you want more challenge, try the Downward Facing Dog variations on pages 351–352.

MOON SALUTE

(Chandra Namaskar)

1. Stand with the feet hip-width apart. Inhale as you bring the hands into Prayer Position and gently press the palms together.

2. Exhale as you slowly lower the hands to the sides. Inhale and sweep the arms out and overhead, scribing the circumference of an imaginary full moon. Bring the palms together and fingers into Steeple Position. Press the index fingers toward the ceiling to elongate the spine.

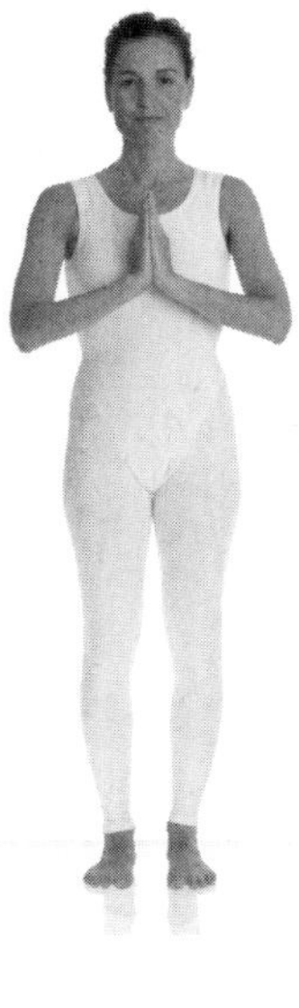

1

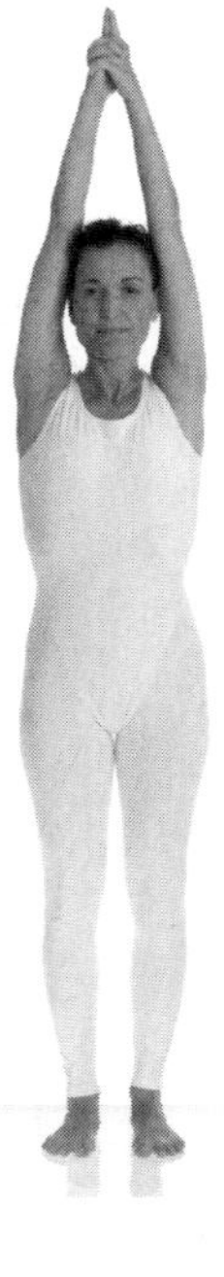

2

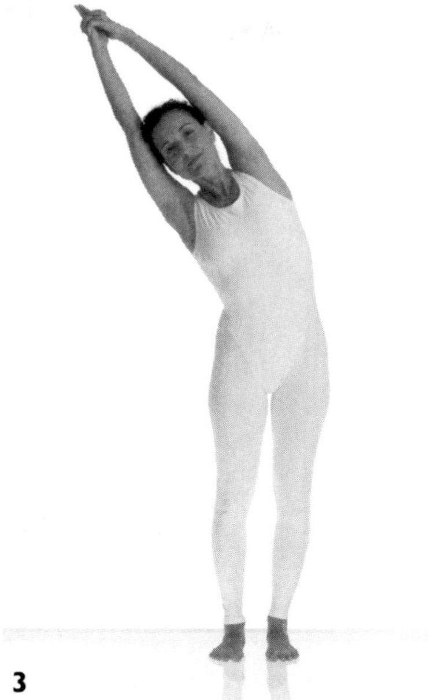

3

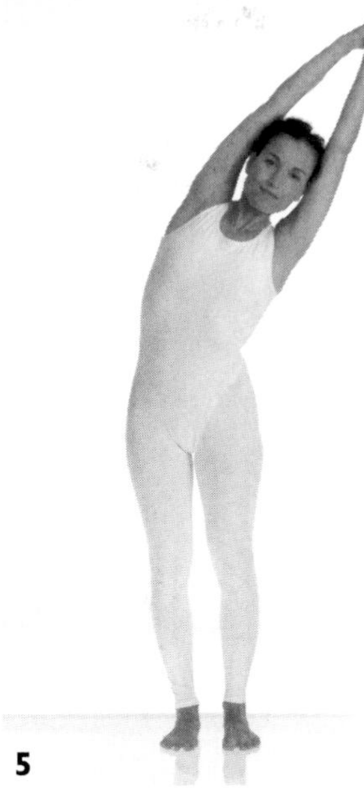

5

3. Exhale as you gently press the left hip out to the side and come into the Half Moon posture to the right.

4. Inhale back to center and elongate the spine.

5. Exhale as you gently press the right hip out to the side and come into the Half Moon posture to the left.

6. Inhale back to center and elongate the spine.

7. Exhale, stepping wide and turning the feet out slightly. Bend the knees and bring the arms out to the sides at shoulder height, elbows bent and palms facing inward. Press the tailbone down and pubic bone forward to level the pelvis, and extend through the crown to elongate the spine. This is Goddess Pose.

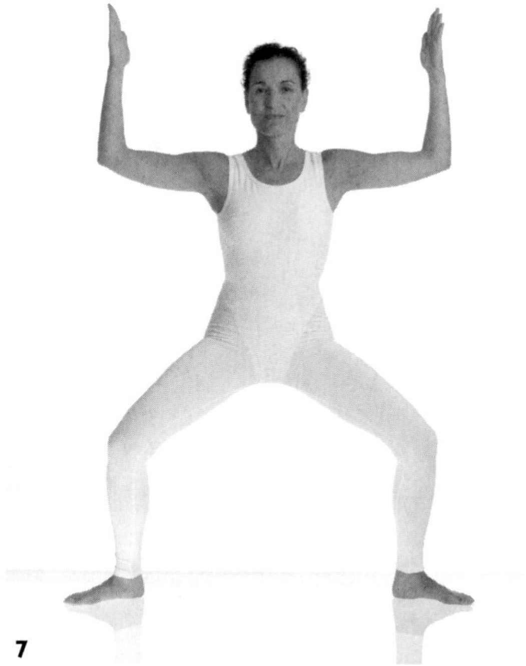

7

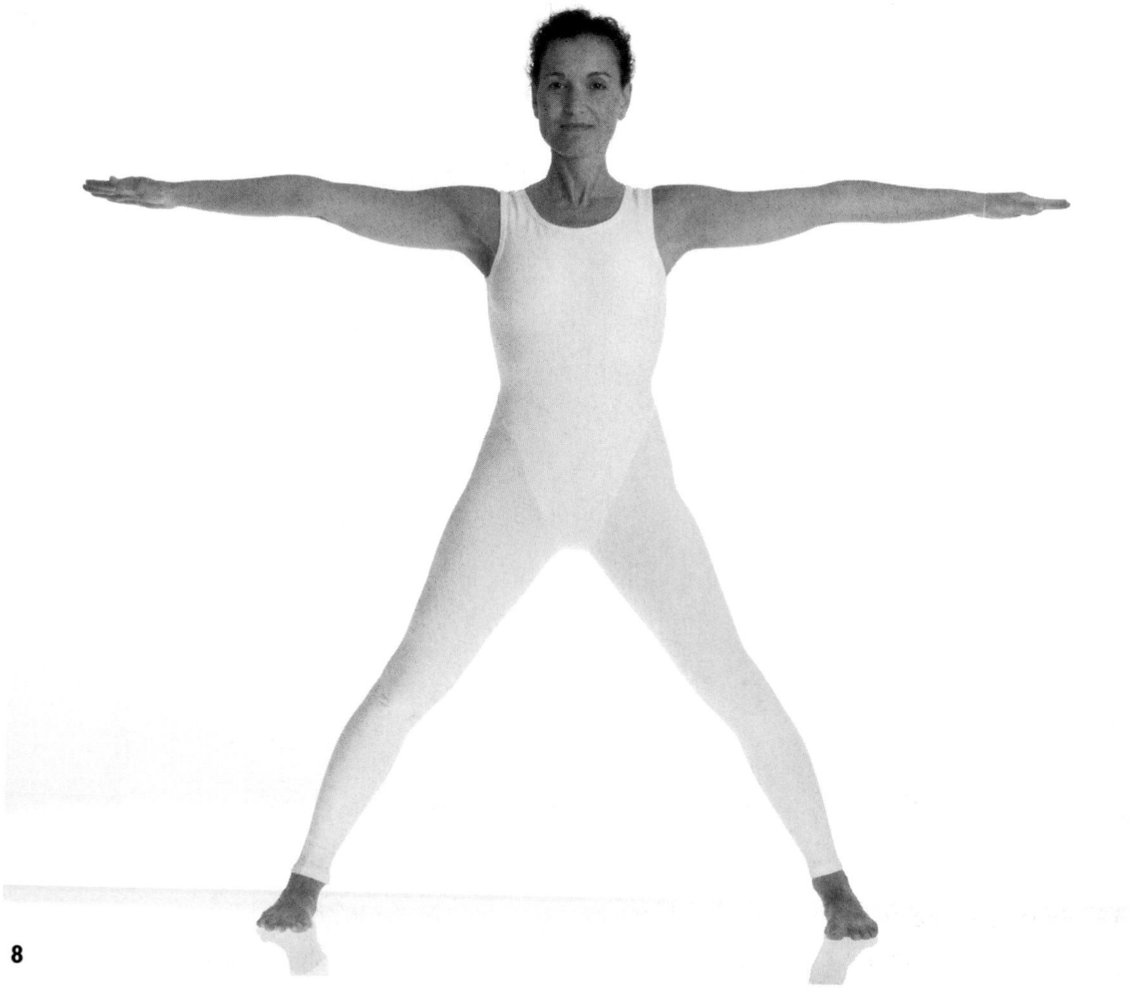

8

8. Inhale as you straighten the legs and arms, coming into Five Pointed Star. Turn the feet to face forward and press out through the fingertips.

9. Exhale and reach the right hand down toward the right knee, lifting the left arm up and coming into a side stretch. Keep the hips and shoulder facing forward.

10. Inhale back up to Five Pointed Star.

11. Exhale as you reach the left hand down toward the left knee, lifting the right arm up and coming into a side stretch. Keep the hips and shoulders facing forward.

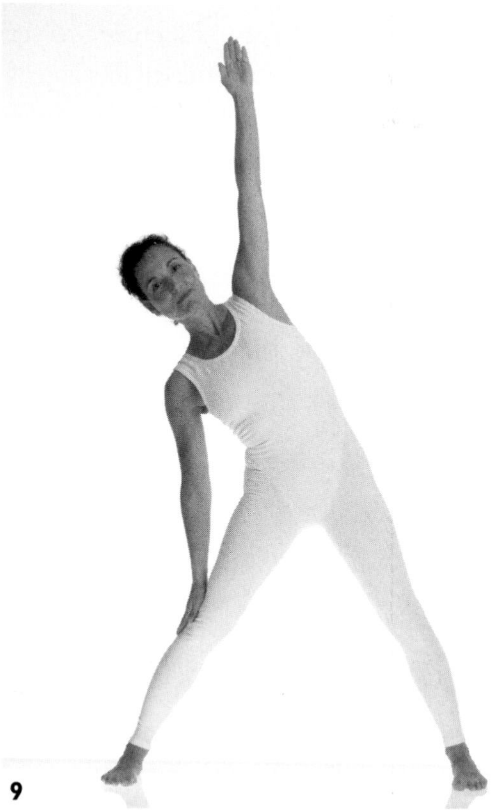

9

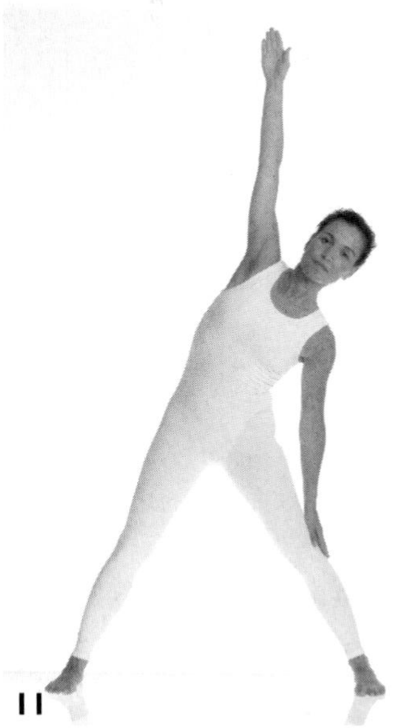

11

12. Inhale back up to Five Pointed Star and press out through the fingertips.

13. Exhale, rotate the hips and shoulders as you reach the left hand down to the right foot and lift the right arm up, coming into a standing twist. Bend the knees as necessary to avoid strain.

14. Inhale back up to Five Pointed Star. Press out through the fingertips.

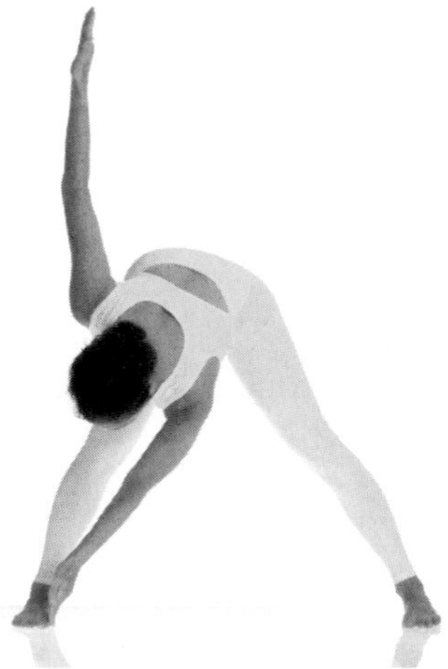

13

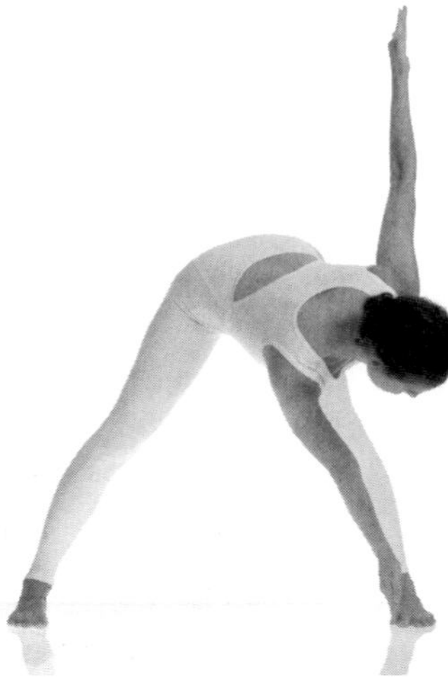

15

15. Exhale, rotate the hips and shoulders as you reach the right hand down to the left foot and lift the left arm up, coming into a standing twist. Bend the knees as necessary to avoid strain.

16. Inhale back up to Five Pointed Star.

17. Exhale, turn the feet out slightly and bend the knees and elbows, sinking back into Goddess Pose.

18. Inhale as you straighten the legs and step the feet back to hip-width while bringing the arms overhead with palms together and fingers in Steeple Position. Press the fingers toward the ceiling to elongate the spine.

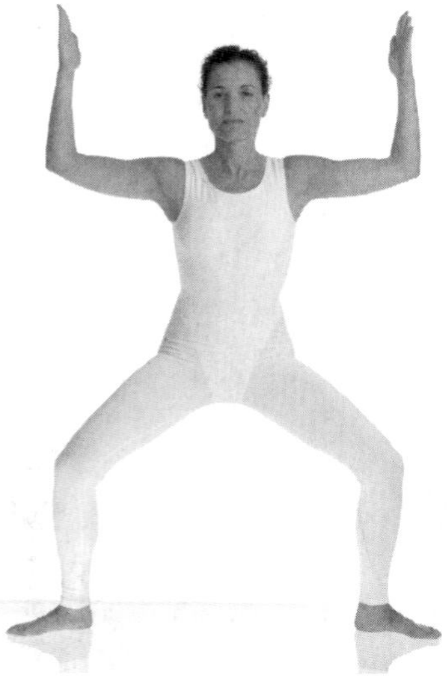

17

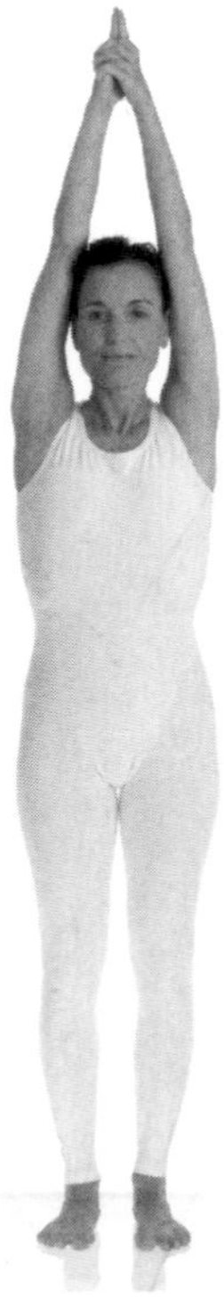

18

19. Exhale as you gently press the left hip out to the side and come into Half Moon posture to the right.

20. Inhale back to center and again elongate the spine.

21. Exhale as you gently press the right hip out to the side and come into Half Moon posture to the left.

22. Inhale back up to center and again elongate the spine.

23. Exhale, slowly sweep the arms out to the sides, scribing the circumference of an imaginary full moon. Inhale as you bring the palms together in Prayer Position and slightly bow the head.

24. Release the arms down to your sides.

Be Aware:

There are many variations of Moon Salute. This one is a flowing warm-up that provides the body with a series of side stretches and twists. It is a nice complement to the Sun Series, which is a flow of forward and backward bends.

If it is difficult for you to raise the arms overhead, you can place the hands on the hips and come into Quarter Moon. If you have knee or low back sensitivity, be sure to bend the knees as you reach your hand to the opposite foot to come into the standing twist. You can also leave out this movement. If you find Moon Salute easy, you can do several repetitions in succession.

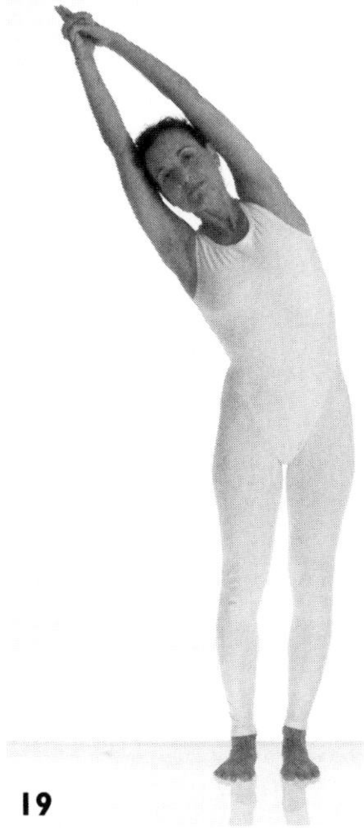

19

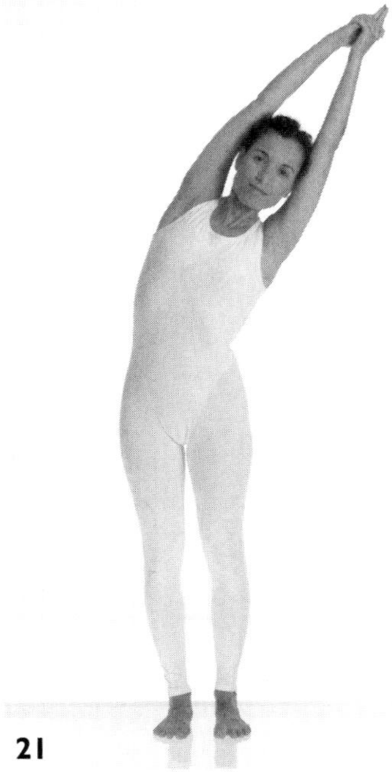

21

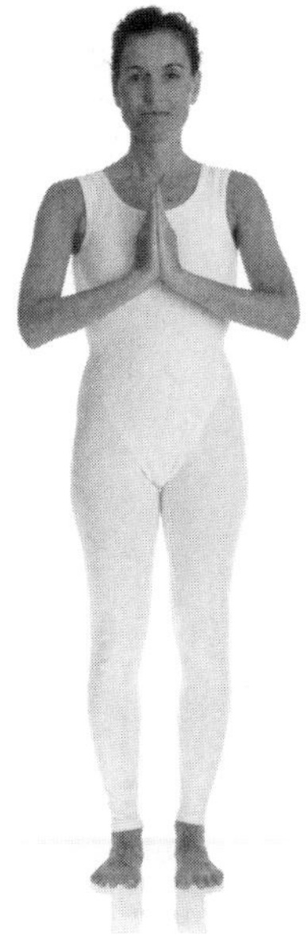

23

PULLING PRANA

1. Stand with the feet parallel, hip-width apart, and knees slightly bent.

2. Inhale as you reach the arms in front of you, fingers spread, thumbs pointing down, buttocks slightly jutting out behind you.

3. Allow the pelvis and hips to rock forward as the hands are pulled back toward the body, exhaling with a "ha" sound, fingers closing into loose fists.

4. Start to move and breathe in rhythm. Inhale as you extend the arms in front of you and let the hips and buttocks rock back. Exhale as you draw both hands back into the sides and rock the pelvis forward.

5. Visualize yourself reaching out to grasp some invisible prana from the atmosphere and pulling it into the core of your body. Let the pace of the breath, hip, and arm motion steadily build over twenty-five repetitions.

6. Inhale as you come back to standing and let out a long, slow exhale. Feel the effects.

Be Aware:

This is a dynamic breathing exercise that activates the body in many ways. Start slowly

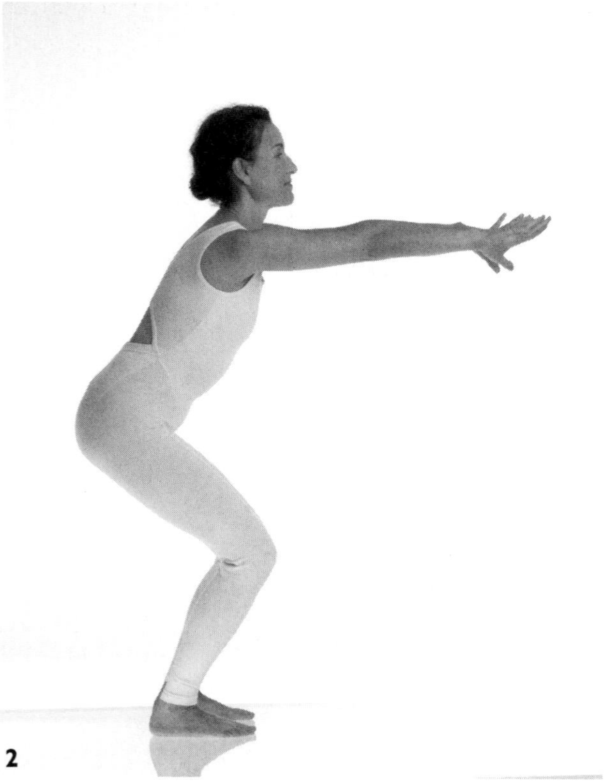

2

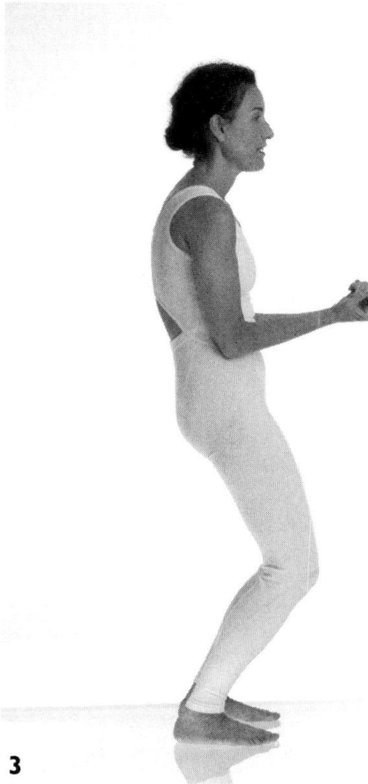

3

and emphasize the breath versus the motion. Let the breath and movement awaken your body's energy.

Skip this exercise if you are pregnant, menstruating, have a fever or unmedicated high blood pressure, become light-headed, dizzy, or experience other unpleasant symptoms. For a less challenging alternative, do Sun Breath.

HALF MOON

(Ardha Chandrasana)

1. Stand in Mountain Pose. Spread the toes and press down into all four corners of the feet to engage the legs. Stabilize the core, elongate the spine, and press the sternum forward to open the chest.

2. Inhale and sweep the arms out to the sides and overhead. Bring the hands into Steeple Position by interlacing the fingers and pointing the index fingers up. Extend through the fingertips.

3. Keeping the arms straight and spine long, exhale and soften the muscles of the shoulders, upper back, and neck. Let the top of the shoulders drop away from the ears. Allow the shoulder blades to move down and back. Squeeze the hands together and press the index fingers up to keep the spine long.

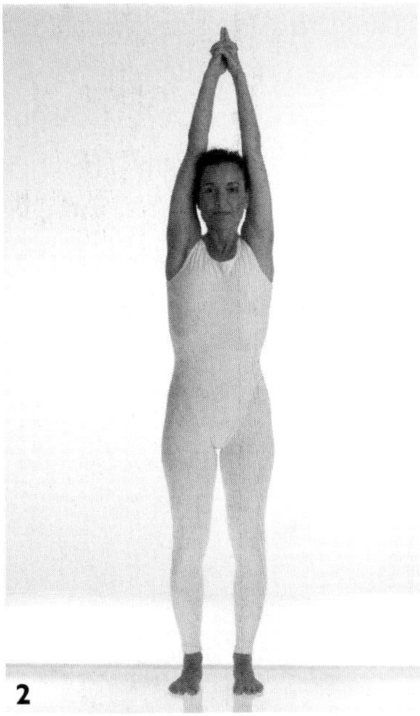
2

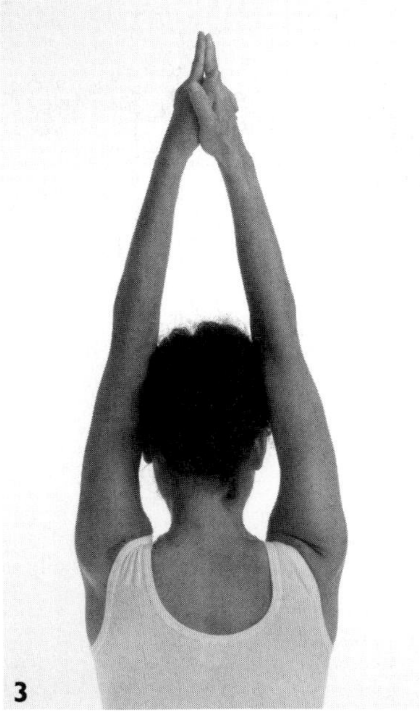
3

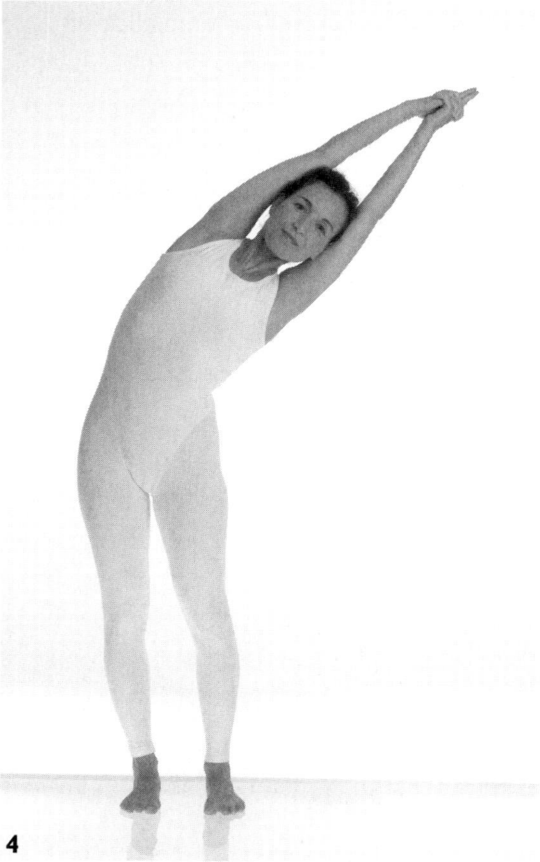

4

4. Take a deep breath in. Exhale and press the hips to the right, keeping hips and shoulders facing forward. The right hip bone lifts slightly, and the left hip bone lowers slightly, but the body stays in one plane. Emphasize the side stretch by resisting the tendency of the hips and shoulders to twist. Press the fingertips away, lengthening both sides of the body.

5. Allow the posture to create space between the ribs and stretch the intercostal muscles. Keep the chin lifted, neck long, and crown extended. Let the breath flow as you hold.

6. Inhale as you press into the feet and bring the arms back to center, pressing the fingertips toward the ceiling to elongate the spine. Exhale into the posture on the opposite side.

7. To release, inhale as you press into the feet and bring the arms back to center. Slowly lower the arms to the sides.

Be Aware:

While Half Moon appears simple, it is not easy to isolate the side stretch and gain the flexibility needed to practice properly. That's why it is done as warm-up in the Moon Salute and again as a posture. As you come into the side stretch, imagine that your body is pressed between two panes of glass. This will help you avoid the tendency to twist the hips or shoulders, targeting the often inflexible intercostal muscles.

If you want less challenge, practice Quarter Moon. If you want more challenge, try Half Moon with the feet touching. Bringing the feet closer together enhances the side stretch, but your stance must be stable to prevent the hips and shoulders from twisting.

STANDING SQUAT

(Utkatasana)

1. Stand in Mountain Pose.

2. Inhale and lift the arms in front of you to shoulder height, palms down, fingers and thumbs together. Press out through the fingertips to engage and lengthen the arms.

3. Exhale and slowly bend the knees, letting the buttocks lower. At first the spine remains erect, but as the knees bend deeper the buttocks jut out and the torso angles slightly forward. The crown of the head remains lifted and the spine long.

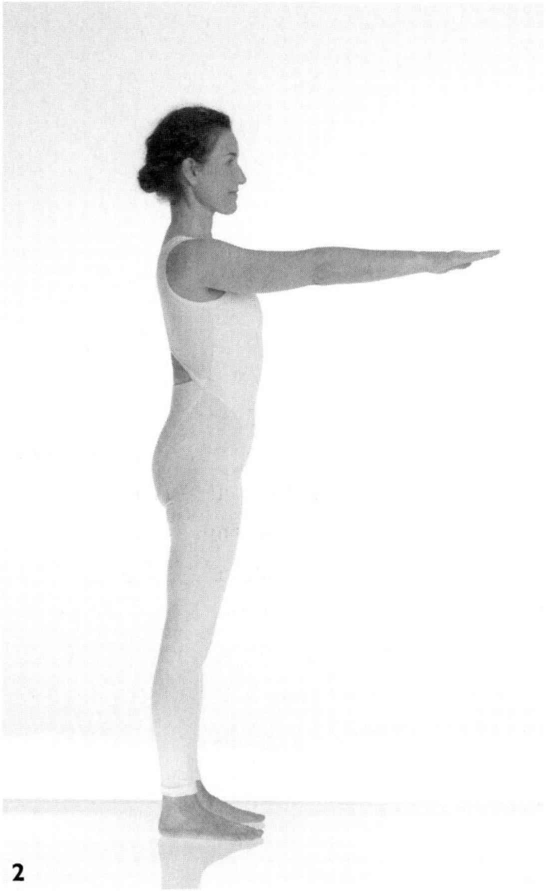

2

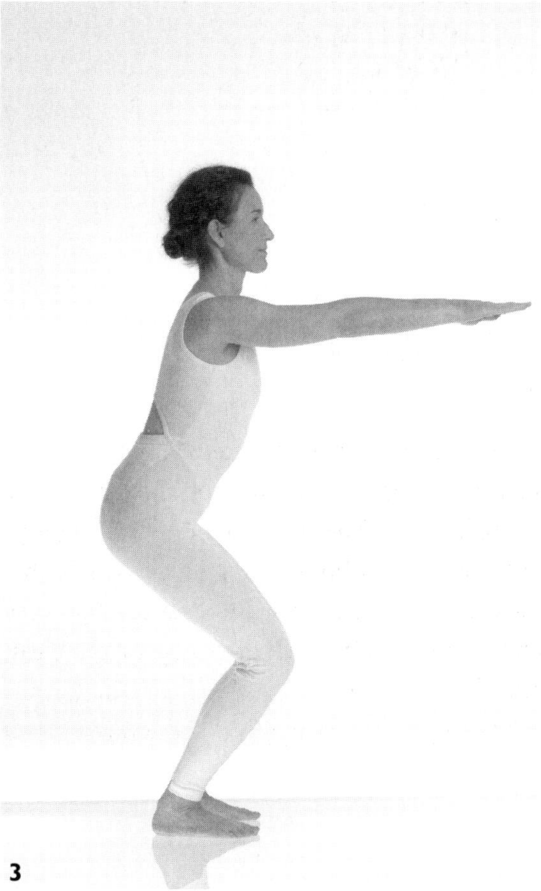

3

4. Continue to lower the buttocks, coming deeply into a squatting posture. Let the weight shift onto the heels, pressing the fingertips forward to find a point of dynamic balance without rounding the shoulders forward. The tailbone reaches out behind you and the back has a slight arch. Work to bring the thighs parallel to the floor.

5. Breathe deeply as you hold the posture, pressing into the feet, lifting the crown, and pressing the fingertips away.

6. To release, inhale and press into the feet, slowly straightening the legs and gradually coming back to standing. Lower the arms to the sides and let the breath flow freely in and out.

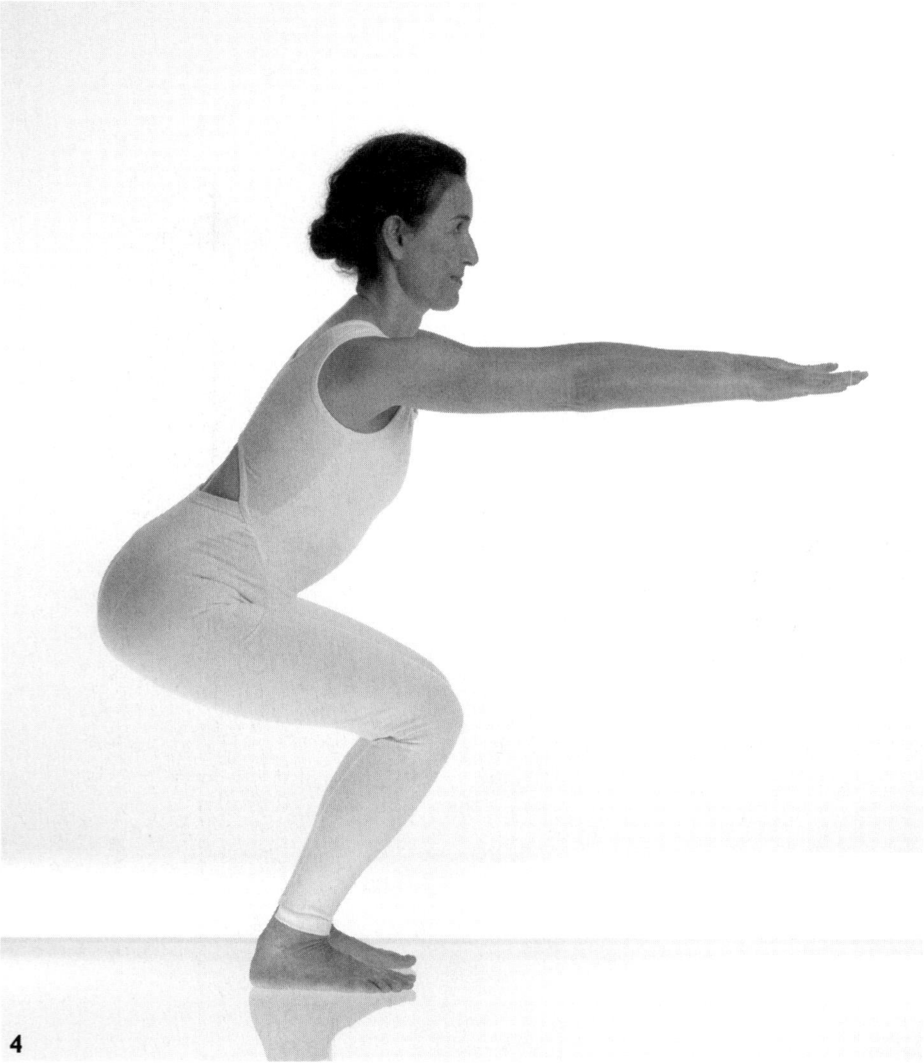

4

Be Aware:

Standing Squat strengthens the lower body and arms and stretches the low back.

Move into the posture slowly to allow the body to adjust to the work required of the legs, buttocks, abdomen, and arms. Moving slowly helps stretch and strengthen a broader range of muscles and connective tissues.

If you want less challenge, come into the partial expression of the posture described in step 3. With regular practice the legs will gain strength and your squat will deepen. If you want more challenge, come slowly into the full expression of the posture while breathing deeply. Hold the posture to the healthy limit of your endurance, and release in slow motion.

STANDING RUNNER'S STRETCH

(Parshvottanasana)

1. Stand in Mountain Pose. Bring the hands to the hips.

2. Take a step forward with the left foot, keeping hip distance between the feet by stepping the foot directly forward from the hip. Angle the right foot slightly out so the heel rests comfortably on the floor. Depending on your height, the feet will be between twenty-four and thirty inches apart.

3. Square the hips, bringing the right hip forward and the left hip back, so both hips face forward.

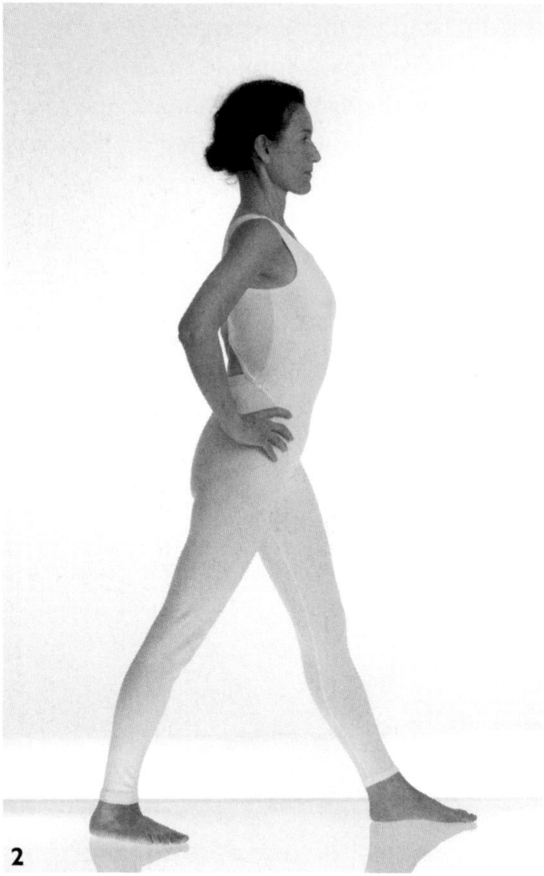

2

4. Press into the feet to engage the muscles of the legs, while avoiding the tendency to lock the front knee. Stabilize the core of the body by pressing the tailbone down, leveling the pelvis, and gently contracting the muscles of the pelvic floor. Elongate the spine by lifting out of the waist and extending through the crown of the head.

5. Take a deep breath in. As you exhale, lift the tailbone and hinge forward from the hips. Press the front foot firmly into the floor, slightly bending the front knee if necessary to avoid strain. Come forward with a straight spine until the torso is parallel to the floor. Pause here for a moment, letting the gaze rest on the floor, and extending through the crown to elongate the spine and neck. Let the breath flow freely in and out.

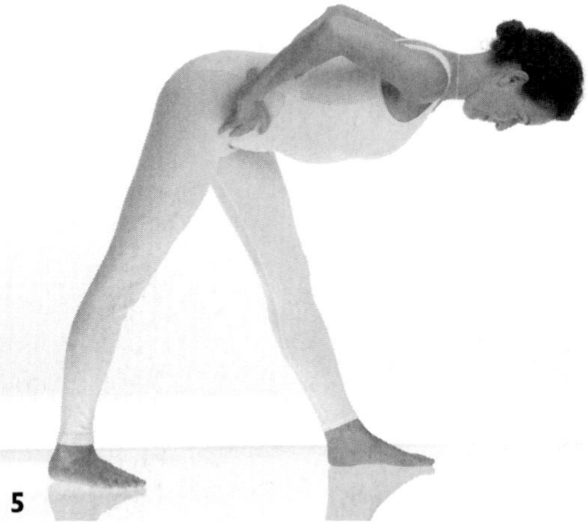

5

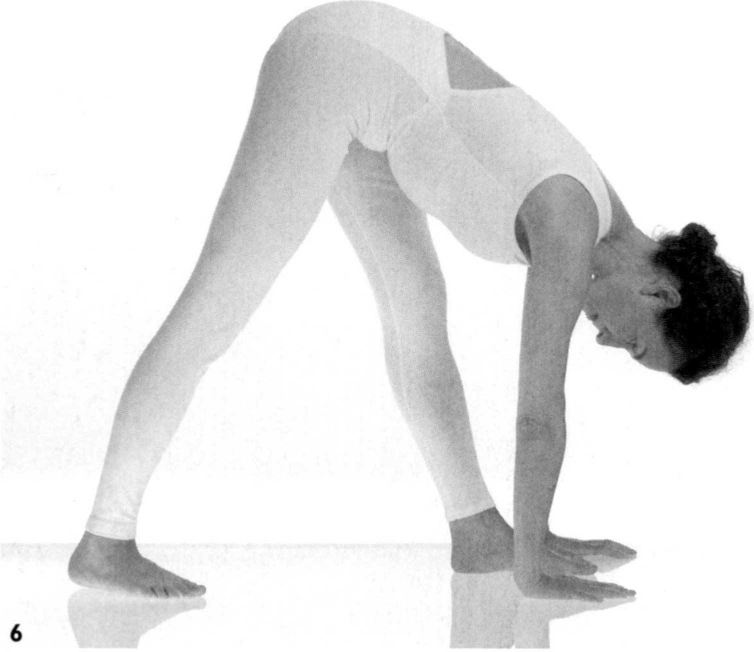

6

6. Continue to hinge at the hips and come forward, reaching the fingertips down to rest on the shin, foot, or floor. Extend the crown of the head toward the floor in front of you. If your hands are on the floor, press gently into the palms or fingertips to enhance the stretch.

7. Breathe deeply as you hold.

8. To release, bring the hands onto the foot or leg. Inhale and press into the feet, engaging the hips to come up with a straight spine and sliding the hands up the leg.

9. Step the left foot back to the starting position. Receive the posture, feeling the effects and taking several long flowing breaths.

10. Step the right foot forward and repeat on the opposite side.

Be Aware:

Standing Runner's Stretch deeply stretches the hamstrings. If you want less challenge, keep the hands on the hips and just do steps 1–5. Placing two cushions or blocks on either side of the front foot is a nice intermediate step toward the full posture.

If you want more challenge, you can explore several hand and arm variations. You can bring the hands behind the back, resting the back of the hands on the sacrum. This heightens the sensation of lifting the tailbone to hinge forward from the hips. You can also grasp opposite elbows or bring the palms behind the mid-back in Reverse Prayer Position. As you stretch forward, you can choose to either keep the hands behind the back or release them to the floor.

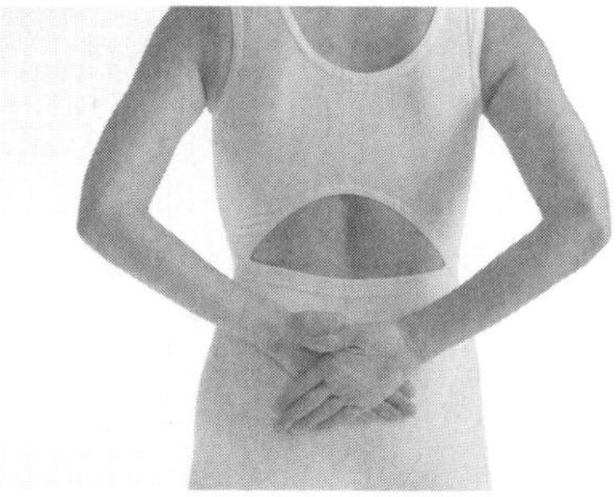

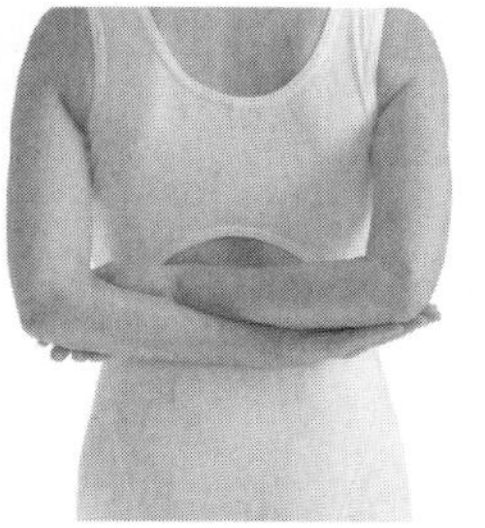

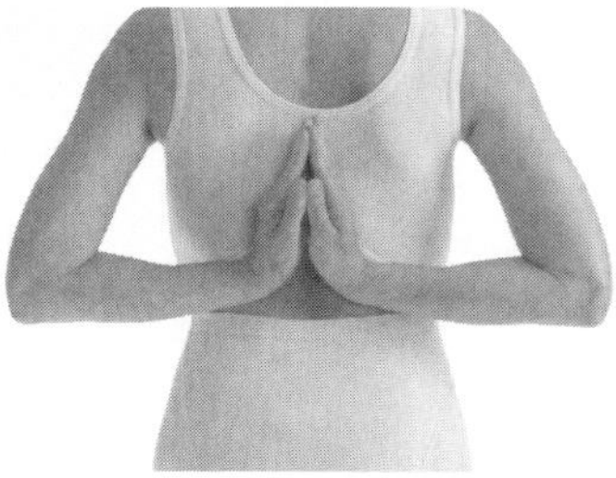

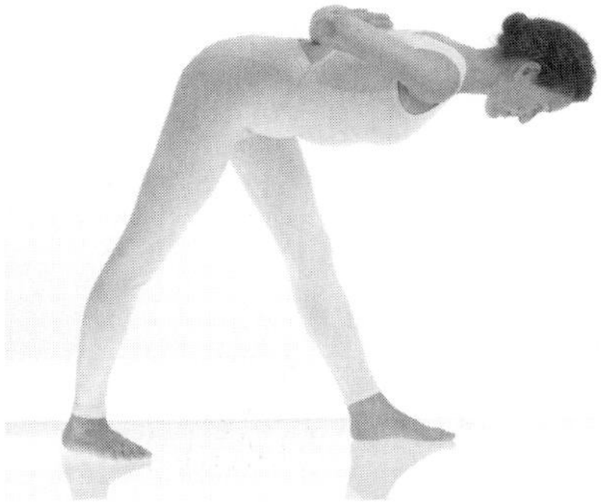

SIDE WARRIOR

(Virabhadrasana)

1. Step the feet slightly wider apart than your legs are long. Turn the left foot out a full turn of ninety degrees, and turn the right foot in a quarter turn. Press into the feet to engage the muscles of the legs.

2. Stabilize the core of the body by pressing the tailbone down, leveling the pelvis, and gently contracting the muscles of the pelvic floor. Elongate the spine by lifting out of the waist, lifting the sternum and extending through the crown.

3. Inhale as you sweep the arms out to the sides and up to shoulder height. Press out through the fingertips to open the chest.

4. Exhale as you slowly bend the left knee, letting the torso sink while keeping the hips and shoulders facing forward. The left thigh moves toward parallel as the left knee comes over the left ankle. Resist any tendency to lean in the direction of the bent knee by pressing into the outside of the back foot, which keeps the weight equally distributed between the feet and also keeps the torso vertical.

5. Turn the head to the left, gazing over the center of the extended left hand. Keep the shoulders facing forward. Breathe deeply as you hold.

6. To release, inhale and slowly straighten the left leg.

7. Lower the arms, reverse the direction of the feet, and repeat on the opposite side.

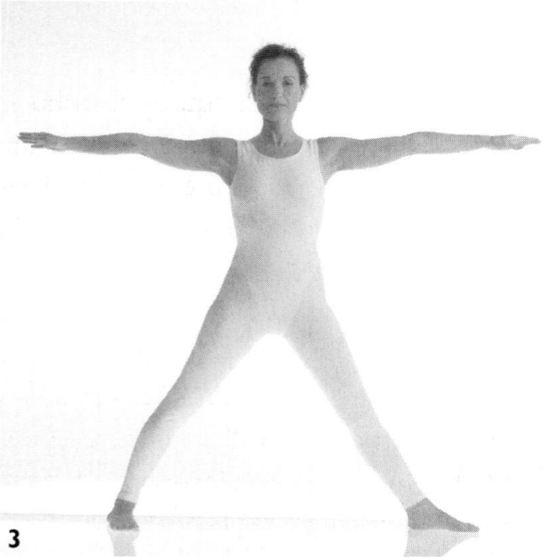
3

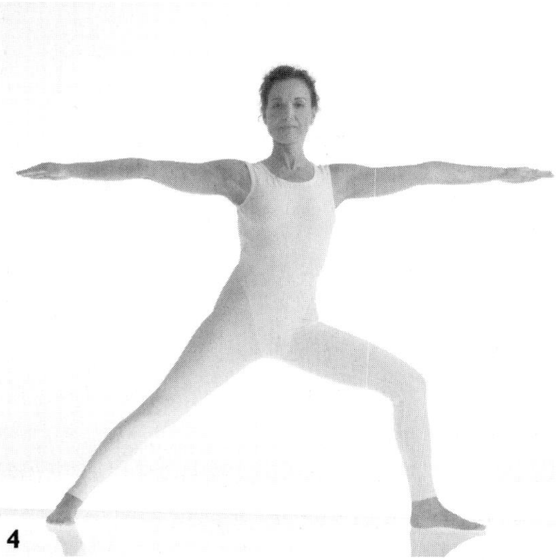
4

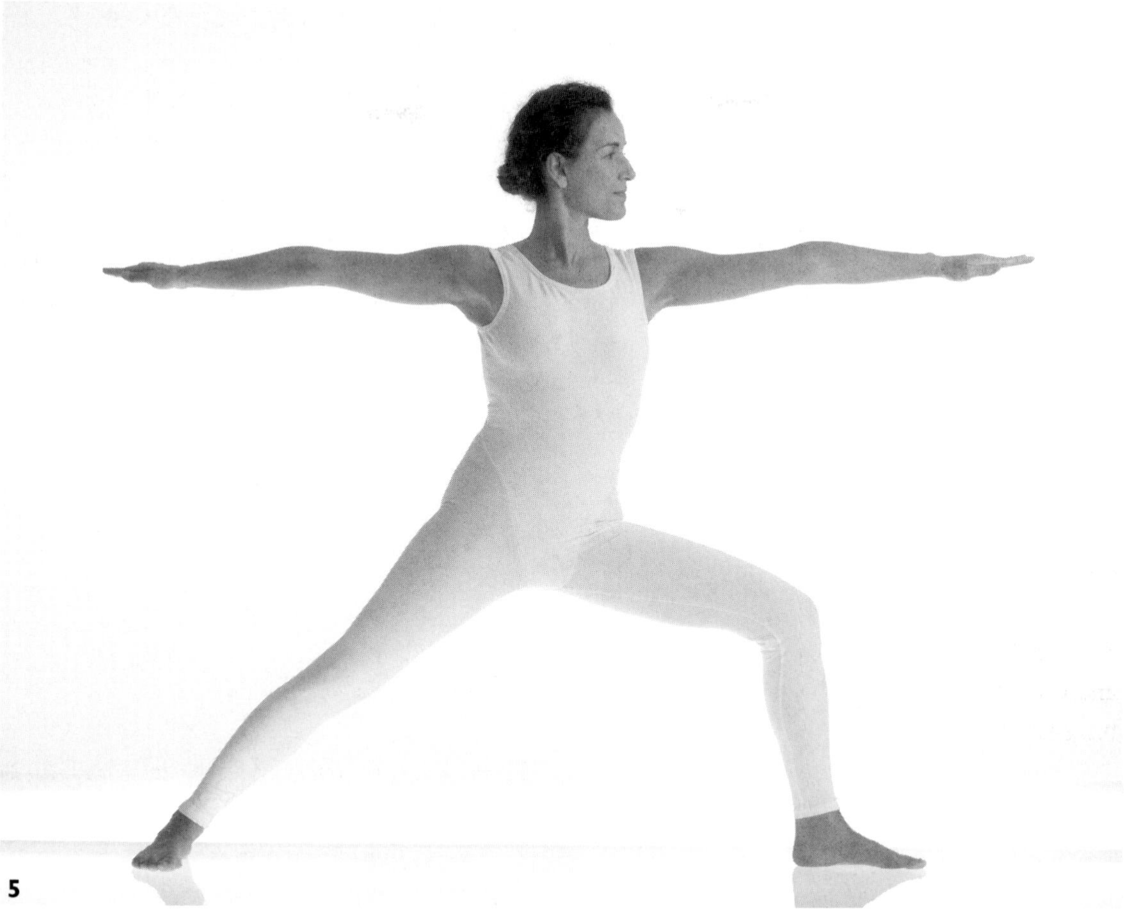

5

Be Aware:

Side Warrior strengthens the legs and opens the hip joints and groin. Do not extend the knee beyond the ankle, as this position can stress the knee joint. If your knee needs to move beyond the ankle in order for the thigh to reach parallel, either slide the feet a little farther apart or come out of the posture and take a wider stance.

When learning this posture, it is common to lean the torso in the direction of the bent knee. By pressing into the outside of the back foot, you keep the weight equally distributed between the feet and the torso vertical. The bent knee tends to collapse inward. Keep the knee pointing in the same direction as the foot.

If you want less challenge, do not bring the front knee over the ankle or thigh parallel to the ground, coming into a partial expression of the posture. Your legs will gain strength and your Side Warrior will deepen over time. If you want more challenge, explore the Bent Knee Side Stretch or Lateral Angle.

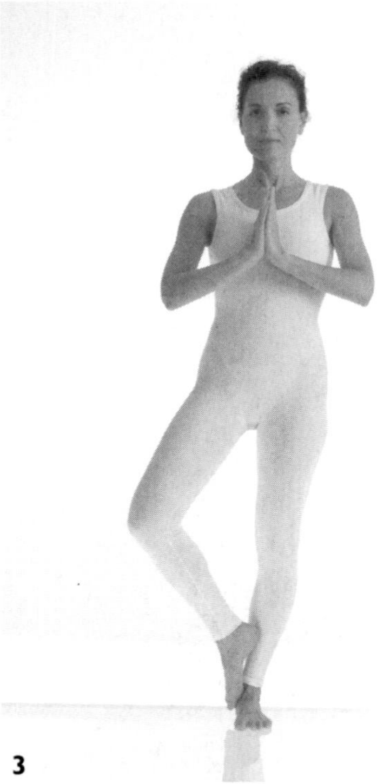

3

TREE

(Vrikshasana)

1. Stand in Mountain Pose.

2. Shift the weight onto the left foot, keeping it pressed firmly into the floor without locking the knee. Bring your gaze to rest at a point on the floor about ten feet in front of you to enhance your balance.

3. Lift the right foot, bringing the sole of the foot to rest on the ankle, calf, or inner thigh of the standing left leg. You can also place the right foot on the top of the left thigh in Lotus Pose. Never position the lifted foot on the in-

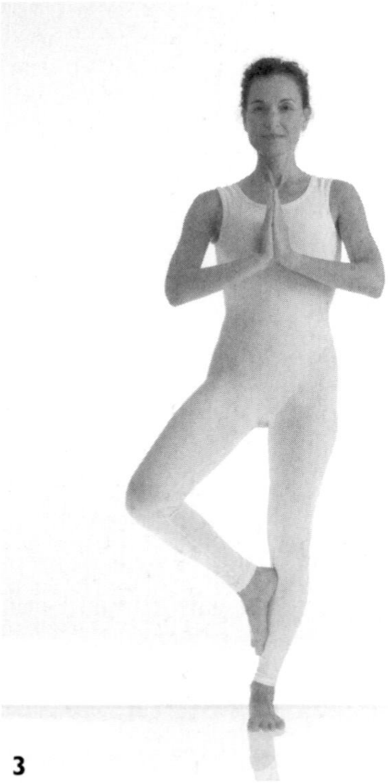

3

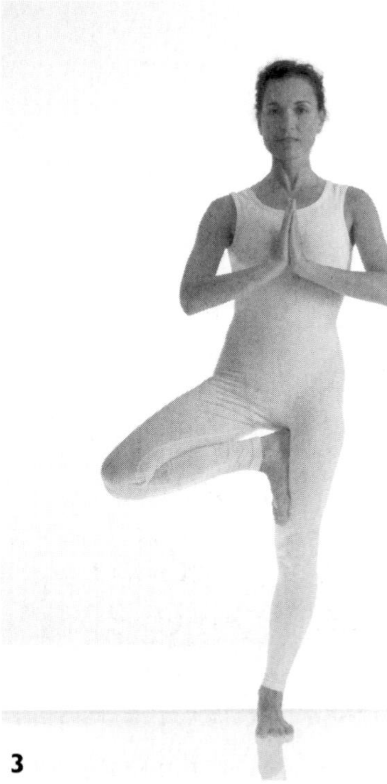

3

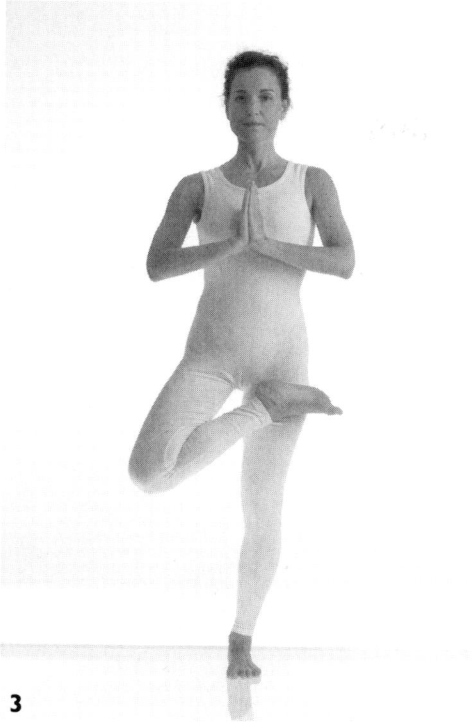

3

side of the knee, which exerts a lateral pressure on the joint. Use your hands as needed to assist in positioning the foot, then bring them into Prayer Position.

4. Work to fully engage the thigh muscle of the standing left leg. Adjust the hips so they face forward and are level. Press gently down and back on the right knee. Hold this position for several flowing breaths to establish your balance.

5. Inhale and sweep the arms out to the sides and overhead, bringing the palms together or interlacing the fingers and extending the index fingers in Steeple Position. The elbows and arms are straight, upper arms framing the ears.

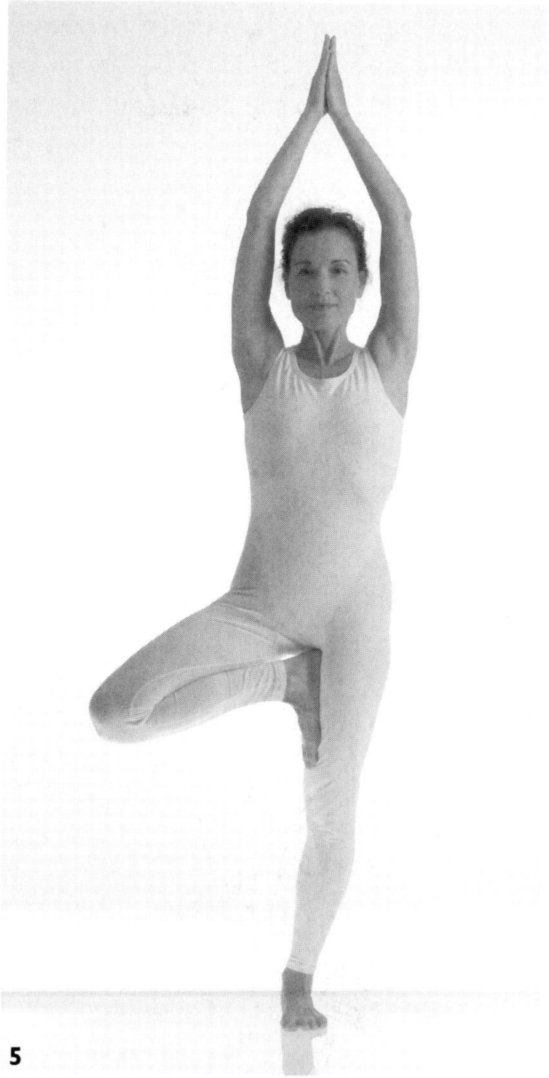

5

6. Press up through the fingertips to elongate the spine. Exhale and let the top of the shoulders drop and shoulder blades move down and back. While keeping the arms straight, relax the shoulders, upper back, and neck. Breathe deeply as you hold.

7. To release, take a deep breath in. Exhale and slowly lower the hands back down into Prayer Position. Take another deep breath in, and as you exhale release the leg back down to the ground and the hands to the sides.

8. Integrate the posture, feeling the effects and taking several long flowing breaths.

9. Repeat on the other side.

Be Aware:

The Tree brings both body and mind into balance. While learning to balance, you will have many opportunities to practice self-acceptance. As you become able to hold the posture, the body will become still and the mind peaceful.

Multiple factors work together to allow you to remain balanced on one leg. The first is focusing the gaze on a point. The second is working to keep the standing leg straight and thigh muscle contracted. The third is the position of the lifted knee, which in all variations presses gently down and back. The last is the elongation of the spine, which begins with the leveling of the pelvis and continues to the pressing of the fingertips to the ceiling. When all these come together, balance results.

SINGLE LEG LIFTS

(Pavana Muktasana)

1. Lie on your back with the legs extended. Reach the arms overhead on the floor, palms up. Wriggle from side to side, stretching the arms overhead and walking the shoulder blades up to elongate the spine, shoulders, and arms. Then flex both feet and press away one heel, and then the other, moving from side to side and lengthening the sacrum, hips, and legs. Stretch your body to its full length using the support of the floor.

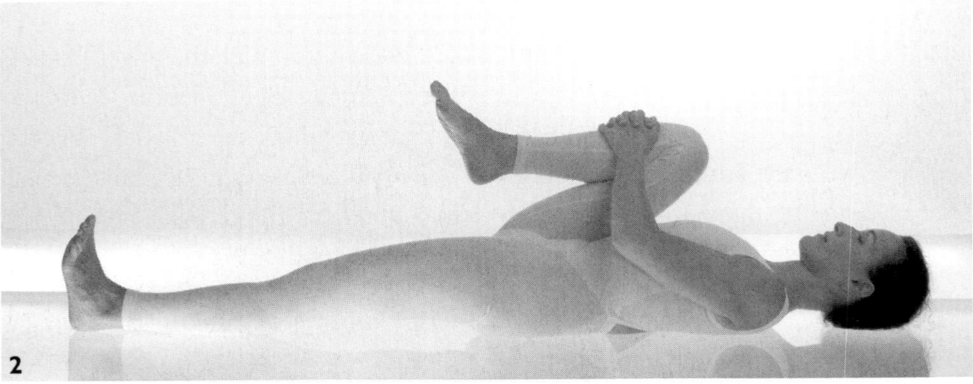

2

2. Draw the right knee up and toward the right side of the chest. Interlace the fingers just below the knee. Using your hand and forearm strength, exhale and draw the knee firmly into the right side of the chest, feeling the massage to the right side of the abdomen. Breathe deeply as you hold for five or more breaths, letting the entire body and especially the right hip joint relax as much as possible.

3. Inhale and lift the left leg, raising the foot toward the ceiling. Pause with the foot lifted. Rotate the ankle joint and foot several times in one direction, and then the other. Then point and flex the foot, squeezing the toes into a tight "fist" as you point, and opening them wide as you flex.

4. Take a deep breath in. As you exhale, lower the left leg toward the floor, stopping at hip height. Inhale and again lift it toward the ceiling. Repeat this Single Leg Lift several times, coordinating breath and movement. End by lowering the left leg to the floor, and taking a deep breath in. As you exhale, release the right knee and extend the leg out onto the floor.

5. Draw the left knee up and toward the left side of the chest, interlace the fingers just below the knee, and repeat steps 2–5 on the opposite side.

6. Draw both knees up into the chest and bring them close together. Wrap the arms around the knees, grasping the elbows if possible, or the forearms or wrists. Elongate the neck by slightly tucking the chin, then pressing the back of the head into the floor, and extending through the crown. Press the sacrum toward the floor to stabilize the low back. Using your hand and forearm strength, draw both knees firmly into the chest, feeling the stretch to the low back and massage to the abdomen. Keep the sacrum pressed into the floor. Breathe deeply as you hold for five or more breaths.

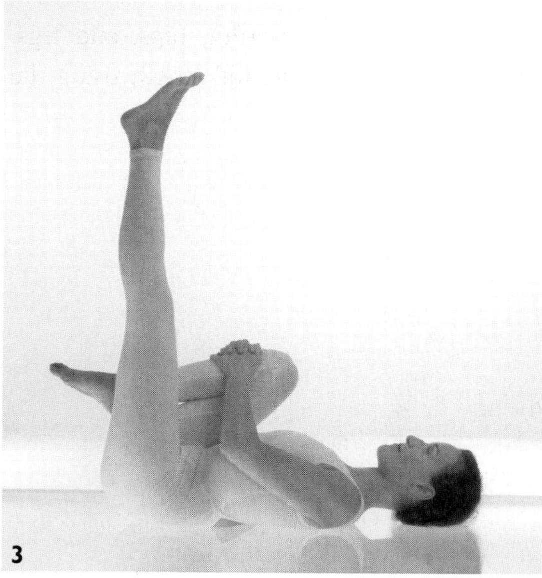
3

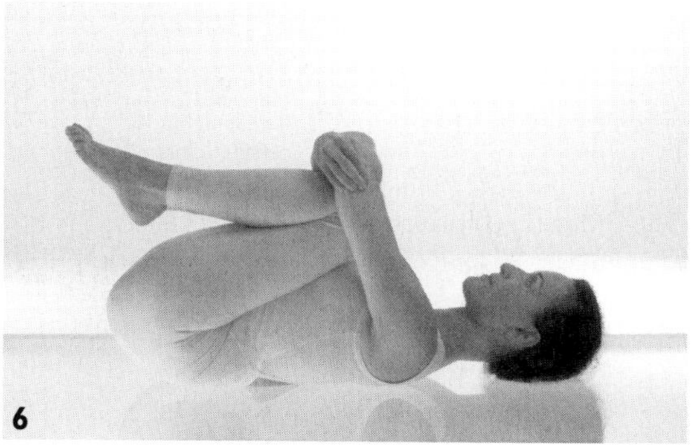
6

7. Release the knees and extend the legs, coming into Corpse. Close the eyes and notice if you feel energy moving in your body.

Be Aware:
Single Leg Lifts are a safe and effective core strengthener. Work to keep the low back and iliac crest resting solidly on the floor as the leg lifts and lowers. Do not allow the low back to tip, buckle, or otherwise become unstable. To accomplish this, you may need to limit your range of motion, especially in the first few repetitions, by not bringing the leg down to hip height. If you want more challenge, slow the motion down and move with the breath, which enhances the strengthening. This version of Single Leg Lifts incorporates the Wind Relieving Series, a basic abdominal massage routine that helps maintain digestive health.

HALF SHOULDERSTAND

(Ardha Sarvangasana)

1. Lie on the back with legs extended, arms at the sides, palms down. Rock the head gently from side to side to relax the muscles of the neck. Bring the head back to center, and elongate the neck by slightly tucking the chin. Relax the chin tuck and rest the back of the head solidly on the floor.

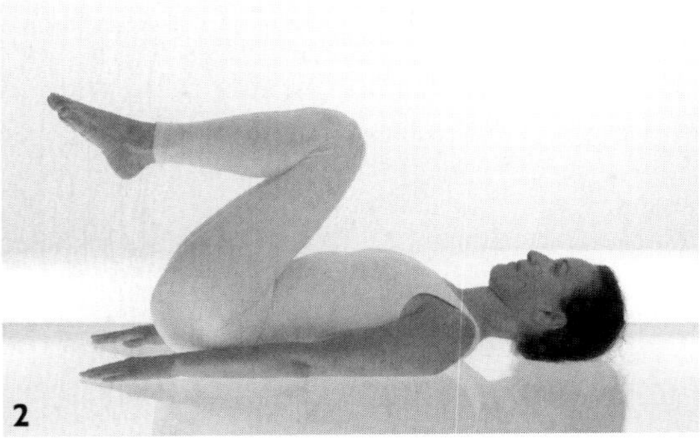
2

2. Draw both knees into the chest. Press down through the fingertips to lengthen the arms, and bring the elbows to rest against the sides of the body.

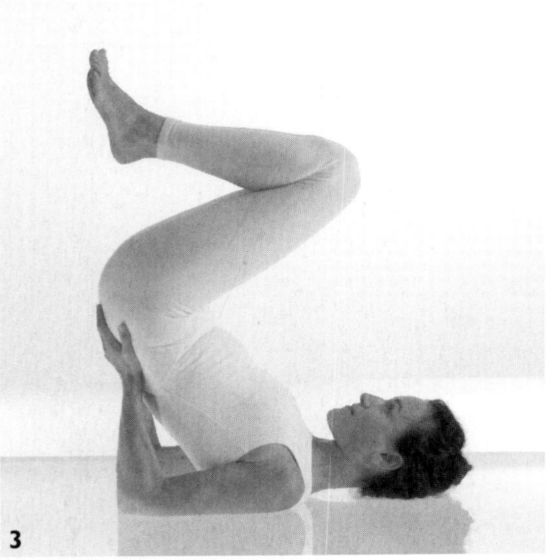
3

3. Press the elbows into the floor to keep them from spreading apart, and gently roll the hips up, bringing the hands to the hips. Adjust the position of the hands so they are either holding

the hip bones or spread out across the low back. The majority of your body weight should be supported by the elbows, with a little resting on the shoulders. If there is more than nominal weight on the back of the neck, come down and try again, keeping the elbows pressed into the floor and closer together. Take a few breaths as your body adjusts to being upside down.

4. Slowly extend the legs. Touch the big toes together, letting the heels fall apart. Find a comfortable position in which you can relax and hold. The angle between the legs and torso varies from person to person. For some, bringing the shins or knees directly over the eyes results in a balanced posture. For others, the toes are directly above the eyes. Whatever your leg and torso position, your body weight comfortably rests on the elbows and shoulders and you can breathe deeply as you hold.

5. Hold the posture with deep, flowing breathing. Slow motion movement with the legs makes it considerably easier to hold. Let one leg fall a little forward, and the other fall a little back. Reverse leg position and explore the stretches that result. Then slowly rotate both legs out to the sides and into a split. Staying in slow motion, explore the full range of motion in the hips and legs.

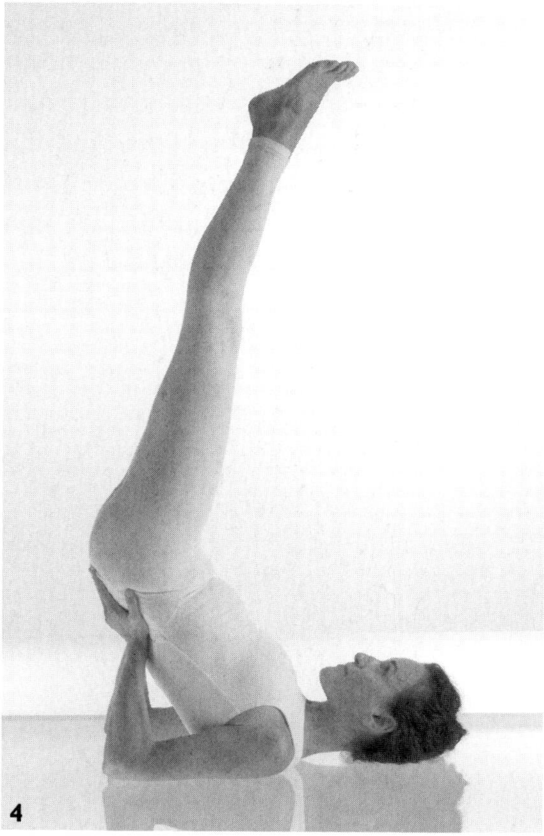
4

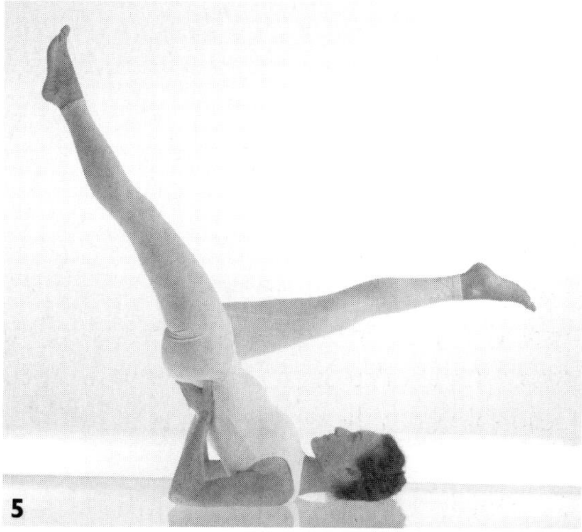
5

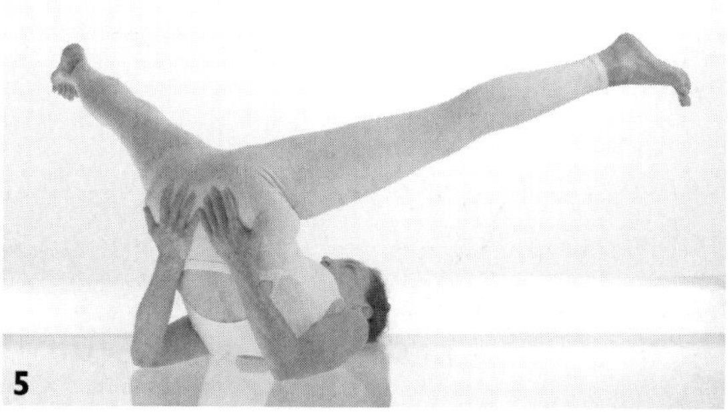
5

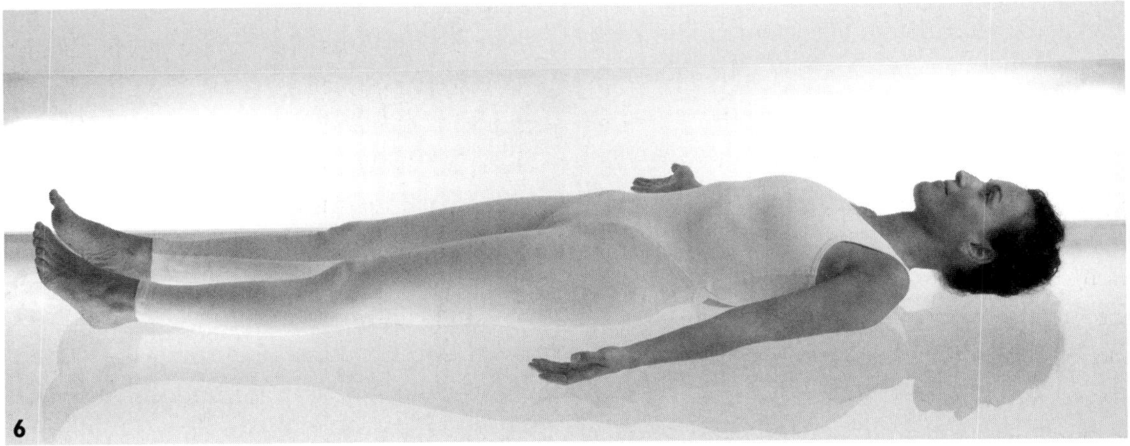
6

6. To release, bring the feet overhead, big toes touching. Take a deep breath in. As you exhale, slowly lower the knees into the chest. Then let the hands slide from the hips or low back across the buttocks as you gently roll down and out of the posture, bringing the low back onto the floor one vertebra at a time. Extend the legs into Corpse.

7. Rock the chin from side to side once or twice to release any neck tension that may have arisen. Close the eyes and don't miss a sensation as your body rebalances.

Be Aware:

Half Shoulderstand is a safe inversion that provides many health benefits. Being upside down reverses the pull of gravity on the body, encouraging blood to flow out of the legs and into the torso and head. All the organs and glands are turned upside down and gently stimulated. Half Shoulderstand is also said to stimulate and balance the function of the thyroid and parathyroid glands critical to health. Traditional guidance suggests Half Shoulderstand is not to be practiced during menstruation.

If your body is heavy, it may not be advisable for you to bear its full weight on the elbows, upper arms, and shoulders. If you find this posture challenging, substitute Dead Bug Pose or Shoulderstand Modifications. Do not practice Half Shoulderstand if you have unmedicated high blood pressure, glaucoma, detached retina, or other eye problems.

Gradually work up to holding for three minutes with deep breathing. Learning how to come into slow motion variations with the legs makes holding the posture more enjoyable. It also allows you to deeply stretch and release tension from the hips while they are not bearing weight. If you want more challenge, explore Three-Quarters Shoulderstand and Fish.

SPHINX

1. Lie on your belly with the forehead on the floor. Reach the arms overhead, palms down. Wriggle from side to side, stretching the arms overhead and walking the rib cage forward to elongate the spine. Then lift one leg and then the other, pressing the toes away to lengthen the legs and open the hip joints. Stretch your body to its full length using the support of the floor.

2. Bring the arms parallel and shoulder-width apart, hands resting palms down on the floor. Bring the legs and feet hip-width apart. Exhale fully.

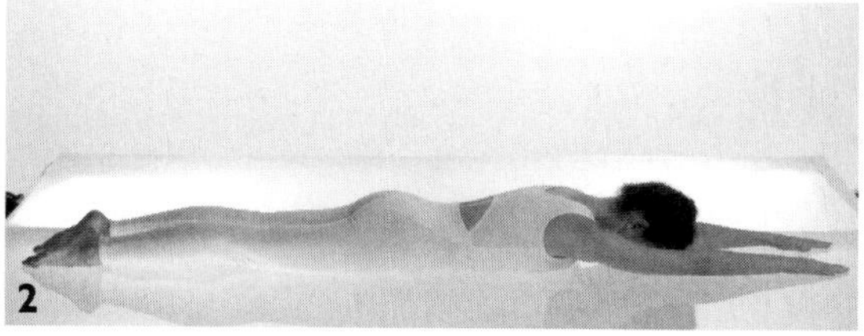
2

3. Inhale and press the pubic bone, hip bones, and lower abdomen into the floor, stabilizing the core of the body. Use the press as a base to lift the head and then the torso by engaging the back muscles. As the torso lifts, slide the elbows back under the shoulders and close to the ribs. The navel, lower abdomen, legs, and top of the feet remain on the floor.

4. Elongate the spine by pressing the pubic bone, hip bones, and elbows down to lift out of the waist. Keep the back of the neck long by slightly tucking the chin and extending through the crown. Press the sternum forward and roll the shoulders back and down. The backward bend of the spine should be a smooth curve, without any sharp bends in the low back or neck. Breathe deeply as you hold.

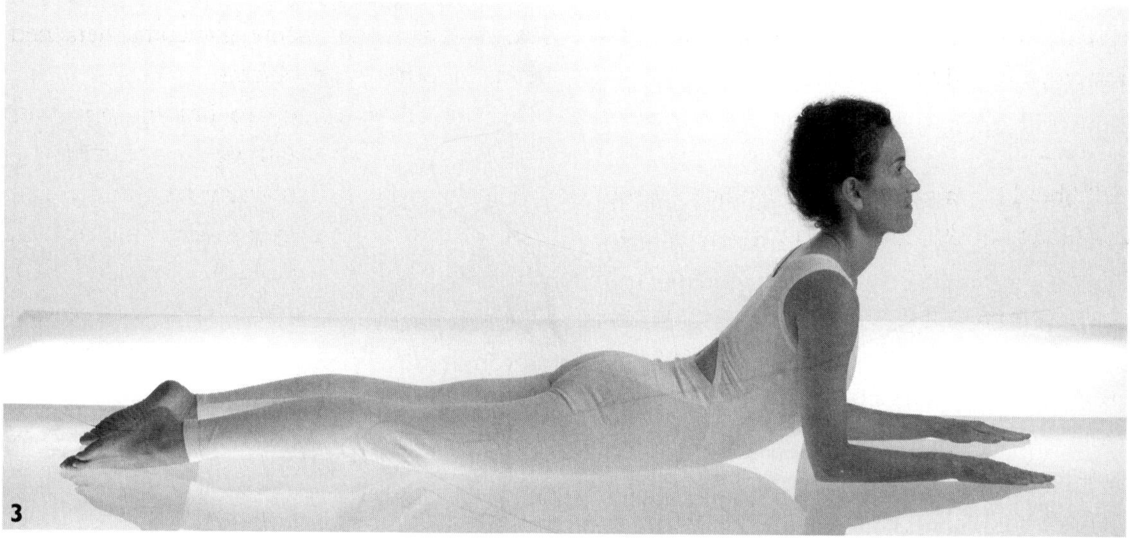
3

5. To release, exhale and slide the hands forward to the starting position, slowly lowering the torso and head. Turn your head to one side and overlap the fingers to form a small pillow under the temple. Bend the legs at the knees and bring the heels toward the buttocks. Release any tension that may have built up by gently waving or circling the feet, feeling the sensation of release in the sacrum and low back.

Be Aware:
The Sphinx is a variation of the Cobra that utilizes the elbows to elongate the spine and stretch the chest. If you are not able to slide the elbows close to the ribs, pause and walk them the last few inches.

By restricting the movement of the diaphragm, the Sphinx makes you breathe in and out of the upper chest. At first, practice the Sphinx and other belly down postures with the feet hip-width apart. These postures were traditionally taught with the legs together and feet touching. Once you become comfortable with the basic posture, experiment to see what leg and foot position works for your body.

BOAT

(Navasana)

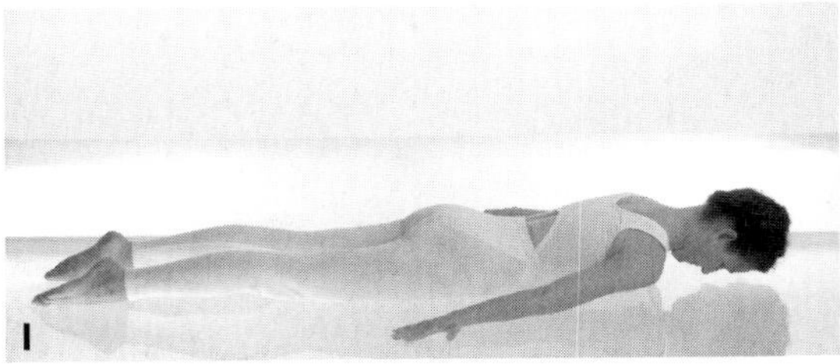

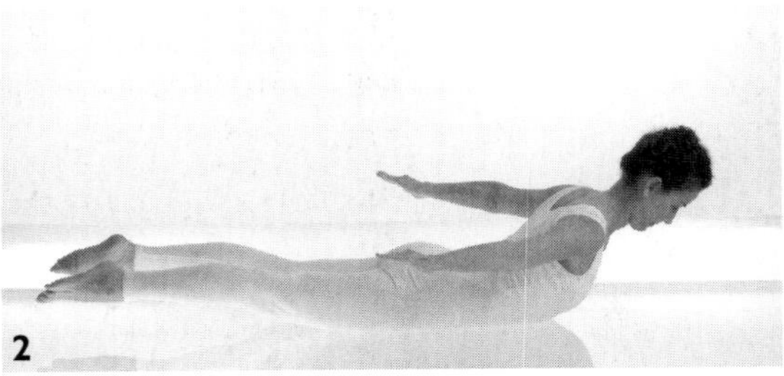

1. Lie on your belly with the forehead on the floor. Stretch the arms out to the sides at a forty-five-degree angle like airplane wings, hands resting palms down on the floor. Bring the feet hip-width apart. Exhale fully.

2. As you inhale, press the pubic bone, hip bones, and lower abdomen into the floor to stabilize the core of the body. Use the press as a base to lift the head, upper torso, legs, and arms. Only the pubic bone, hip bones, and abdomen remain on the floor.

3. Press the toes back and heels up to raise the legs a little higher. Press the fingertips back to help lift the shoulders, back, and torso. Extend through the crown to keep the spine elongated and lift the back of the head toward the ceiling. The backward bend of the spine should be a smooth curve, without any sharp bends in the low back or neck.

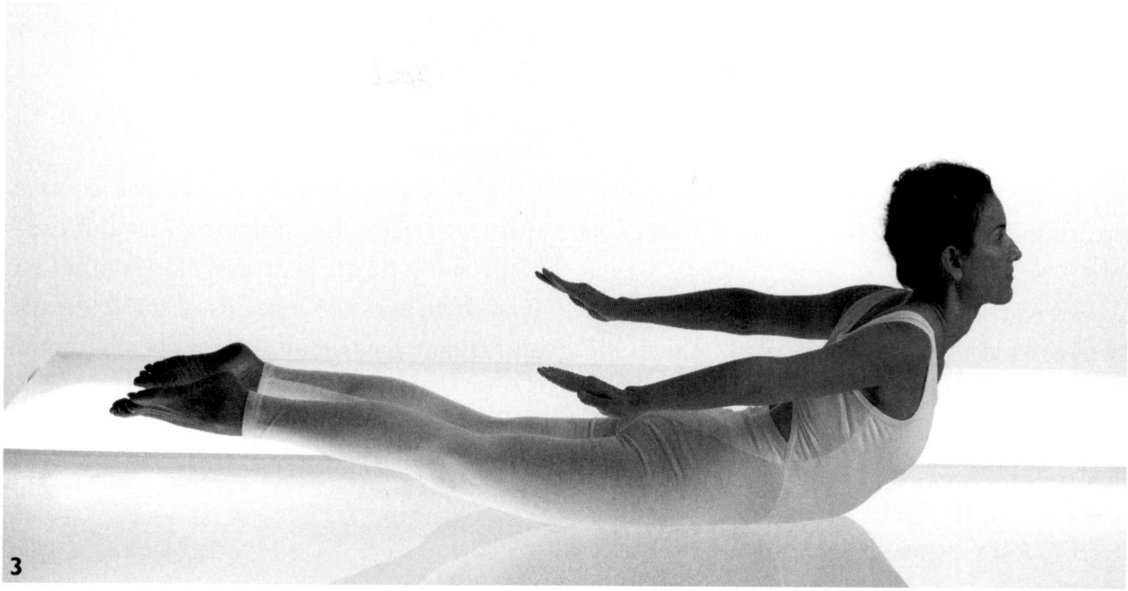

3

4. Breathe deeply as you hold.

5. To release, exhale and let the forehead, torso, legs, and arms slowly return to the floor. Turn your head to one side and overlap the fingers to form a small pillow under the temple. Bend the legs at the knees and bring the heels toward the buttocks. Release any tension that may have built up by gently waving or circling the feet, feeling the sensation of release in the sacrum and low back.

6. Receive the posture, taking several long flowing breaths and feeling the effects.

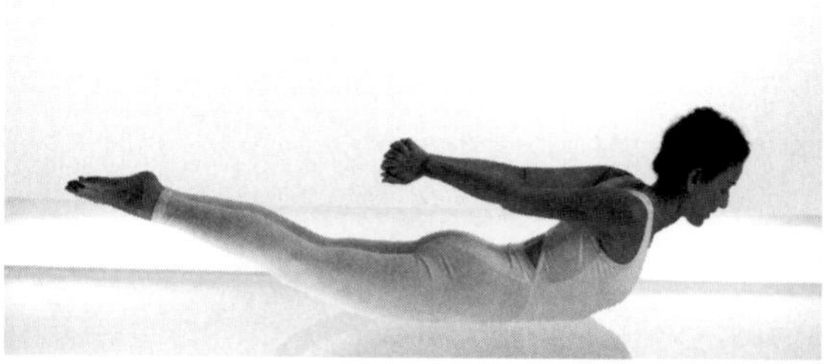

Be Aware:

The Boat strengthens the major muscles of the back, while massaging the abdominal organs, kidneys, and adrenals. If you want less challenge, lift only the torso and legs, keeping the arms on the floor. If you want more challenge, try this variation. Come into the posture as described above. Then reach the arms around behind the back, interlacing the fingers. Press the knuckles behind you, drawing the shoulder blades down and wing points together. Press the sternum forward to open the chest. Breathe deeply as you hold.

CHILD

(Garbhasana)

1. Come into Table Pose. Take a deep breath in.

2. As you exhale, slide the hips and buttocks back toward the heels. The palms remain on the floor and the arms overhead. Let the torso extend over the thighs, the buttocks sit on the heels, and the forehead rests on the floor.

3. Bring the arms down to the sides, hands palms up.

4. Relax and let the breath flow freely as you hold for a minute or more.

5. To release, bring the hands under the shoulders and press up into Table.

Be Aware:

Child is a resting pose and a nice complementary stretch for all backbends and especially belly down postures like Sphinx and Boat. It relaxes the muscles of the low back, and encourages blood flow to the abdominal

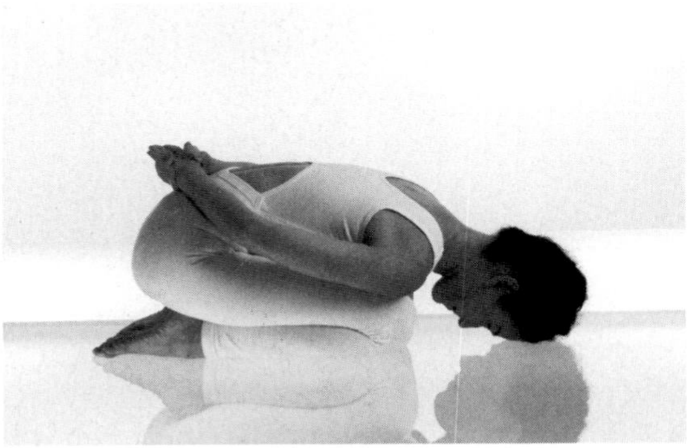

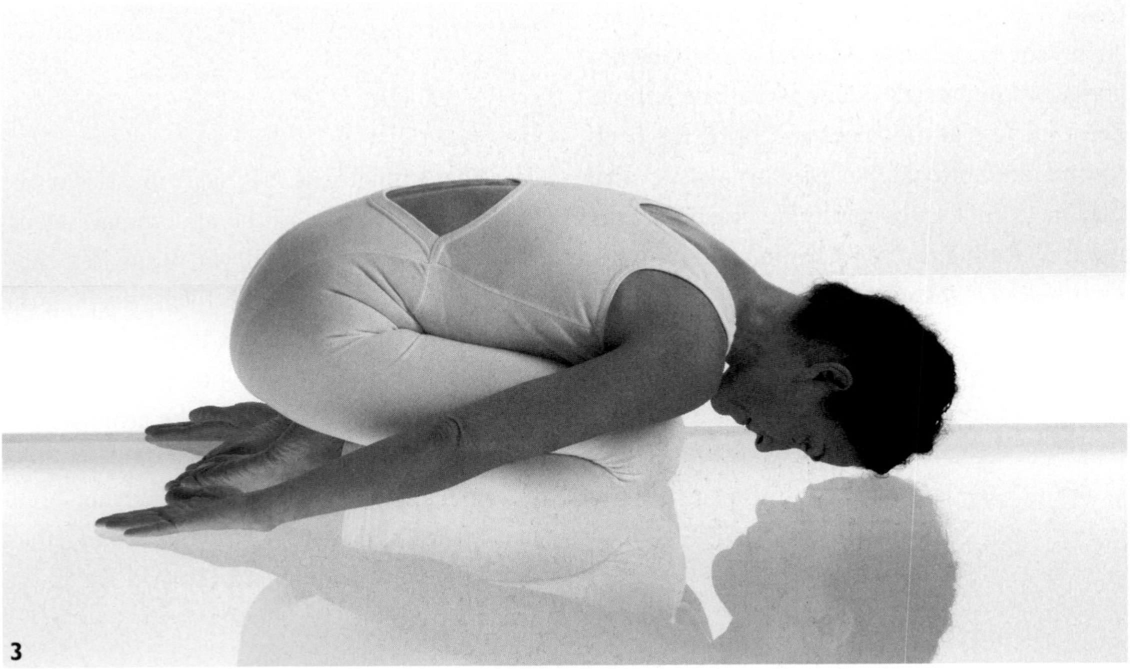

3

organs, kidneys, and adrenal glands. Remain in Child Pose for a minute or more to drink in its benefits.

If you find this posture easy, you can simply press the buttocks back into Child from Boat without going through Table. For more variety, come into Child as above and circle the arms behind your back, holding one wrist with the opposite hand.

POSTERIOR STRETCH

(Paschimottanasana)

1. Sit with the legs extended and feet together, hands resting on the floor in front of you. Press the heels away and slightly flex the feet to engage the muscles of the legs. Walk the sides of the buttocks back a few inches, rotating the pelvis forward. Press the sitz bones into the floor to create a stable base for your sitting posture. Gently contract the muscles of the pelvic floor. Elongate the spine by lifting out of the waist and extending through the crown.

2. Inhale as you sweep the arms out to the sides and overhead, palms facing. Extend through the fingertips to further elongate the spine. Exhale and relax the top of the shoulders down away from the ears. Allow the shoulder blades to move down and back.

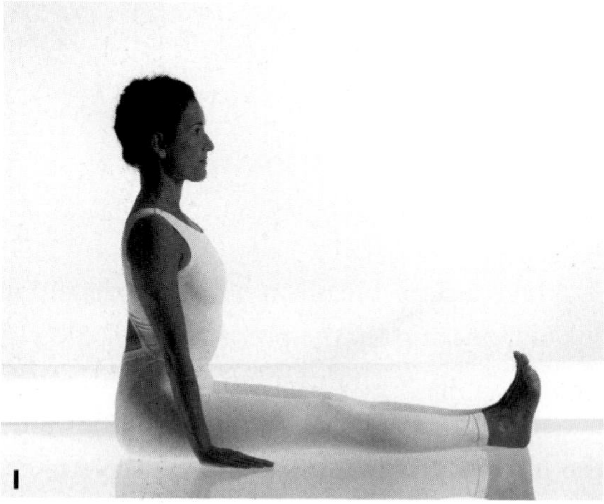

1

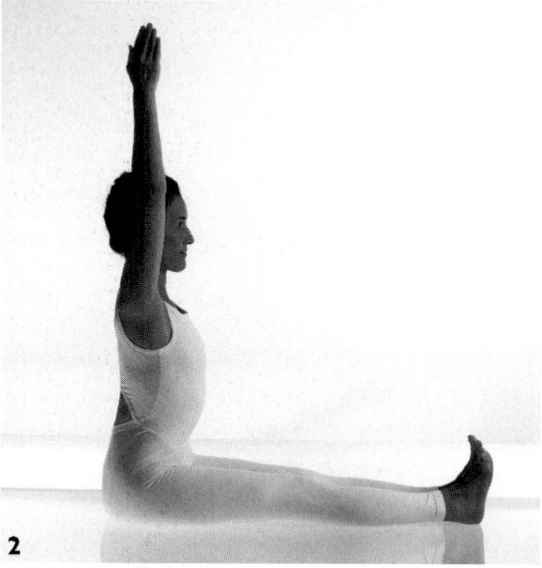

2

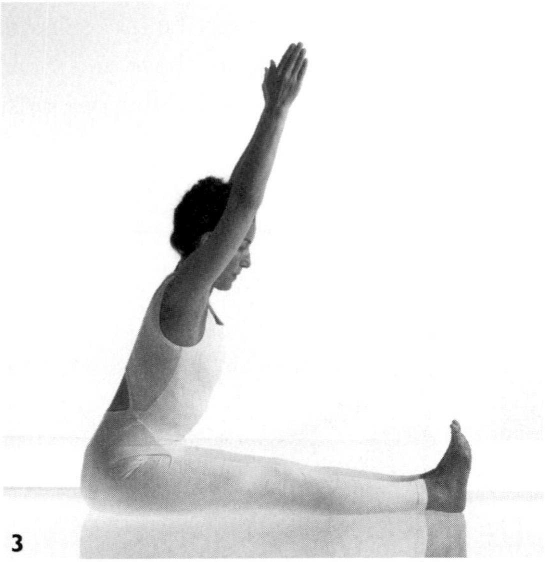

3

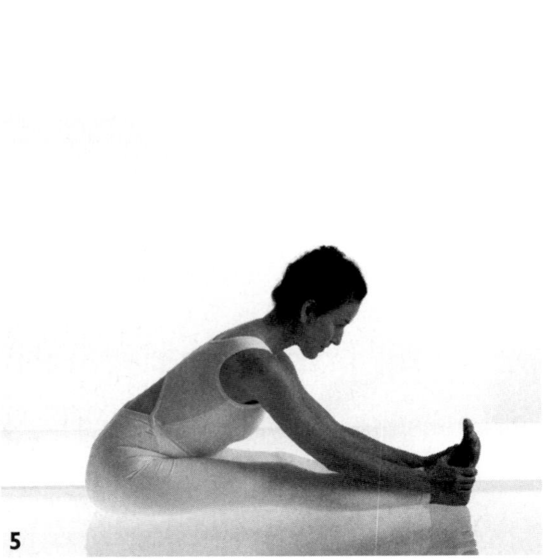

5

3. Take a deep breath in. As you exhale, lift the tailbone and tip the pelvis forward. Slowly hinge forward with the spine elongated, rotating the hip joints rather than rounding from the lumbar spine. You should feel the stretch in the back of the legs and hamstrings rather than the low back.

4. Come to your full forward extension with a straight spine. If your hamstrings or hips are tight, you may not come very far forward. Pause for a moment to let the breath flow and feel the legs stretch.

5. Allow the upper spine to gently round and lower the hands to rest on the legs or feet. Relax the back of the neck but continue to extend through the crown to keep the spine elongated.

6. If you want more stretch, you can use your hands to gently enhance the forward rotation of the hips, bringing the belly toward the upper thighs, the sternum toward the knees, and extending the crown toward the toes. Do not use excessive hand strength to round the spine forward from the waist and low back. Breathe deeply as you hold, emphasizing a long exhalation in which residual air is actively squeezed out of the lungs by a gentle contraction of the abdominal muscles.

7. To release, bring the hands to rest palms down on either side of the legs. Rotate the hip joints to bring the torso back to vertical. As you come up, do not raise the arms overhead. Allow the hands to slide along the floor and come to rest by the hips. Integrate the posture, feeling the effects and taking several long flowing breaths.

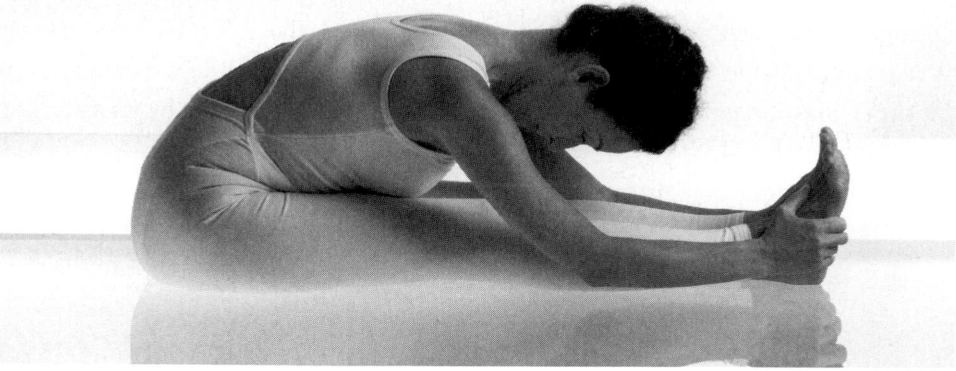

6

Be Aware:

As in Great Seal, coming down with the arms overhead can strain the low back. Another way to enter the posture is by lifting the arms overhead as described in step 2 to elongate the spine to its maximum length. Then bring the hands palms down on either side of the extended legs. Continue with the instructions, sliding the palms along the floor as you come forward with a straight spine. You can also place a cushion under the buttocks if your hamstrings are tight and you cannot come forward easily.

If you want more challenge, you can reengage the arms after holding and come out of the posture the same way you came into it. Reach the arms forward, pressing out through the fingertips to straighten the arms. Then rotate the hips to lift the torso and return the arms overhead. Press up through the fingertips to elongate the spine a final time, and sweep the arms back down to the sides.

Posterior Stretch is an excellent posture for holding. Come into the posture and hold for an extended period of time by relaxing and letting gravity do the work of stretching the body forward. Emphasize a long exhalation and notice how simply breathing in this way brings you more deeply into the posture.

INCLINED PLANE

(Purvottanasana)

1. Sit with the legs extended and feet together. Bring the arms behind you, placing the heels of the hands on the ground directly behind the hip joints, fingertips pointing away from the buttocks. The arms are straight, with the upper arms touching your sides.

2. Press the heels away and slightly flex the feet to engage the legs. Gently contract the muscles of the pelvic floor. Elongate the spine by lifting out of the waist and extending through the crown. Open the chest by pressing the sternum forward.

3. Touch the sides of the big toes together, and tuck the chin slightly into the chest. Inhale as you lift the hips by pressing down on the heels of the feet and hands, letting the torso straighten. Press the soles of the feet toward the floor. Maintain a slight chin tuck, extending through the crown to lengthen the neck. Lift the hips as high as you can without straining.

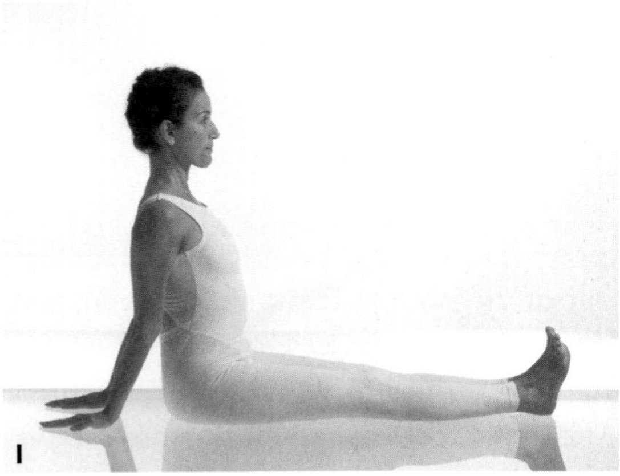
1

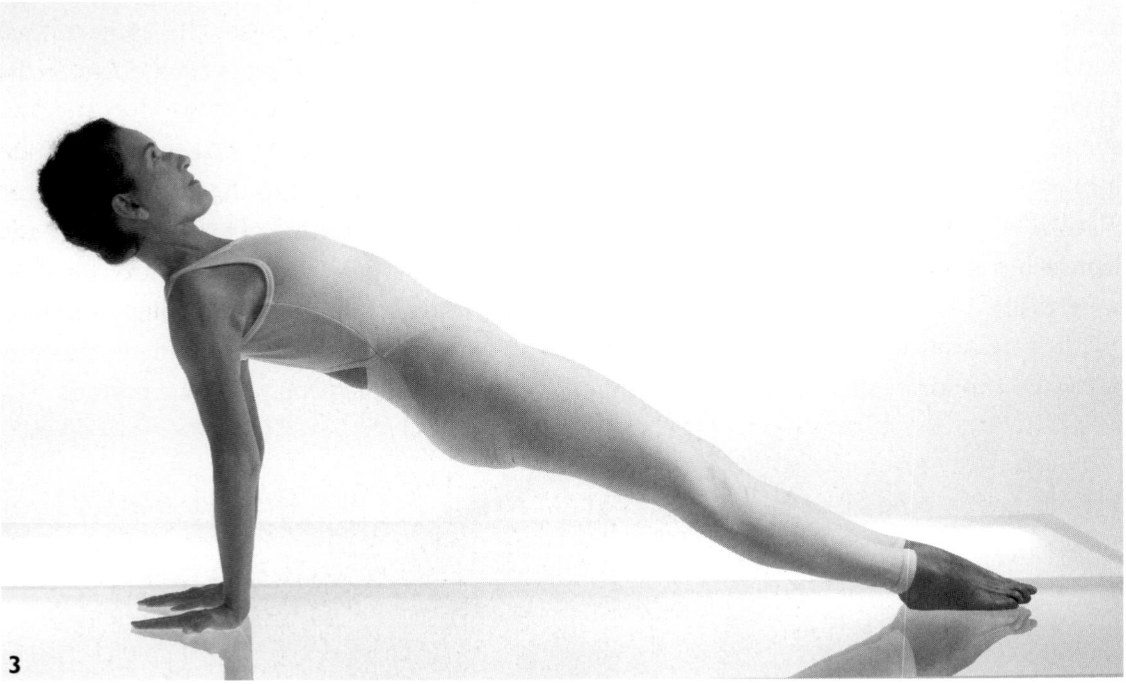
3

4. Breathe deeply as you hold.

5. To release, exhale and lower the hips down to the floor, then bring the torso back to vertical.

Be Aware:
Inclined Plane provides a needed complementary stretch after intensive forward bending. It is also a great core strengthener. If you experience discomfort in the hands or wrists, you can make the hands into fists and press the knuckles into the floor. You can also try the posture with the hand position reversed, fingers pointing toward the body. After coming out of the posture, release the wrist by grasping the opposite hand with the thumb and forefinger and squeezing between the wrist bone and the base of the hand. Then gently shake out the hands. This technique can be used for any postures in which the wrists bear significant weight.

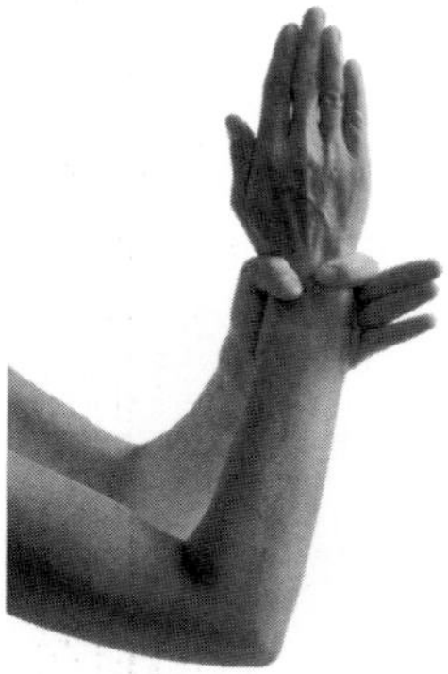

BRIDGE

(Setu Bandhasana)

1. Lie on your back with the legs extended. Reach the arms overhead on the floor, palms up. Wriggle from side to side, stretching the arms overhead and walking the shoulder blades up to elongate the spine, shoulders, and arms. Then flex both feet and press away one heel, and then the other, moving from side to side and lengthening the sacrum, hips, and legs. Stretch your body to its full length using the support of the floor.

2. Bring the arms to the sides, palms down. Bend the knees, bringing the feet close to the buttocks, feet and knees hip-width apart. Rock the head gently from side to side to relax the muscles of the neck. Bring the head back to center, and elongate the neck by slightly tucking the chin. Relax the chin tuck and rest the back of the head solidly on the floor.

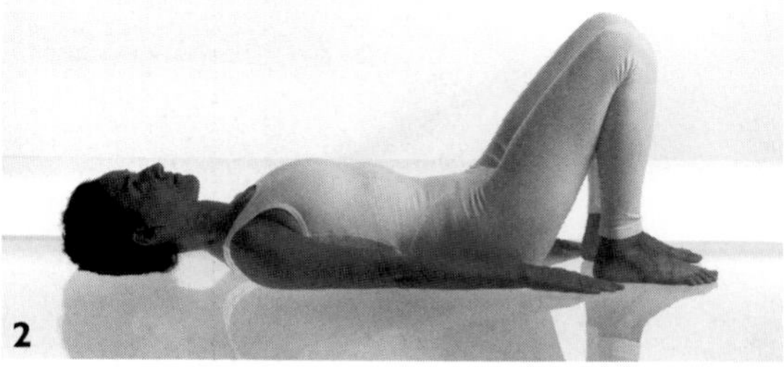

2

3. Take a deep breath in. As you exhale, press into the feet to lift the hips. Allow the shoulders to rest solidly on the floor. Pause for a moment and breathe as the body adjusts to this position.

4. Bring the hands together underneath the buttocks, interlace the fingers. Squeezing the palms together, walk the shoulder blades a little closer together, straightening the arms as much as possible. Your weight should now be resting on the feet and shoulders, with only minimal weight on the neck.

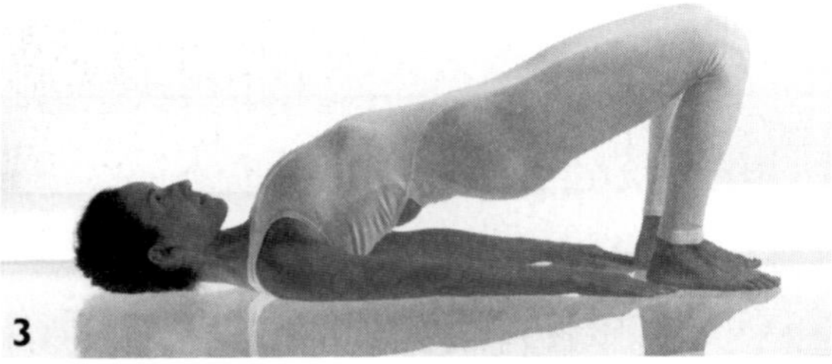
3

5. Press the hip bones and pubic bone toward the ceiling. Allow the sternum to move slightly toward the chin. Breathe deeply as you hold, letting the diaphragm move freely and the belly balloon in and out.

6. To release, take a deep breath in. As you exhale, separate the hands, slide the arms out to your sides, and slowly lower the spine and buttocks to the floor.

Be Aware:

The Bridge is a supported backbend that opens the abdominal area. While in the posture, the diaphragm can move freely. Let the breath flow, watching the belly balloon in and out as you hold. If you want less challenge, come into a simple Bridge by following steps 1–4. You can also substitute Angels in the Snow.

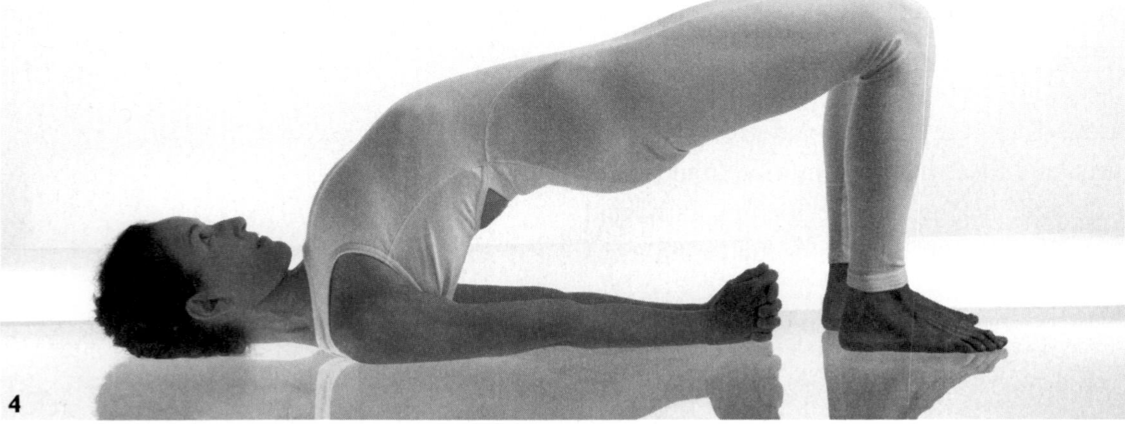
4

If you want more challenge, come into the Bridge as described above. Then release the interlaced fingers and slide the hands under the feet, grasping the heels. This handhold will help you come deeper into the posture. The Bridge is an excellent posture for prolonged holding as detailed on page 375. If you find the basic posture easy, try Bridge variations.

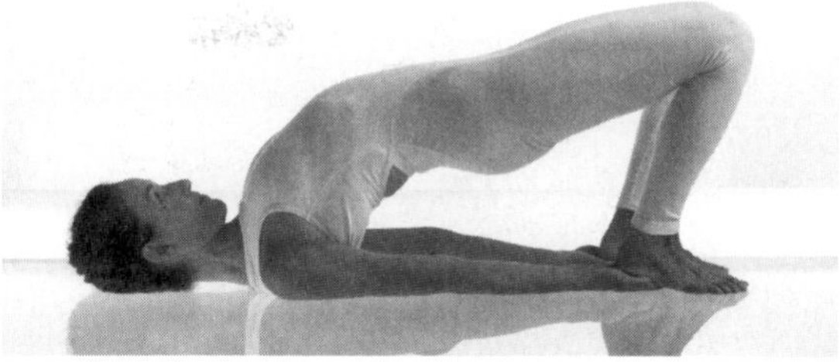

KNEE DOWN TWIST

(Supta Matsyendrasana)

1. Lie on your back with the legs extended.

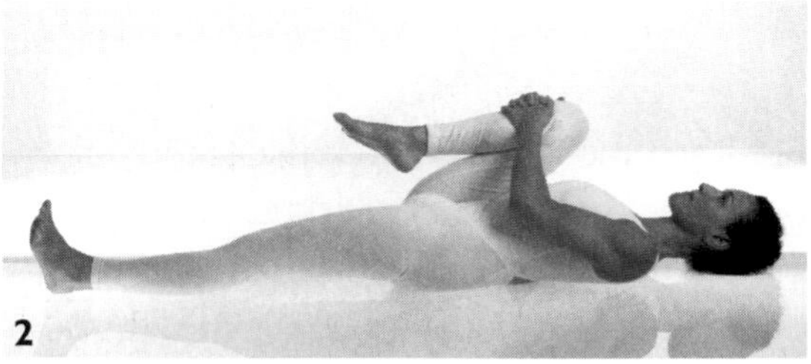

2

2. Draw the right knee up and toward the right side of the chest. Interlace the fingers just below the knee. Using your hand and forearm strength, exhale and draw the knee firmly into the right side of the chest. Take several deep breaths in and out, letting the right hip joint relax as much as possible.

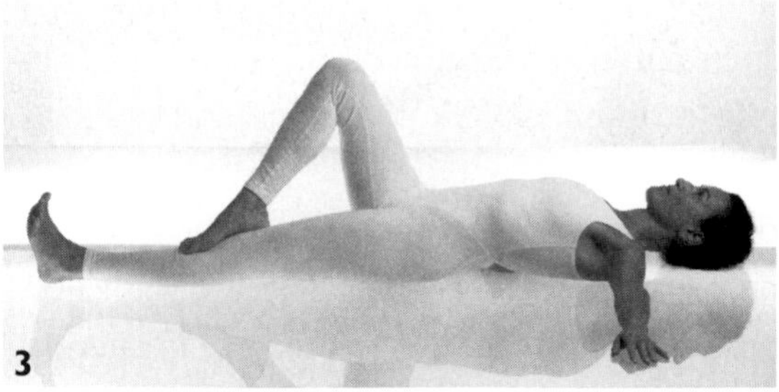

3

3. Keeping the knee raised, reach the arms out to the sides at shoulder height in a T position, palms down. Place the arch of the right foot directly over the left kneecap. The heel of the foot is just above the knee, and the toes are just below the knee.

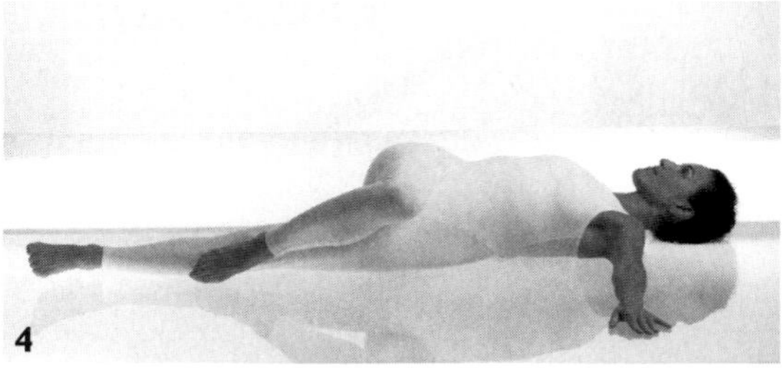

4

4. Take a deep breath in. Exhale and press the right knee across the body and toward the left, rolling the right hip off the floor. Keep both shoulder blades resting on the floor, pressing the right knee toward the floor to rotate the hips and twist the spine.

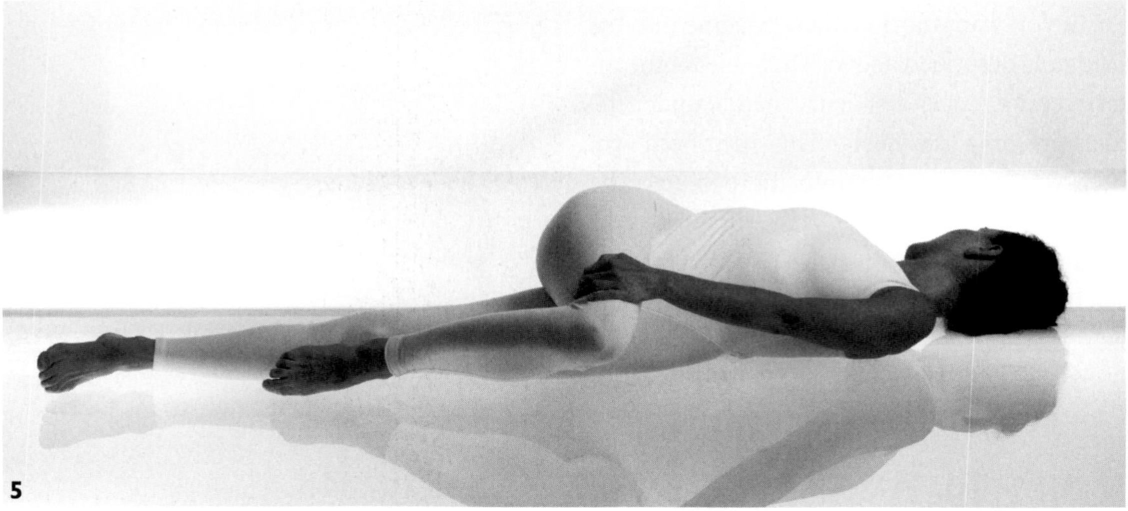

5

5. Bring the left hand onto the outside of the right knee. Keeping the right shoulder blade resting on the floor, gently press the right knee toward the floor with the left hand. Turn the head to look right, bringing the twist into the upper spine and neck. Breathe deeply as you hold, letting the muscles of the back, hips, and legs relax.

6. To release, inhale and rotate the knee and head back to center. Elongate the right leg out on the floor and let the breath flow in and out.

7. Repeat this series of movements on the other side.

Be Aware:

This series uses Single Wind Relieving to compensate for Bridge and prepare to move into Knee Down Twist. If you find Knee Down Twist challenging, substitute Supine Twist. If you experience low back tension after Knee Down Twist, try bringing both knees into the chest and rocking gently side to side to massage the muscles of the low back. This movement is also a nice transition into deep relaxation. If you find Knee Down Twist easy, you can deepen the stretch by placing the foot as high on the thigh as comfortable. The higher you place the foot, the deeper the stretch.

DEEP RELAXATION IN CORPSE

(Yoga Nidra in Shavasana)

1. Lie on your back with the legs extended. Rest the hands lightly on the lower belly. Adjust the feet so they are a comfortable distance apart, and let the toes fall out to the sides.

2. Close the eyes to facilitate feeling. Let the whole body relax and sink into the floor.

3. Focus your attention on the flow of breath, simply watching and feeling the breath rebalance after postures.

4. Gradually move into Relaxing Breath. Allow the inhale to happen naturally, then let the exhalation roll out long, slow, and smooth. Over time, the exhalation will grow approximately twice as long as the inhalation. Stay with Relaxing Breath for three minutes or more. Feel the heartbeat grow slow and steady. Notice the state of introversion that naturally arises from breathing in this way.

5. Release any conscious control of the breath and begin any of the relaxation techniques detailed in chapter 6.

6. Let go into deep relaxation, allowing worries, concerns, and defenses to fall away.

Be Aware:

As your body relaxes, its surface temperature tends to drop, so put on an extra layer of clothing or cover yourself with a blanket prior to entering Corpse. If it is uncomfortable to lie flat on the floor, a pillow beneath the knees helps relieve low back tension. If you experience neck tension, place a folded towel or blanket under the head. Don't use a large pillow, which will cramp the neck and obstruct the free flow of breath. For more relaxation tips, see page 65.

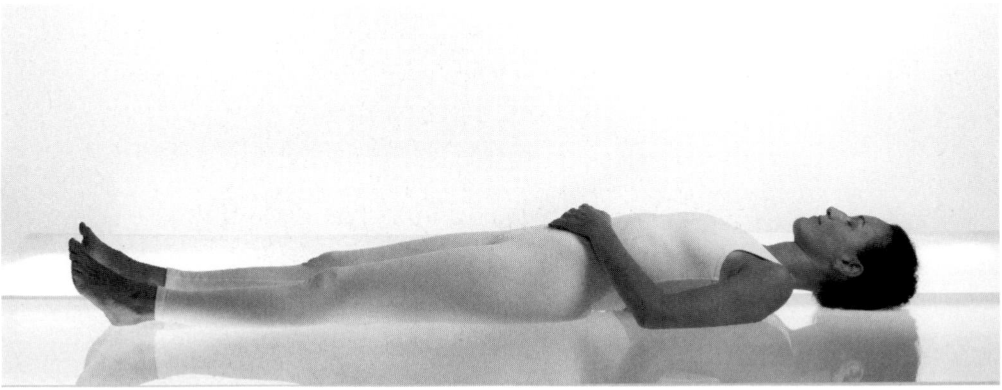

3. YOGA AND HEALTH

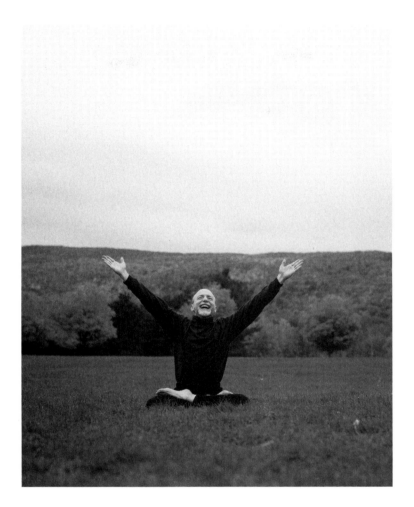

CHAPTER EIGHT

NURTURING THE ROOTS OF HEALTH

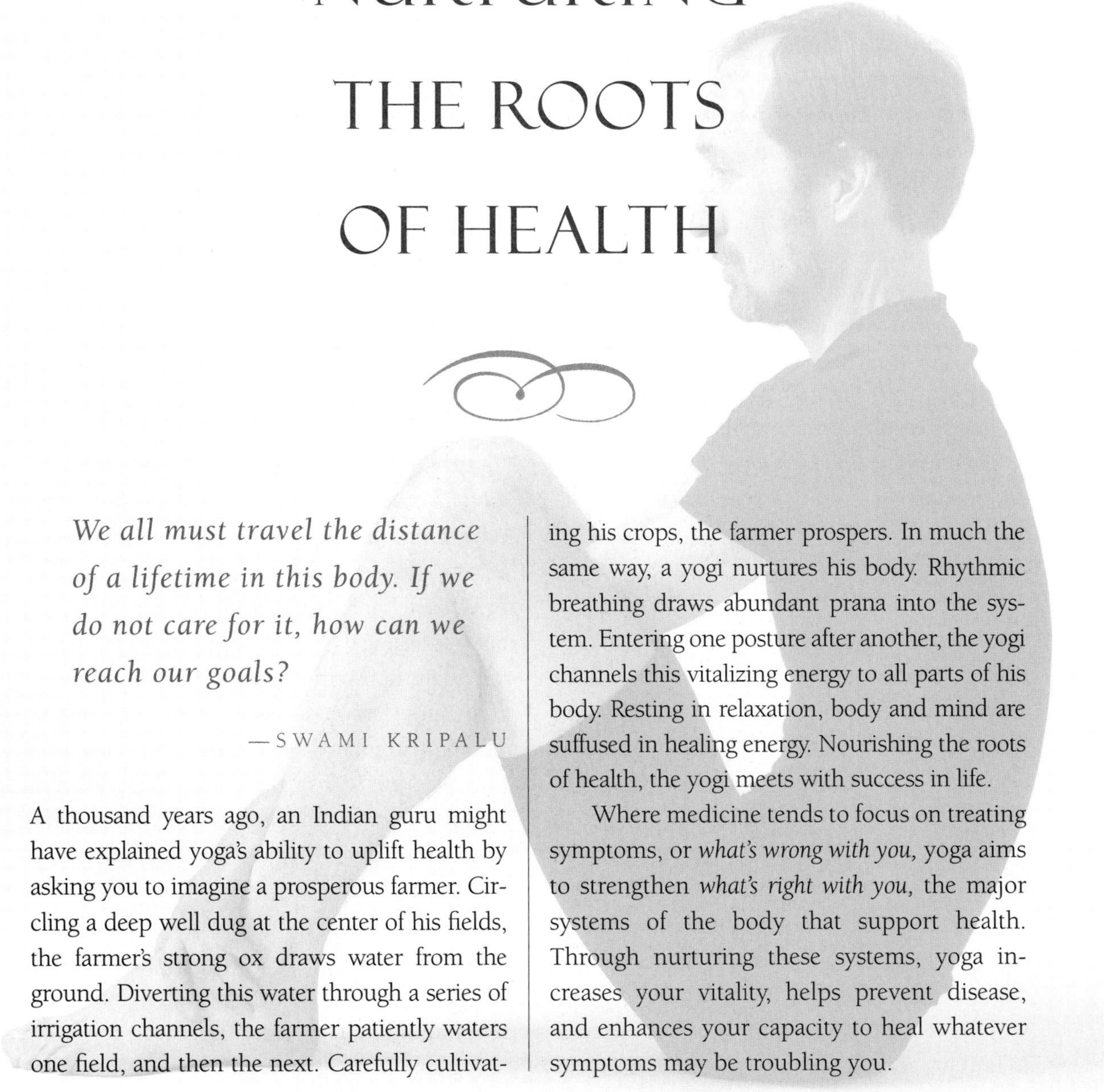

We all must travel the distance of a lifetime in this body. If we do not care for it, how can we reach our goals?

—SWAMI KRIPALU

A thousand years ago, an Indian guru might have explained yoga's ability to uplift health by asking you to imagine a prosperous farmer. Circling a deep well dug at the center of his fields, the farmer's strong ox draws water from the ground. Diverting this water through a series of irrigation channels, the farmer patiently waters one field, and then the next. Carefully cultivating his crops, the farmer prospers. In much the same way, a yogi nurtures his body. Rhythmic breathing draws abundant prana into the system. Entering one posture after another, the yogi channels this vitalizing energy to all parts of his body. Resting in relaxation, body and mind are suffused in healing energy. Nourishing the roots of health, the yogi meets with success in life.

Where medicine tends to focus on treating symptoms, or *what's wrong with you,* yoga aims to strengthen *what's right with you,* the major systems of the body that support health. Through nurturing these systems, yoga increases your vitality, helps prevent disease, and enhances your capacity to heal whatever symptoms may be troubling you.

Seven years ago at age fifty, I was diagnosed with Ewing's sarcoma, an aggressive form of cancer usually found in teenage boys. After extensive surgery, fourteen months of chemotherapy, and a "lifetime allotment" of radiation, I was on my way to recovery. But I had lost some lung and shoulder function, suffered nerve damage that produced chronic pain, and was thirty-eight pounds underweight. Physical therapy helped me get stronger and more symmetrical, but it was only when I went back to Kripalu Yoga that my husband said, "You're beginning to look like yourself again!" And it was true: the woman looking back at me from the mirror was no longer gray and listless. I had regained the radiance of vitality.

—Jane Collins

Most of us grew up with a limiting conception of health as the absence of disease or chronic pain. Actually the word *health* comes from the Old English word *hal*, which means *whole* and is also the root of the words *hale* and *holy*. Health is much more than the absence of disease; it's a positive state of wellness. Through nurturing the roots of health, Kripalu Yoga keeps the body in good repair and optimizes its ability to respond to routine challenges and occasional times of stress. It also works to maintain the mental and emotional balance needed to find joy and meaning in life.

How Kripalu Yoga Nurtures the Roots of Health

- Restores the capacity to breathe freely
- Attunes mind and body
- Counters the negative effects of stress
- Enhances immune response
- Fine-tunes gland and organ function
- Improves cardiovascular health
- Aids digestion and elimination
- Preserves structural integrity
- Improves balance and prevents falls
- Creates an abundance of energy
- Bestows beauty from the inside out

• Restores the Capacity to Breathe

It's easy to take breathing for granted, to overlook its amazing power to increase your energy, calm your mind, and help you perform at peak levels. The life of the body depends upon the breath. Each inhalation brings oxygen into your body, sparking the metabolic process that transforms nutrients into energy. Each exhalation eliminates carbon dioxide and other wastes. Taking just a few deep breaths noticeably amplifies alertness. A single long exhalation helps let go of tension. Improve your breathing, and you literally uplift the health of each and every cell in your body.

A free and rhythmic breath is natural for babies, but most people have lost the ability to breathe freely and deeply by the time they reach adulthood. Unfortunately learning how to regain this natural breath is not so easy. The lungs cannot breathe on their own. They depend on the muscles of the diaphragm, abdomen, and chest to move air in and out. These muscles must be strong, flexible, and free of tension to smoothly fill and empty the lungs. Yoga's prescription to regain this ability is the regular practice of postures that stretch and strengthen all the muscles of the torso, coupled with breath awareness and physical relaxation.

I didn't come to yoga until my early forties. By then, life had tossed me around and I was bruised. Without even being aware of it, I walked around in a thick veil of fear and sadness. The final blow came on Mother's Day 1996, two weeks before my twentieth wedding anniversary, when my husband announced he was leaving. With two teenage sons counting on me, I didn't think I could shoulder the burden and crashed.

For years, I had racewalked for exercise. One day I was walking and a powerful gut feeling told me to go to a yoga class. I asked around and found a Kripalu Yoga teacher. From the first class, I felt like I was home. Slowly the veils lifted. Colors became vibrant again. It felt wonderful to be in my body. My breath became sweeter and deeper. I learned that life could be lived, one breath at a time.

—Lynne Greene

Life is the breath. He who half breathes, half lives.

—Ancient proverb

Medical research has shown that the breath is intimately tied to heart rate, blood pressure, brain wave activity, and mood. How you breathe affects the autonomic nervous system, with shallow chest breathing arousing its sympathetic branch and increasing the amount of stress chemicals like adrenaline and lactic acid in the bloodstream. Deep diaphragmatic breathing stimulates the parasympathetic branch, triggering an opposite response that decreases stress chemicals, calms the mind, and relaxes the body. For all these reasons, regaining the ability to sustain a deep and flowing breath is the single biggest health benefit of yoga. Better breathing on the mat gradually alters your breathing patterns off the mat, and breathing freely and easily once again becomes second nature.

• Attunes Mind and Body

All day long you are engaged with the world around you, mental awareness focused externally to meet life's challenges. At the same time, your involuntary nervous system is maintaining the delicate balance of your inner world. Monitoring respiration and heart rate, circulating the blood, and digesting your food, your autonomic nervous system is engaged twenty-four/seven in sustaining the internal homeostasis essential to well-being. And while the conscious mind is juggling the practical details of your personal and professional life, the subconscious mind is busy processing your deeper thoughts and feelings.

With so much going on at once, it is easy for a split to develop between mind and body. The outer-directed part of the mind focused on action tends to lose touch with the inner-directed part of the mind focused on being. The result is a sense of being fragmented and cut off from your deeper self. Often this self-alienation also leaves you feeling isolated and separate from others.

For as long as I can remember, I had a love/hate relationship with my body. Always the last to be picked for any athletic team effort, I was busy sucking in my stomach to look trim and holding my breath against what I experienced as life's continuing assaults. Then a good friend of mine became a Kripalu Yoga teacher. With her encouragement, I decided to use yoga to get to know my body in a completely new way. For the first time, I felt at home in my body. That's where I have remained ever since.

—Ava Wolf

This split between body and mind is the root cause of many problems. To live like the proverbial Zen master who simply eats when he's hungry and sleeps when he's tired, a strong connection to the body is required. If you are out of touch with your body, it is impossible to attend to the intuitions and urges that signal its basic needs. Yoga provides quality time when your attention is not divided between the inner and outer worlds, time dedicated to feeling, listening inside, restoring inner balance, and healing. It offers a practical way to get back in touch with the wisdom of your own body and heart.

Yoga's approach to healing the body-mind split is simple and exceedingly direct: you focus the mind on the sensations that arise in the body from breathing, stretching, and moving. Without a host of competing external demands, the nervous system is able to rebalance your biochemistry and attend to health maintenance and healing. Then the focus of practice shifts to building strength, deepening your connection to self, and remaining connected as you flow and grow through life. Ultimately yoga is meant to weave the separate strands of body, heart, and mind into the whole cloth of a deeply integrated life.

One day, while stopped at a traffic light, I was rear-ended by a pickup truck. I didn't seem hurt and was able to drive home. But the next morning, I couldn't lift my head off the pillow. I had to roll onto my side and support my head with my hands to sit up. It was then that I realized I had whiplash.

As the day progressed, my neck felt worse and I wondered what to do. In the early evening, I felt drawn to Kripalu

Yoga. I lay down on the floor and began to take some relaxed breaths. I noticed an urge to move different parts of my body, and allowed it to happen. Without direction from my mind, my body began to move on its own in very simple, gentle ways. The movements didn't look like yoga postures, but they felt good, so I continued. I allowed them to keep going until they naturally stopped.

I went to bed and was amazed in the morning to discover that the whiplash was almost completely gone. The posture flow of the night before had a powerful, healing effect. My mind hadn't known what to do, but my body obviously did.

—Shantipriya Marcia Goldberg

• Counters the Negative Effects of Stress

There is no such thing as a "stress-free" life. A certain amount of challenge is stimulating and healthy. But when demands rise to a level where they are interpreted as a threat, the body prepares for action by entering a state called *fight-or-flight arousal*. Fight-or-flight is a reflexive response that quickly empowers us to confront or escape danger. It is activated when a portion of the brain called the *hypothalamus* stimulates the adrenal glands to secrete the hormone adrenaline, which dramatically increases the activity of the sympathetic nervous system. Within seconds a stunning number of physiological changes take place. Respiration and heart rate increase two to three times their normal rate. Blood pressure soars. Functions not essential to meet the anticipated threat are suppressed, including digestion and the immune response. The abdomen tightens to protect the vital organs. Blood flow is directed to the muscles of the arms and legs. Attention is focused externally as vision and hearing become more acute, and the entire body is poised for action.

What we call *stress* is the deep exhaustion that results when relentless psychological demands keep us stuck in a state of low-grade fight-or-flight arousal. Unable to sleep, digest our food, or heal our bodies, we gradually become stressed-out. Stress undermines our ability to concentrate and be creative, which can lead to problems at work. It subjects us to mood swings and compromises our ability to be empathic, which often leads to problems at home. Underlying all these symptoms is a chronic state of biochemical arousal that is extremely damaging to the body. Over time it leads to the condition called *burnout*. Stress is the invisible epidemic of our times, predisposing us to common complaints such as insomnia, backaches, headaches, digestive disorders, and major illnesses such as cancer, heart disease, and strokes. Studies estimate that 80 percent of all health conditions and 60–90 percent of all physician visits are stress-related.

Fortunately for all of us, the body has a

MEN, WOMEN, AND STRESS

Recent research indicates there are important differences in the biochemical response of men and women to stress. Both men and women secrete adrenaline to trigger the *fight-or-flight response.* New studies suggest that women under stress get a quick burst of adrenaline followed by the secretion of oxytocin from the pituitary gland. Oxytocin is a hormone and mood regulator released during childbirth, now believed to be the biochemical source of the *tend-and-befriend response.* When confronted with danger, females of all species are inclined to protect their young and bond with other females. Males are more likely to exhibit aggressive behavior.

Yoga provides men with a way to break the stress cycle by turning on the relaxation response. For women who care for others and may neglect their own needs, yoga provides time for focused self-nurturance.

second reflex mechanism that is the mirror image of fight-or-flight. While studying traditional healing practices, Dr. Herbert Benson and a team of Harvard colleagues identified the *relaxation response.* When activated, it causes the levels of adrenaline and other stress hormones in the bloodstream to drop. Respiration, heart rate, and blood pressure decrease. Muscles relax, blood is directed into the vital organs, and the activity of the immune and digestive systems is stimulated. Attention is drawn inward as slower alpha brain waves, associated with feelings of well-being and heightened creativity, become predominant. In the state of deep relaxation that results, the body is able to apply its full energy to the task of healing. Groundbreaking in its time, the relaxation response has become a standard element of body-mind medicine.

In 1986, I had a wonderful and responsible job but was living an unhealthy and unhappy life. Watching myself slowly lose my mind to addiction and depression spurred me on to sign into drug and alcohol rehab for a month. When I got out, a friend took me to a Kripalu Yoga class. That was the beginning of a wonderful and courageous journey for me. I have been sober for nineteen years now, and Kripalu Yoga has been an integral part of my recovery. It has helped me learn, in a very gentle way, who I really am, and to positively embrace that.

—Evelyn Zak

If you pay attention, you can feel the relaxation response gently rise and sweep over you during yoga practice. It begins as Ocean Sounding Breath encourages you to soften the abdomen. It continues as postures and micromovements help you release excess muscle tension. It builds as your focus deepens, enabling you to let go of external distractions and become absorbed in a flowing state of inner awareness. It culminates as you enter deep relaxation. By providing you a way to turn off the fight-or-flight response and turn on the relaxation response, Kripalu Yoga is an effective tool to break the vicious cycle of stress.

• Enhances Immune Response

The AIDS epidemic painfully raised awareness of the role played by the immune system in preventing disease. While medical science continues to explore how the immune system functions, and what causes it to fail, it seems clear that a number of alternative health modalities, including yoga, boost immune response. To anyone steeped in the yoga tradition, this comes as no surprise. Yoga has always viewed disease as an offensive force that attacks the body. In the same way a walled city with a strong army can resist a siege, the body of a person practicing yoga is described as able to repel the onslaught of disease into old age.

Until recently, Western medicine remained skeptical of claims that body-mind techniques like yoga could enhance immune function because there was no known connection between the nervous and immune systems. Then a previously unknown network of nerves was discovered that is a hardwire link between the central nervous system and key components of the immune system: bone marrow, thymus gland, lymph nodes, spleen, and blood vessels. Continuing studies revealed a second biochemical link, showing how the brain directs the immune system by releasing neurotransmitters that deliver chemical messages to receptor sites on the surface of immune cells. This biochemical exchange is actually a two-way conversation, as chemicals released by the immune cells feed back to the brain.

With hardwire and biochemical links between the brain and immune system established, it became much easier for physicians to accept the profound role the mind can play in the healing process. Yoga, meditation, biofeedback, deep relaxation, visualization, guided imagery, prayer, music and art therapy, psychotherapy, and support groups are quickly becoming accepted treatments in contemporary medicine. Techniques like yoga that calm the mind and focus it inward are believed to facilitate the inner dialogue between mind and body, fine-tuning the interaction of the nervous and immune systems to help us stay well.

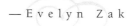

Yoga also enhances immune response in a mechanical way through dramatically increasing the flow of lymph. The *lymphatic system* is the circulatory system of the immune response. You may be surprised to learn that your body has more lymphatic fluid than blood, and more miles of lymph ducts than blood vessels. A complex network of fluid, vessels, and nodes that parallels the circulatory system, the lymphatic system is constantly killing infectious organisms and sweeping metabolic wastes and other toxins from around the cells and carrying them back to the bloodstream to be cleansed by the liver and kidneys. One key component of the lymphatic system is its hundreds of lymph nodes, meshlike tissues loaded with immune cells that kill invading germs. Another is its systems of ducts that keep the lymph flowing. Chief among these is the thoracic duct, located in the center of the chest, into which all the lymph vessels eventually drain.

Where the circulatory system has the heart, the lymphatic system relies upon movement to pump the lymph. All movement increases lymph flow to some extent, but yoga appears to increase it in dramatic ways. By fostering relaxation, yoga releases hormones that dilate the lymph vessels. Deep diaphragmatic breathing and backbending postures keep the large thoracic duct open and the river of lymph flowing freely. Through a variety of positions, and especially through inversions, yoga uses gravity to move lymph to places it might not otherwise flow so freely. Lymph glands are concentrated in the armpits, neck, and groin. By stretching these areas, yoga facilitates their elimination of infectious invaders. All of these effects together help the lymphatic system accomplish its task of keeping the body free of wastes, germs, and toxins.

• Fine-Tunes Gland and Organ Function

The nervous system has a close ally in its task of integrating the functions of the body into a synchronized whole. The endocrine system is a network of glands that secrete powerful biochemical messages called *hormones* into the bloodstream to coordinate the multitude of tasks carried out by organs. Hormone balance is critical to health, with disorders resulting from excessive or deficient levels. Yoga enhances endocrine function by increasing blood circulation to glandular tissues.

Yoga can be understood as a form of self-massage. Stretching or contracting an area of the body that contains glands or organs applies a gentle pressure. This pressure forces blood to flow out of the tissues, facilitating the release of waste products into the bloodstream. As the posture is released, fresh blood flows in carrying needed nutrients. The analogy of wringing out a sponge is often used to describe this process, which yoga calls *rinsing and soaking*. To intensify the effects, a posture that applies pressure to an area is often followed by a complementary stretch that opens it up to circulation, soaking the organ or gland in fresh blood. The belly down postures are a good example of this technique, applying significant pressure to the abdominal or-

EXPERIENCE: KEEP YOUR RIVER OF LYMPH FLOWING

Puppy Stretch is a simple posture that stimulates lymph flow, opening the thoracic duct and massaging lymph nodes in the armpits, neck, and chest. It also stimulates the thymus gland, another key component of the immune system.

1. Come into Table Pose, hands directly under the shoulders, and knees directly under the hips.

2. Take a deep breath in. As you exhale, slowly slide the palms forward on the floor until you feel a good stretch to the chest and armpits. Inch the fingers forward on the floor, stretching through the rib cage and coming to your full expression of the stretch. Then let the back of the neck relax and the forehead come onto the floor. Gently press the sternum down, keeping the hips high and tailbone lifted. Breathe deeply as you hold, allowing the chest to open.

3. If you want more stretch, press the elbows into the floor and bring the hands into Prayer position behind the head. Feel the stretch stimulating and massaging all the lymph nodes located in the neck and armpits.

4. To release, slide the hands back into Table Pose. You can also release by pressing the buttocks back onto the heels and resting in Child Pose.

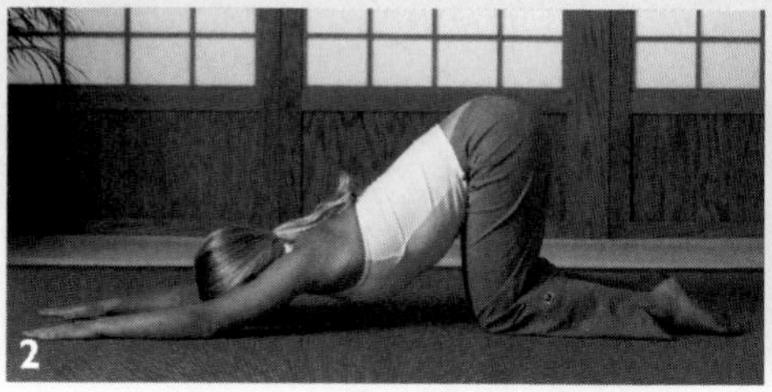

2

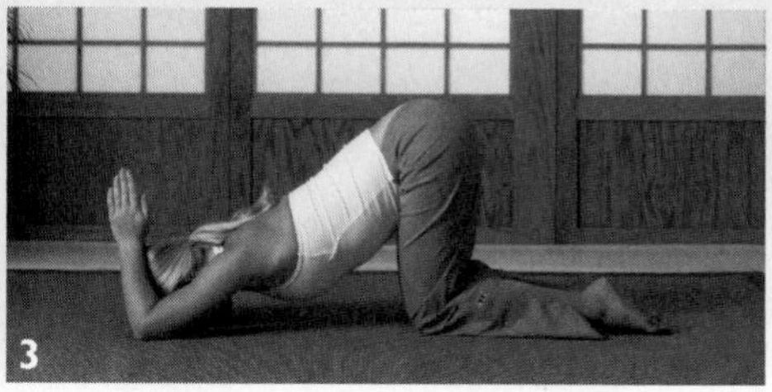

3

gans and strongly contracting the muscles surrounding the kidneys and adrenal glands. The complementary posture is Child Pose, which increases blood flow to the belly and low back.

Massage can do more than increase circulation. Applying pressure to certain areas of the body stimulates various nervous system reflexes that activate organs and glands. Yoga shares this healing technique with reflexology, a contemporary healing modality that works with reflex points on the feet, hands, and ears. Acupuncture and acupressure, more traditional systems developed in China, also work by stimulating carefully mapped energy pathways in the body. While therapeutic applications of reflexology and acupressure may be employed by yoga therapists to activate organs and glands believed to have grown lethargic, full-body stimulation is built right into the basic postures.

Yoga also increases circulation through the skillful use of inverted postures like Half Shoulderstand. Being upside down reverses the pull of gravity, encouraging blood to flow out of the legs and into the torso and upper body. All the vital organs are turned upside down and forced to shift positions in the abdominal cavity. As the posture is held, gravity directs blood flow to the neck area where the thyroid and parathyroid glands are located. A slight chin tuck is an important part of Half Shoulderstand, as it helps blood pool in surrounding tissues. When the posture is released by moving into Corpse Pose, circulation shifts again as blood flow returns to normal. Cobra or Fish Pose (taught in part 5) finishes the traditional sequence, arching the neck in the opposite direction. Although this description is specific to Half Shoulderstand, the same idea applies to every posture. Each posture changes the body's position and relationship to gravity, enhancing circulation to certain parts and limiting it elsewhere. Moving from posture to posture rejuvenates the whole body.

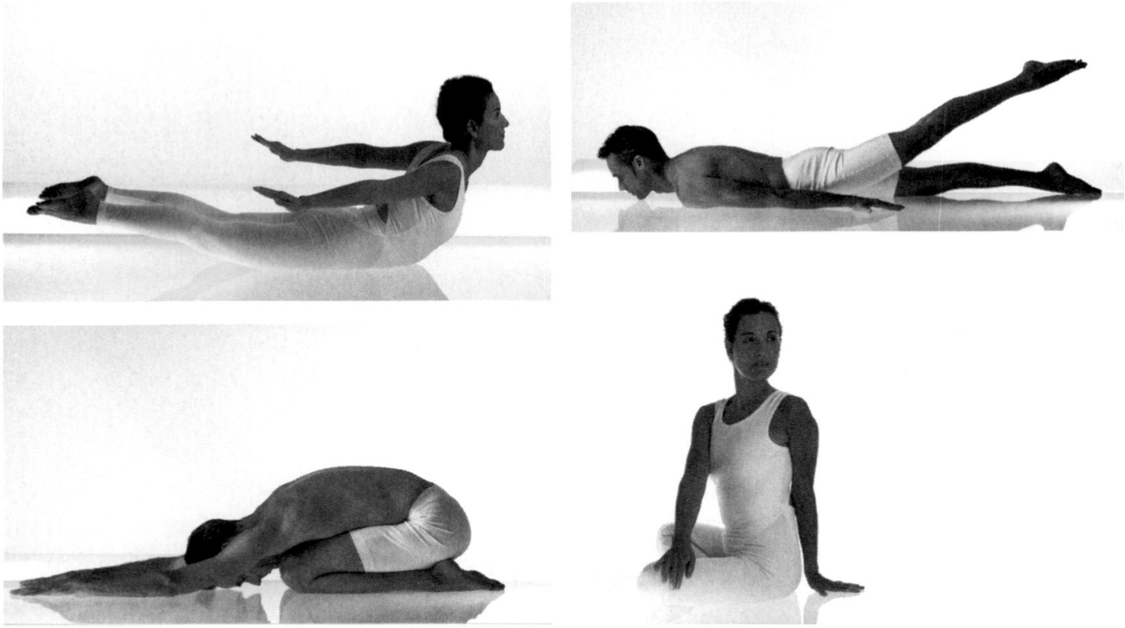

Some yoga postures apply gentle pressure to areas of the body containing organs and glands. This pressure forces blood and waste products to flow out of the area. When released, fresh blood and needed nutrients return. It also stimulates nervous system reflexes that activate organs and glands that have grown sluggish.

• Improves Cardiovascular Health

Dr. Dean Ornish made headlines by proving that a lifestyle regimen of yoga, meditation, a low-fat vegetarian diet, aerobic exercise, and support groups can reverse coronary artery disease. Since then, numerous researchers have confirmed yoga's ability to reduce high blood pressure. Without a doubt, yoga is good for your heart.

Combining flowing movement with deep breathing, yoga provides a mild cardiovascular workout. More important, yoga stimulates the relaxation response known to dilate blood vessels and lower blood pressure. Ornish and many others believe that regaining the ability to access emotion is an integral part of the healing process for cardiovascular disease. Yoga "opens the heart" by helping us regain the ability to feel.

The yoga practices integral to the Ornish program were developed by Nischala Devi. Nischala encourages heart patients to listen to their bodies, to move slowly in yoga postures, and to stop before they feel pain. She reminds participants that yoga is not a competitive

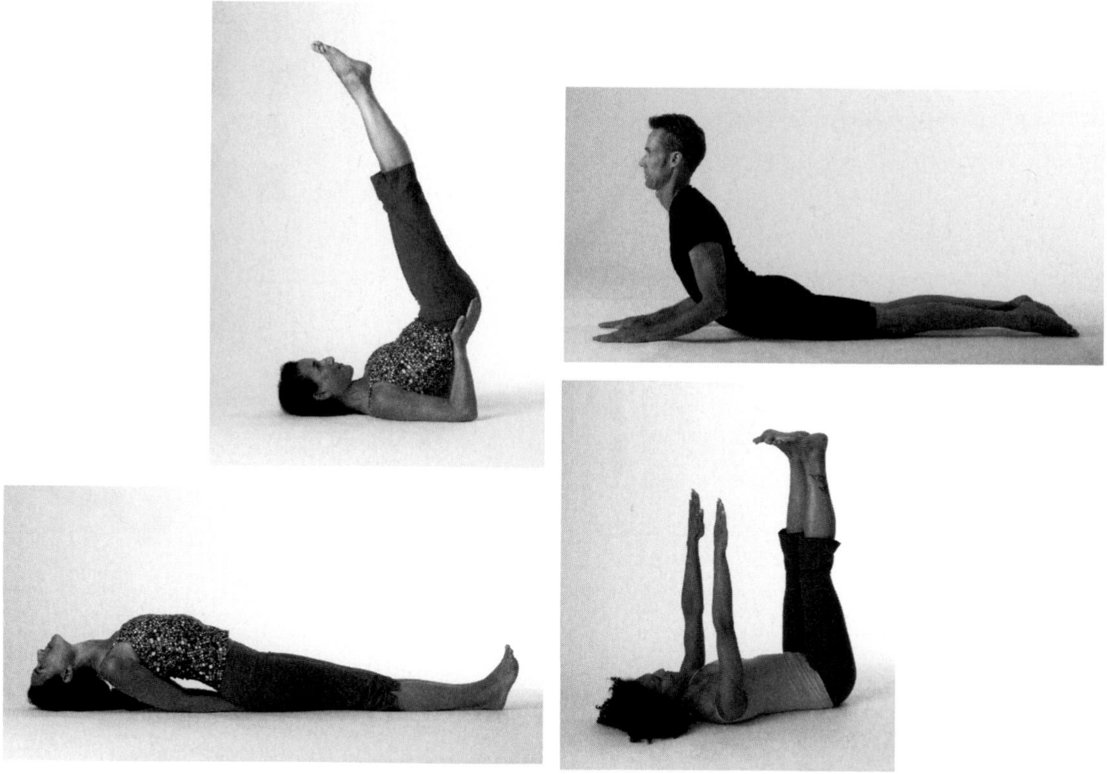

Yoga postures use gravity to facilitate circulation to all parts of the body. Certain postures are targeted to increase circulation to specific glands and organs.

EXPERIENCE: FIRST AID FOR INDIGESTION

If your digestive tract feels clogged or bloated, Wind Relieving Series can work wonders. Done daily, it's a powerful tonic that promotes digestive health.

1. Lie on your back with the legs extended. Draw the right knee up toward the right side of the chest. Interlace the fingers just below the knee and draw the elbows in close to the sides. Take a deep breath in. Using your hand and forearm strength, exhale and draw the knee into the right side of the chest with a firm and steady pressure. Let the right hip joint completely relax.

2. Resist the tendency of the knee position to render the breath shallow. Breathe freely and deeply, letting the movement of the diaphragm accentuate the massage to the right side of the abdomen.

3. To release, take a deep breath in. As you exhale, release the hands and extend the leg into Corpse Pose. Close the eyes and feel any sensations of flow or movement in the belly.

4. Draw the left knee up and repeat steps 1–3 on the opposite side.

5. Draw both knees up into the chest and bring them close together. Wrap the arms around the knees, grasping the elbows if possible, or the forearms or wrists. Elongate the neck by slightly tucking the chin, then resting the back of the head on the floor. Press the sacrum toward the floor to stabilize the low back. Using your hand and forearm strength, draw both knees firmly into the chest.

6. Keep the sacrum pressing toward the floor and the breath moving, feeling the massage to the abdomen.

7. Release the knees and extend the legs into Corpse Pose. Close the eyes and let the breath flow freely. Attune to the belly, noticing if you can feel any effect of Wind Relieving Series on the abdominal organs.

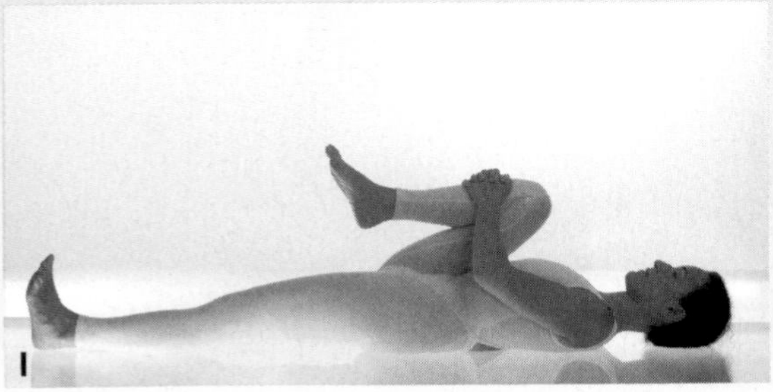
1

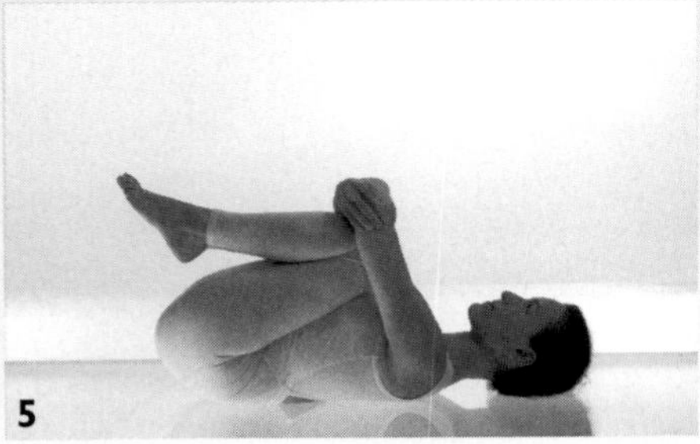
5

sport, and that doing fewer postures and relaxing more is often a winning combination. For those with serious medical conditions, learning how to use yoga to enjoy moments of inner peace and harmony is especially important, as this breaks the cycle of stress and anxiety that often contributes to heart disease. If you have a heart condition, check with your physician before beginning a yoga practice. If possible, find a yoga instructor trained to work with heart patients to ensure a safe and effective practice.

• Aids Digestion

The health of the body depends on its ability to assimilate nutrients and dispose of wastes. Yoga enhances this twin process of digestion and elimination in many ways. Deep breathing increases metabolism, stoking the digestive fire yoga calls *agni*. Managing stress keeps the digestive processes from being suppressed by the fight-or-flight response. On a more mechanical level, yoga postures stretch, strengthen, and massage the abdomen in a way that supports the smooth flow of digestive matter through the intestines and colon.

Wind Relieving Series targets the digestive system. Drawing the right knee into the chest massages the right side of the abdomen, applying a steady pressure to the ascending colon that supports the clockwise movement of peristalsis. It also massages the small intestines, gallbladder, and liver. Drawing the left knee into the chest applies a similar pressure to the descending and sigmoid colon and massages the small intestines, stomach, pancreas, and spleen. Then both knees are brought into the chest, applying pressure to the transverse colon, rectum, and all the vital organs. Done regularly, this routine helps prevent digestive matter from becoming compacted in the two ninety-degree bends that separate the ascending, transverse, and descending colon. Numerous other postures tone and massage the abdomen to help maintain full digestive health.

• Structural Integrity

Structural integrity refers to the healthy condition of the skeleton, joints, and soft tissues of the body. As you age, preserving structural integrity becomes increasingly important because the compromised condition of any single component can make movement painful and reduce your activity level. Beyond allowing you to stand tall and move gracefully, structural integrity promotes deep breathing, minimizes joint wear, and supports the efficient functioning of organs and glands.

The spinal column is the central axis of the skeleton, housing the spinal cord, the vital link between body and brain. The spine also bears the weight of the body; even while bending or rotating it must protect the delicate spinal cord. Branching off the spinal column and exiting through small openings between the vertebrae are the nerve roots, the origin points of the peripheral nerves that carry electrical messages to every cell

YOGA AND CHIROPRACTIC ADJUSTMENTS

Chiropractic is a health care modality almost entirely built on the idea of restoring structural integrity to the body. Chiropractors believe that many diseases are caused by ***subluxations***, misaligned vertebrae that place pressure on nerves exiting the spine. Nerve tissue is soft and pliable. Chiropractors believe that pressure impairs nerve function, compromising the nervous system's ability to sense the body and maintain health.

In a chiropractic adjustment, the chiropractor applies manual force to the spine to correct a subluxation, restoring normal nervous system function and allowing the body to heal itself. Essentially, an adjustment "turns the power back on" to a part of the body. Adjustments often produce a cracking or popping sound as the joint surfaces separate. The source of this sound is actually the release of gases from joint fluids and tissues. Similar sounds happen in yoga practice, as stretching allows the vertebrae and joints to return to proper alignment. Many chiropractors find that yoga and chiropractic are complementary. Chiropractic adjustment restores spinal alignment. By strengthening the musculature and supporting good posture, yoga helps the patient hold the adjustment.

---

of the body. Flowing through the nerves and spinal cord is an unceasing dialogue between body and brain. Nerve impulses carry information about the functioning of every organ and gland to the brain, allowing it to coordinate their activities. If the spine's integrity is compromised and pressure applied to a nerve root, the flow of impulses through that nerve is impeded. This "pinched nerve" not only causes painful muscle spasms, it compromises information flow, dulling self-awareness and limiting the brain's ability to sustain the health of the tissues.

Kripalu Yoga helps you develop the muscular strength in the torso required to keep the spine elongated during movement. A balanced yoga session articulates the twenty-four movable spinal vertebrae, flexing the spine forward and back, side to side, and twisting it left and right. Regularly performing these six

EXPERIENCE: CHILL OUT WITH THESE SHOULDERSTAND MODIFICATIONS

Two simple modified versions of the Shoulderstand make it possible for anyone to experience the power of inversions, at any time of the month. For Legs on a Chair pose, you can use any type of chair or sofa. To come into Legs Up the Wall pose, position the side of your body against the wall. Then bring your knees into the chest, turn your buttocks toward the wall, and extend your legs.

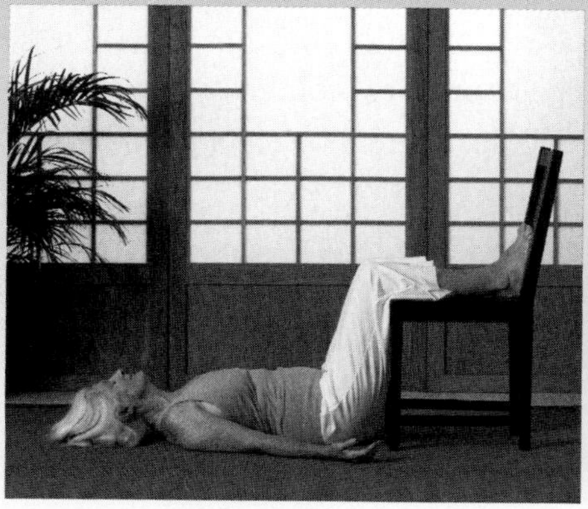

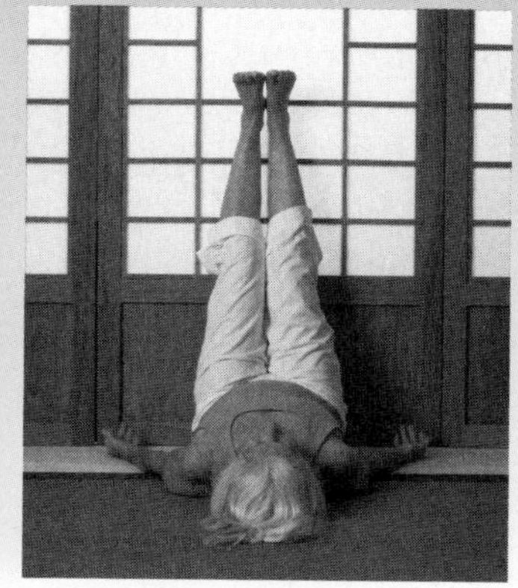

movements of the spine helps keep the spine both flexible and aligned. Blood circulation to the spinal column and nerve roots is increased, pinched nerves are avoided, and the full functioning of your nervous system is maintained.

Preserving the suppleness and resiliency of the shock-absorbing vertebral disks is another facet of structural integrity that grows increasingly important as you age. By increasing the circulation of interstitial fluid within the disk, which imports nutrients and exports wastes, yoga keeps the spine young. Of course the most obvious benefit of a flexible spine is that it preserves your capacity for full and free movement, allowing you to engage in all the activities of a fulfilling life.

- **Improves Balance**

It is easy to take your ability to balance for granted—until you lose it. Aging and inactivity can compromise our kinesthetic sense of balance, leaving us prone to the kind of falls that often prove devastating to otherwise healthy senior citizens. Yoga works to improve balance in two ways. Posture practice creates the whole-body strength that makes it easy to maintain good posture and move gracefully. By including postures that require good balance to perform—like the Tree and Crane—yoga also fine-tunes the inner ear function and muscular coordination underlying our ability to balance.

• Creates an Abundance of Energy

Your energy is strong when respiration is deep, metabolism is steady, and the organs are doing their job. Your energy is balanced when the nervous and endocrine systems are finely tuned. Your energy is available for productive use when not being drained by muscle tension or chronic pain. By fostering all these things, yoga produces a great by-product: abundant energy.

Better yet, yoga improves your appearance. Smooth skin, bright eyes, shiny hair, and a firm figure are really nothing more than the outward signals of a healthy body. By nurturing the roots of health through a regular Kripalu Yoga practice, you enjoy the best cosmetic of all: that natural blush of good health.

CHAPTER NINE

ACCESSING BODY WISDOM

My challenge in shaping the ashram's yoga curriculum was to find creative ways to enable each learner to access the impulses and intuitions arising from the body and to rely on his or her direct experience as the ultimate source of authority.

—DON STAPLETON

Kripalu Yoga came of age in the dynamic ashram community that flourished from the early 1970s to the mid-1990s. If you had walked through the doors of Kripalu Center as a guest in the ashram's heyday, your first impression would have been one of entering a Hindu religious community. Three hundred ashram residents lived on-site, almost all of whom were known by Sanskrit names. White clothing was worn to symbolize a commitment to purification, an endeavor made real by a strict vegetarian diet and a weekly fast day. Mornings started before dawn with yoga, pranayama, and meditation. Long hours of selfless service to the community were punctuated by an extended lunch break designed to encourage vigorous exercise. After dinner, the community gathered to chant, dance, and listen to spiritual discourses by the guru in residence Yogi Desai, along with senior residents and a steady stream of visiting luminaries.

A sizable cohort lived this ashram lifestyle for twenty years. Others spent a decade or more as residents, or left after shorter stints to join the sizable lay community of "householders" living a parallel life in society. Yes, we were an idealistic group of American youth adopting the garb of a foreign culture, but just beneath the Indian veneer, something of greater consequence was happening. The entire Kripalu community was engaged in a deep inquiry, exploring the traditional yoga lifestyle through personal practice and discovering what aspects worked—and which didn't.

Over the years, yoga was coupled with running, aerobics, and weight lifting in a pursuit of body-mind fitness. In a quest for optimal nutrition, the kitchen evolved from the granola-based diet that was 1970s health food to explore sophisticated systems such as Macrobiotics and Ayurveda that seek to create a refined balance in body and mind. Psychotherapy and other tools adapted from self-help psychology were combined with introspective pursuits like meditation to deal with the rapid shifts and changes wrought by ashram living. In this rich interaction of East and West, something altogether new was arising: a contemporary yoga lifestyle.

Although the cross-fertilization of diverse approaches made the ashram a hothouse of innovation, there was another element in the mix that ultimately proved seminal. The keystone teaching of Kripalu Yoga is a call for each individual to use the techniques of yoga to access the innate evolutionary intelligence lying dormant in the body. Any practice learned from an external source, no matter how refined or intensively done, is only a preliminary discipline clearing the way for the emergence of *body wisdom*.

I look back on my twenty years in the ashram with gratitude. It was exciting to be engaged in such a noble experiment, and we actually steered the organization by what created vitality and life force in the individual, the community, and the retreat center business—all three bundled in an integrated whole. My wife and I left with little money and few possessions, but we were whole people with the skills and confidence needed to build a healthy, successful life. My life remains focused on the fascinating question of what makes individuals, organizations, and communities thrive. That's why I am still connected to Kripalu.

—Dinabandhu Garrett Sarley

Body wisdom became the North Star used by the ashram community to navigate a profound journey. In the spirit of the 1960s, most began with a hearty renunciation of the prevailing Western lifestyle. Habitual patterns were confronted and broken by adopting the precepts of yoga. As inner wisdom emerged, the traditional yoga lifestyle was freely adapted to meet current needs. Slowly and at times painfully, the whole community learned the important lesson that "one size fits all" approaches don't work in the long run. Individual differences are too great for everyone to benefit from doing, eating, and believing the same things. At some point, each individual has to find his or her own way through trial and error.

Kripalu Yoga's current teachings on lifestyle are sourced in this understanding of the pivotal role played by body wisdom in the search for true health.

> *I learned a lot about the principles of a good diet when I became Macrobiotic. But only by going through the process of becoming macro-neurotic and eventually macro-psychotic did I get my most valuable lesson on eating: I need to listen to my own body.*
>
> —Sudhir Jonathan Foust

Body Wisdom

Your body is constantly speaking to you, communicating what it needs to be happy and healthy through its language of instinctual urges and feelings. By bringing you more in touch with your body, yoga helps you hear and honor its messages. Practiced regularly, yoga begins to exert a powerful effect on lifestyle. It is not uncommon for people to stop smoking or break other harmful habits after years of trying, simply as a result of practicing postures, conscious breathing, and relaxation.

Body wisdom is one component of intuition, the ability to know without conscious reasoning. The ability to feel, and the capacity to derive meaning from the subtle textures of feeling, vary markedly among individuals, but both can be dramatically increased by training. Kripalu Yoga is designed to hone body wisdom by deepening your capacity to feel and ensure that in matters of diet, exercise, and lifestyle you are guided by something more than disembodied rational cognition.

> *Yoga and meditation made me more sensitive to my physical needs, and this changed my life in many ways. Most of the time, I am aware of what foods my body needs and have grown to prefer them. Whenever I stray too far from balance in any area, I just turn back to yoga to reestablish harmony and health.*
>
> —Shantipriya Marcia Goldberg

More Than a Felt Sense

Accessing the wisdom of your body is not difficult. You simply feel what is true for you, momentarily giving up the need for things to make logical sense. Instead of being logical or verbal, body wisdom is preference-based and especially strong when choosing from available options. When your companion asks if you want to eat Italian or Chinese, the cognitive mind tends to seesaw back and forth between what you enjoyed in the past and your best guess of what the other person wants. Body wisdom is automatic and immediate. It responds free of concerns over social acceptability. It just knows what it wants.

A simple technique to access body wisdom is to imagine a gyroscope revolving inside your belly. As you picture alternatives, comparing a garden salad with lots of brightly colored vegetables and a side of whole wheat toast to a steaming piece of broiled salmon with a baked potato, notice how the gyroscope reacts. Does it spin faster when presented with one option, gaining energy and momentum? Does it slow down and start to wobble in response to the other? Does an entirely different and unexpected idea pop into your mind? Another technique is to visualize yourself in a situation, like the office of a new job you've been offered, and notice how your body feels in that setting. If you take the time to experiment by tuning in and asking your body what it wants, you are likely to be amazed at how much it tells you.

Because it is simply a felt sense, body wisdom can easily be negated and overridden by the conscious mind. Understanding its source in the *adaptive unconscious,* an aspect of the psyche under scrutiny by research psychologists, may help you trust its guidance. The adaptive unconscious is a set of sophisticated mental processes that operate below the threshold of consciousness yet are proven to influence judgments, feelings, and behaviors. Its purpose is to help us quickly size up our environment and initiate behavior. If you close your eyes and get quiet, you can sense the ceaseless working of the adaptive unconscious as part of the resonant hum we call our *being*. Research shows that these nonconscious functions are indispensable in making our way through life. In some tasks, such as recognizing faces, sensing danger or opportunity, and detecting complex patterns in the environment, the adaptive unconscious far outperforms the conscious mind.

Back in 1988, I was living in Boston and working in human services. Drinking several cups of coffee a day, I spent my time reading three newspapers, worrying about the state of the world, and completely ignoring my body. At night, anxiety attacks would awaken me. I heard about yoga and found a class that enabled me to dissolve layers of tension and relax for the first time in my life. A few months later, I went to a weekend program at Kripalu Center. On the last day, a staff member demonstrated a posture flow, moving with awareness of her own body and breath, animated by an inner rapture of sorts. That experience touched a primal and ancient place inside of me. I returned home, gave up coffee, and started sleeping better and worrying less. I began to eat more vegetables, less sugar, and feel more hopeful about the world. Kripalu Yoga started me on the path of yoga by teaching me how to befriend my feelings and trust body wisdom.

—Ann Greene

While a bit mysterious because we've lost touch with it, body wisdom is not mystical or infallible. It is instinctive and primal, even primitive. Along with an automatic knowing, we surely need conscious decision-making to

WHY TRUST BODY WISDOM?

The idea that the body has a wisdom all its own is supported by current thinking in neuroscience. The human brain evolved over millions of years, with distinct layers that developed at different times and correspond to different types of mental function. The brain stem and cerebellum, sometimes called the *reptilian brain*, regulates a host of involuntary functions. The emotional brain, or limbic system, is similar in both humans and primates. Both of these layers evolved long before the cerebral cortex, the cognitive brain that makes language and speech possible. It is likely that *body wisdom*, which is described in the Kripalu Yoga tradition as an instinctual intelligence common to both humans and animals, arises from the more primitive layers of the brain. Relying on higher cognitive faculties to decide what to eat or how to exercise may not be the best strategy, as they are often divorced from the body's basic needs.

meet the mix of biological, psychological, and social needs we face daily. But if you are cut off from the simple and direct wisdom of your own body, you have lost an important compass on the journey toward greater health and wellness.

Body Wisdom or Habit?

While we like to emphasize our capacity for free will, humans are largely creatures of habit. We easily become accustomed to routines and rituals. Past choices become inclinations, which grow into unconscious rules for living, and ultimately become ingrained habits. Habit is not by nature a negative force. Habits are efficient, a kind of automatic pilot that helps us maneuver through life without actually thinking our way through each and every action. But habit also drives us to repeat actions over and over again, so that we become dull to the moment and caught in ruts of self-destructive behavior.

Listening to body wisdom will compel you to closely examine your habits. The first habits you are likely to encounter are your so-called bad habits, the ways you repeatedly act to undermine your health and vitality. The most effective way to break any habit is to establish a new one. Attuning to body wisdom, you can explore positive routines that support your health. Most people discover they thrive within a schedule of work, exercise, meals, and rest.

EXPERIENCE: ACCESSING BODY WISDOM

- Bring yourself present in your body: breathe, relax, feel, watch, and allow.
- Let your attention drop from the head into your belly. Rest the attention there for a few deep breaths and then feel the awareness spread out until it permeates each and every cell.
- Attuning to the felt sense of your body, ask what it needs right now. If body wisdom is obvious, move to the next step. If not, consider the following and notice your body's response:

  Is any part of your body tense?
  If so, how can you move to release it?
  Is your body too hot or too cold?
  Does it need something to eat or drink?
  Is it time for a stretch or bathroom break?
  Does your body need exercise or rest?
  What is your body asking for right now?

- Resist any tendency to try to understand or make sense of sensations and urges. Just feel them and allow the knowing that comes with them to surface in your conscious awareness.
- Give yourself what you need. Don't skip this step! Responding to body wisdom builds self-trust.

Regular mealtimes are especially important, as they lend a rhythm to the body's major tasks of food intake, digestion, and elimination. Finding balance and maintaining it over time is no small feat in today's fast-paced world, and moving from here to there takes self-discipline and a willingness to go through the process of change. Once established, a healthy routine will feel just as natural as your former, less-supportive habits.

Eventually body wisdom will lead you to confront your so-called good habits. While the body likes positive routines, it also needs flexibility and a willingness on your part to be spontaneous. After a few weeks of enjoying a workout before dinner, you may come home from a difficult day and want to take a nap. Your body is not a machine; its needs change from day to day. Routines are best held lightly and must be free to evolve. Body wisdom does not lead you to become a health nut or exercise fanatic; it bestows an ability to sense actual needs. The supportive lifestyle that results is a middle path that allows for structure and spontaneity.

Although it might not sound that way, learning to hear and honor the wisdom of your body is very different than giving in to all your desires. It is a process of growing in self-awareness, observing the consequences that flow from your actions, and strengthening your ability to make conscious choices. As you learn to discriminate between body wisdom and habit, you are free to live with a greater degree of self-trust.

NAVIGATING THE JOURNEY OF CHANGE

Awareness is the first step in lifestyle change. Feelings and insights that arise during yoga practice are important signposts, but life provides constant opportunities to see yourself and grow in self-awareness. As you attune to where you are right now, you often have a strong sense of the direction you want to move.

Acceptance is being at peace with however you are showing up in the moment. Acceptance frees up the energy required to change. Judging yourself for not being better only undermines self-esteem and drains energy. Without acceptance, there is little possibility for true change and absolutely none for enjoying the process.

Adjustment is making a desired lifestyle change to enhance well-being. Start with easy-to-accomplish adjustments you find pleasant. Inspired by success, you will naturally move on to areas of greater challenge. Avoid the trap of wanting to change everything overnight, or feeling that the changes required are so great that it is not even worth starting. The secret to long lasting change is gradual adjustments over time.

Conscious Eating

Learning to eat well is perhaps the most powerful thing you can do to improve your quality of life. It is common knowledge that diet either lowers or raises your risk of major diseases, including type 2 (adult-onset) diabetes, hypertension, heart disease, osteoporosis, strokes, and cancer. Research suggests that diet may also play a role in Alzheimer's and other forms of dementia. Along with preventing future problems, the immediate benefits of eating well are apparent minutes after a meal. You feel better in your body and that good feeling stays with you for hours afterward. Kripalu Yoga's approach to eating well is based on three principles: conscious eating, making healthy food choices, and eating moderately.

Conscious eating is the practice of being present and paying attention to the act of

CONSCIOUS EATING BASICS

- Before eating, take a few deep breaths, relax the body, and be grateful for the food before you.
- Eat slowly and chew your food thoroughly.
- Savor all the sights, smells, and taste sensations.
- Maintain a relaxed and peaceful attitude.
- Change your diet gradually.

nourishing yourself. When hungry, we all have a tendency to enter a feeding frenzy and wolf down our food, which tends to fill the belly but leaves other needs unsatisfied. Each meal offers an opportunity to slow down, breathe, choose your food, and enjoy the sensual experience of eating. Take the time required to set aside other tasks and be conscious of what you are doing. Chew your food thoroughly and savor all the taste sensations. Chewing is essential to healthy digestion. It mixes food with the digestive enzymes contained in saliva. It also mechanically breaks food down to a form that can pass easily through the stomach and intestines, easing the burden of digestion and enhancing the absorption of nutrients.

Your state of mind also plays an important role in eating well. Anxiety and worry inhibit the digestive process. Being grateful you have food to eat helps maintain a peaceful attitude, minimizing stress and maximizing blood flow to the abdominal organs. Because it takes the body about twenty minutes to register that it's full, slowing down to eat consciously is a big help in portion control.

The topic of diet is a maze in which even the most intelligent person can get lost.

— Swami Kripalu

What to Eat

Given that humans have been feeding themselves for a few hundred thousand years, it is baffling that the question of what foods to eat in what proportions remains so controversial. Recent studies indicate that genetics play a crucial role in healthy food choice, and that it is the interaction of foods and genetic makeup that determines whether a particular diet meets an individual's needs. Based on its experiments, the Kripalu ashram community came to a similar conclusion: dietary needs vary widely among individuals. After this insight, the ashram kitchen stopped serving any particular diet in the late 1980s, focusing instead on offering a broad range of foods and dishes that residents could choose from to meet their individual needs.

Dietary systems can play an important

role in helping you learn more about the relationship between food and health. They can lend you a fresh perspective on food choices, wean you from what you have grown accustomed to, and help you change habits that no longer serve you. In the final analysis, your body—and only your body—remains the ultimate authority. Experts, no matter how gifted, can only teach you what has worked for them or others. With that proviso, Kripalu Yoga embraces a short list of dietary principles:

- Eat foods in their whole and natural state. Avoid refined and processed foods, which tend to have more chemical additives and far less nutritional value.

- Avoid saturated fats, which are known to contribute to heart disease, and partially hydrogenated oils and trans-fatty acids. The oils found in vegetables, nuts, and fish are healthy when eaten in moderation.

- Eat plenty of fresh fruits and vegetables. Organic produce lowers the amount of pesticides, fertilizers, and other agricultural chemicals you take into your body.

- Limit your intake of sugar, which for some people triggers mood and energy swings and has an addictive quality. Sugar consumption places a burden on the pancreas and raises the risk of adult-onset diabetes, obesity, and heart disease. Although alternatives like honey, rice and barley malts, molasses, and raw cane juice may provide certain trace minerals, they are all sugars converted to glucose by the body.

- Eat low on the food chain. As you go up the food chain from plants to vegetarian animals to predatory animals, concentrations of harmful chemicals and antibiotics increase.

While working to improve your diet, expect to encounter the emotional and mental patterns that lie beneath your eating habits. Our preferences for certain foods get established in childhood, at a time when food is equated with love and acceptance. As body image becomes an important part of our identity, food can become an area of conflict and confusion. It is impossible to make lasting changes to your eating habits without healing your relationship with food.

The questions I hear most often about diets are: "What should I eat? Which is the best diet to follow?" Behind these questions is the assumption that there is a perfect diet. We take a biological drive that says, "I must eat in the best way possible because a balanced diet is essential for health," and twist it into, "I must eat a perfect diet." Perfect dieters often discuss their way of thinking and eating in much the same way as religious fundamentalists air their doctrines. Instead of using food to celebrate life and share with others, food becomes a source of alienation.

—Marc David,
Nutritionist

To Be or Not to Be Vegetarian

In accord with the principle of nonviolence, the traditional yoga diet is vegetarian, usually with the inclusion of dairy products. There are many good reasons to be vegetarian, the most obvious being that it is a commercial vote against animal cruelty. It also minimizes the damage done to the earth to create grazing land for cattle and helps conserve the considerable resources consumed by factory farming. Because meat production is relatively inefficient and entails feeding grains and legumes to cattle and other animals, vegetarians claim they help make more food available to satisfy world hunger.

Despite these virtues, it is important to recount the actual experience of hundreds of residents with the ashram's strictly vegetarian diet. With spending money scarce, most residents lacked the ability to supplement their diet with restaurant meals or trips to the supermarket. Eating an exclusively vegetarian diet supported a healthy process of physical cleansing over the first few years of residency. As more time passed, it became apparent that the ashram's diet was not meeting the needs of a significant number of individuals. Diagnosed by both alternative and allopathic health care practitioners, common problems included inadequate protein assimilation, certain vitamin and other deficiencies, and intense carbohydrate or sweet cravings. Former residents will remember with amusement the aberrant behaviors evident on "dessert night." As time passed, more and more people were granted special dispensation to eat fish or chicken. Today many former residents continue to practice yoga and eat a plant-based diet, but surprisingly few are vegetarian. As a result of this ashram experience, Kripalu Yoga acknowledges that even conscious people aspiring to eat ethically make different food choices, eating at different places on the food chain.

> *Soon after I began yoga, I found myself becoming a vegetarian without much drama or struggle. I had some close relatives who'd died of colon cancer, and for health reasons I'd been eating less meat anyway. Cutting out meat altogether simply felt like the next step. Over time, that evolved into a vegan diet as I let go of eating any animal products at all. There were forays into Macrobiotics, and into what my husband jokingly called the "no-nothing diet"—no oil, no sweeteners, no salt, no flour. Each experiment with diet had pluses and minuses. What I discovered was that diets were healthy for brief periods, as eating narrowly helped my body detox and cleanse. But rigid ways of eating weren't healthy for me in the long run. After many years of being a strict vegetarian, the diet left me with little energy. I began eating fish again and my body sang, grew stronger, and my energy level soared. Letting go of fixed concepts around diet seems to be part of the path, at least for me.*
>
> —Danna Faulds

SWAMI KRIPALU ON MITAHAR

Mitahar, or moderation in diet, is a foundation of spiritual progress in yoga. Mitahar is eating a wholesome diet in the amount required to keep the body healthy and mind happy. In the same way that an instrument gives music when its strings are tuned neither too tightly nor too loosely, the amount of food should be regulated. Undereating leads to physical weakness and eventual binges. Overeating leads to dullness and eventual disease. Moderation in diet gives rise to alertness, strength, and health.

Many people mistakenly believe that eating moderately means taking only a small, fixed quantity of food per day. When an elephant and ant decide what is moderation, their portions will definitely be different! If a person exercises a little, his appetite is naturally reduced, so he should eat less. On days when he exercises a lot, his appetite is increased, so he should eat more. Young people are growing and active and require more food. Elderly people tend to be less active and eat less. Appetite can also increase or decrease based on one's emotions, for the body and mind are so intricately related. What is moderate eating will differ from one person to another.

Prolonged fasting and dieting purifies the body but also weakens it. Because the attraction to food increases day by day, fasters often do not maintain control of their appetite and tend to resume old patterns of eating. Where abstinence requires suppression, mitahar is a path of moderation that requires discrimination and restraint.

Moderation in diet is easier said than done. If a delicious dish is placed in front of a brilliant orator preaching about the virtues of mitahar, he will want to stop and not resume talking until he has finished eating. If you desire health, happiness, and success in life, learn to eat moderately.

Moderate Eating

Eating too little deprives the body of what it needs, slowing metabolism and leaching minerals. Overeating smothers the digestive fires and produces a buildup of toxic wastes in the system. A person who eats moderately strikes a balance between these extremes by ingesting an amount of food they can easily digest. Traditional yoga texts define moderation as filling half the stomach with food, one-fourth with water, and leaving one-fourth empty.

The tendency to overeat is rooted in humankind's evolutionary past. For the bulk of human history, food was at times abundant and other times scarce. Fat reserves had survival value, helping people live through famine. Although times have changed and food is now plentiful for most of us, our minds and appetites haven't quite caught up. Where many of the health problems that once plagued humans were related to food scarcity, the problems now prevalent in developed countries are diseases of excess.

While food fuels the body with needed calories, it also requires a substantial investment of energy to digest. Eating heavily burdens the body with the task of digestion and elimination, causing you to expend as much energy as you gain in the process and stockpiling extra calories in fat. By eating moderately, or slightly less than your digestive capacity, you derive a net gain of energy and eliminate wastes effectively.

While learning how to eat moderately is admittedly a challenge, it is much more than an exercise in abstinence and self-deprivation. Eating moderately makes you feel better, look better, sleep deeper, and live longer. When you are established in the practice, moderate eating is significantly more pleasurable than overeating. It satisfies you in the moment, and ensures that come time for the next meal you will be hungry. If you stay attuned to body wisdom, it will teach you how to celebrate life and food without eating to excess.

Let the yogi eat moderately. Otherwise, no matter how clever, he cannot attain success.

—Siva Samhita

My journey to a healthier lifestyle started in 1990, when I was thirty pounds heavier. I began working with diet, and then dug out an old bike and pedaled to the end of my road and back. It was three miles, and I about died. So I began running and later added strength training. Eventually my efforts to achieve greater physical fitness brought yoga into my life, and I discovered a whole new world of psychological and spiritual growth to explore.

—Ken Cotton

Get Enough Exercise

Although yoga is often called "the most perfect form of exercise," the ashram experience suggests that a regular yoga practice may not satisfy all of your exercise needs. In many ways, the ashram was a temple of exercise. Rows of shiny bicycles hung neatly on hooks in the basement. A fully equipped weight room was in constant use. As lunchtime arrived, runners and walkers streamed out of their offices and onto the many woodland paths crisscrossing the Berkshire Hills. Others changed into sweats for spirited aerobic dance. In the heat of summer, a short bike ride to the lake followed by a long swim might be just the thing. While it was different strokes for different folks, virtually every ashram resident found the yoga lifestyle benefited from branching out to embrace other forms of exercise.

Some traditional yoga schools downplay the need for any activity beyond postures. Exercising to exhaustion is viewed as an unnecessary depletion of the body's vital energy. Repetitive movements like running are seen as stressing the joints and best avoided. Although it is true that postures can be practiced with sufficient intensity to strengthen the entire body and provide a cardiovascular workout, many people cannot practice with such intensity. It is also good to remember that the yogis of old ate sparingly. In addition to postures, they practiced intensive breathing exercises and spent hours in meditation as part of an overall contemplative lifestyle. While honoring anyone who chooses an exclusive focus on yoga techniques, the ashram experience indicates that the value of additional exercise far outweighs its detriments. The majority of today's Kripalu Yoga practitioners supplement their practice with some form of aerobic exercise. A smaller but still significant number feel a need for additional strength training, usually in the form of weight lifting. While offering a profound range of benefits, Kripalu Yoga considers postures one part of a holistic lifestyle.

I was an exercise enthusiast before the ashram. At first, I focused exclusively on learning the yoga and eventually being trained as a Kripalu Yoga teacher. After a while, I added jogging, swimming, and weights to my routine. Back then yoga experts said lifting would make you tight and hamper your practice, but I found weights helped me a lot with my poses. Truth is, I started swimming because the cars going to the pool were full of female residents and the drive provided time for joking and small talk, but I discovered that swimming also made my yoga deeper. Many years later, I firmly believe that yoga nurtures the joints and has prevented me from getting the knee, ankle, and other injuries that plague so many of my friends.

At 190 pounds, I was a heavyweight by ashram standards. I was a vegan, as were most residents, and was okay with the diet, but I remember finding tuna fish cans in the garbage. Looking back from the vantage point of a holistic health counselor, I see that some of the residents were having problems. I remain a vegan, although if taken out to dinner will go for a salmon steak without showing any mercy on the other person's wallet. I am also careful to supplement my diet with Spirulina, seaweed, minerals, enzymes, and B vitamins.

It was at Kripalu that I met Bikram Choudhury and was exposed to his yoga sequence, which is done in a heated room. This is a more masculine, athletic, grunt and groan style of yoga that appealed to me immediately. I now teach Bikram yoga, but I also bring my Kripalu background into the room. I like to think this adds a little more heart and soul to Bikram Yoga, without taking anything away from its essence.

—Viraj Nelson Santini

Rest for the Weary

Accustomed as we are to burning the candle at both ends, it can be challenging to make the adjustments required to get enough sleep. During sleep the body is freed from other responsibilities to focus its full energies on the tasks associated with health maintenance and healing. Sleep is the time when children grow. Similarly, it is during sleep, and other times of rest and retreat, that adults heal and transform. As science studies sleep and dreaming, a growing body of research is making the connection between inadequate sleep and conditions such as adult-onset diabetes, hypertension, obesity, impaired immune response, mood disorders, and poor cognitive function.

Some traditional yoga schools downplay the need for sleep in favor of nocturnal meditation, going so far as to label sleep as "unspiritual" and saying that realized beings have no need for sleep. This was not the approach of ashram residents, who "laid their body down on the altar of sleep" each night, or for Swami Kripalu, who spent ten hours a day in meditation but also got a good night's sleep each night.

Although the ashram was decidedly an "early to bed and early to rise" community, it is worth noting that a sizable number of resi-

SLEEP AND WEIGHT LOSS

You might wonder how sleep could have anything to do with weight loss or obesity. During sleep, the endocrine system secretes a wide range of hormones that regulate various physiological processes. One of these hormones is leptin, which tells the body when it should feel full and thus directly influences appetite and weight. The inability to sleep deeply may play a role in some forms of binge eating, as lower leptin levels can make a person crave carbohydrates regardless of the number of calories consumed. Similarly, some connective tissues only heal in deep sleep, and chronic soreness or joint pain can also result from sleep disorders.

dents could never get the swing of this schedule. For many years, this was seen as a moral failure and many people flunked out of the ashram because they just couldn't drag themselves out of bed for yoga before dawn. Eventually it became obvious that they just weren't morning people. Many people find that practicing yoga in the afternoons is more enjoyable and better for their bodies.

The Power of Community

In its quest to pioneer a new approach to holistic health and spiritual growth, the ashram engendered a magical feeling of community. It was powerful to be surrounded by other people of like heart and mind, mirroring each other in authentic relationship, and sharing a commitment to healing and growth. In recent decades, the power of support groups to help people survive and recover from major illness has grown apparent to physicians, psychologists, and social workers. It stands to reason that if a strong community helps you heal, it can also help you stay healthy and happy in the first place.

When it comes to creating the balance of work, rest, play, and spiritual attunement that makes for a great lifestyle, the ashram taught that "company is stronger than willpower." People who practice yoga tend to have a lot in common. You might find "your ashram" and a potent source of inspiration and support among the people gathered in a weekly yoga class.

> *My first Kripalu Yoga class opened a window to my life. For the first time, I became embodied. I understood that my body has a wisdom of its own beyond that of my analyzing brain. For a brief moment, everything made sense and all the pieces that I'd tried to get together for years were united. Of course, my problems weren't solved, but I got a glimpse of who I really am, and a sense of possibility that I could get there.*
>
> —Jennifer Cann

CHAPTER TEN

WORKING WITH PROBLEM AREAS

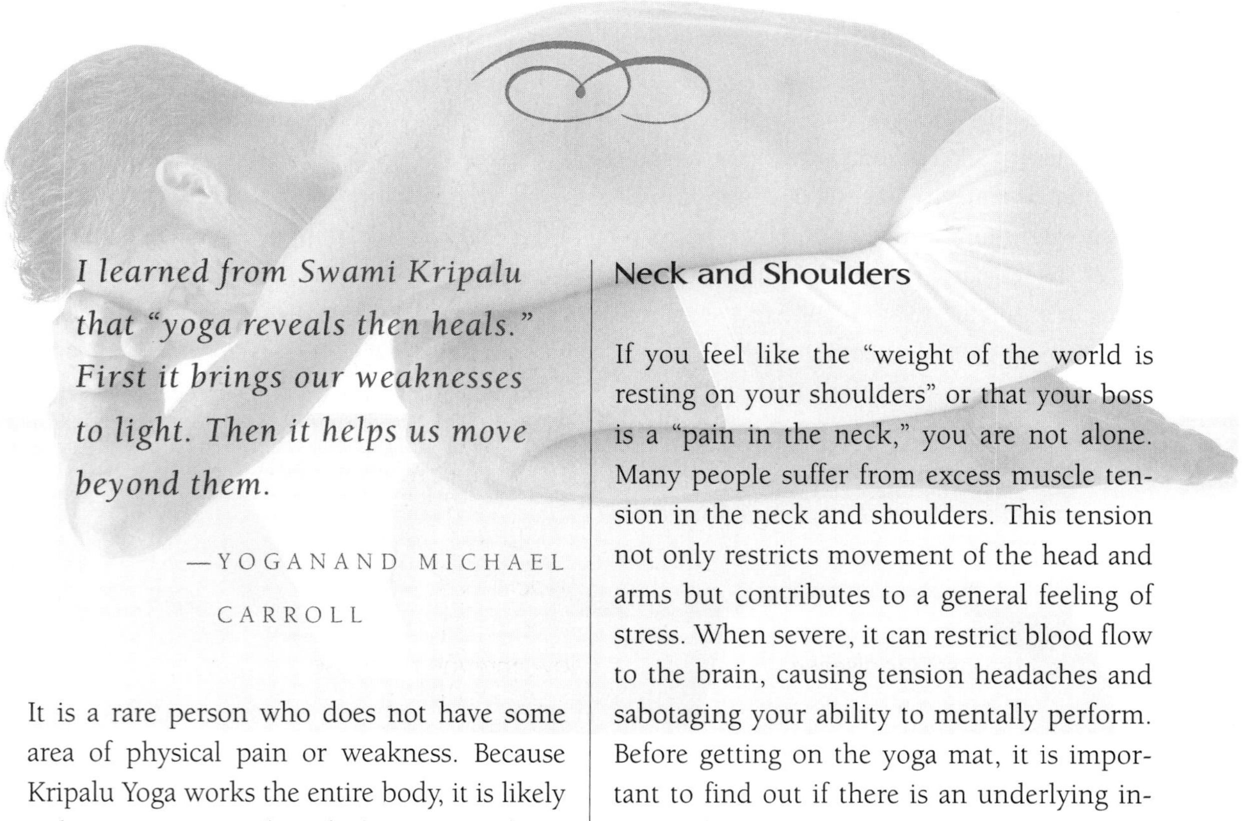

I learned from Swami Kripalu that "yoga reveals then heals." First it brings our weaknesses to light. Then it helps us move beyond them.

—YOGANAND MICHAEL CARROLL

It is a rare person who does not have some area of physical pain or weakness. Because Kripalu Yoga works the entire body, it is likely to bring you in touch with those parts of you that work less than perfectly. Here are some tips to help you work successfully with your problem areas and other health challenges.

Neck and Shoulders

If you feel like the "weight of the world is resting on your shoulders" or that your boss is a "pain in the neck," you are not alone. Many people suffer from excess muscle tension in the neck and shoulders. This tension not only restricts movement of the head and arms but contributes to a general feeling of stress. When severe, it can restrict blood flow to the brain, causing tension headaches and sabotaging your ability to mentally perform. Before getting on the yoga mat, it is important to find out if there is an underlying injury, often some damage to the cervical vertebrae or rotator cuff. If there is numbness or tingling in the arms or hands, sharp or immobilizing pain in the neck or shoulders, see a physician to make sure that yoga does not aggravate your condition.

Once a serious condition has been ruled out, yoga practice is an effective way to work with chronic neck and shoulder tension. The neck connects the head to the shoulders and upper back through a complex network of vertebrae, muscles, and connective tissues. While a multitude of muscles working in concert with the small cervical vertebrae allows the head a wide range of movement, it also makes the neck prone to muscular imbalances and joint misalignments. This can lead to postural asymmetry, such as habitually leaning the head to one side, which eventually causes painful muscle spasms as the neck muscles—instead of the vertebrae—strain to support the weight of the head. Because numerous nerves and blood vessels pass through the neck, spinal alignment is essential for the proper functioning of the brain. Misalignments can pinch nerves and strain other delicate structures, negatively affecting the function of the entire body.

CONDITIONS PROVEN TO BENEFIT FROM YOGA AND MEDITATION

The healing power of yoga and mindfulness meditation is now being scientifically studied in India, the United States, and Europe. Current research suggests that yoga and meditation are beneficial for the following conditions:

- anxiety
- arthritis
- asthma
- cardiovascular disease
- carpal tunnel syndrome
- chronic pain
- depression
- diabetes
- epilepsy
- fibromyalgia
- headaches
- hypertension
- infertility for women
- low immune response
- multiple sclerosis
- obesity
- premenstrual syndrome (PMS)
- psoriasis
- sleep disorders
- stress

While needing to be flexible to provide for arm movement, the shoulders must also be strong. These contradictory functions make its structure complex and prone to imbalance and injury. Holding one shoulder higher than the other, or keeping the shoulders lifted up by the ears in a chronic "startle response" are common types of shoulder asymmetry. While the startle response may be an understandable reaction to a particular situation, chronic asymmetry indicates that the muscles have become accustomed to the imbalance and require some form of therapeutic movement or massage to return to balance.

Neck and shoulder tension is released through the basic yoga approach of gentle stretching accompanied by deep breathing and relaxation. As in all postures, heed the message of pain while exploring areas of discomfort. If your neck or shoulder condition is not remedied by basic practices like those in the following experience, consider consulting a yoga therapist, chiropractor, or other health professional.

You may have noticed that this book does not include the Headstand, Full Shoulderstand, or Plough Poses. These postures require the relatively small cervical vertebrae to bear a significant portion of the body's weight. Misalignments of the cervical vertebrae, or simply doing the posture over time, can lead to injury. Do not practice Headstand, Shoulderstand, or Plough without personal guidance from a qualified teacher.

In January 1988 I slipped on black ice and hit the back of my head on an outdoor slate stairway. I suffered cognitive problems including a short-term memory loss, completely lost my sense of smell, and could barely taste my food. A pinched nerve on the left side of my neck led to a frozen left shoulder. I could barely turn my head and was able to lift my arms only a little distance from my sides. Fatigued all the time, I became quite depressed. My doctors said I would never recover my sense of smell or taste, and recommended arthroscopic shoulder surgery. I tried acupuncture, chiropractic, physical therapy, and cortisone shots, but nothing helped.

At the suggestion of a friend, I tried Kripalu Yoga. I did what I could within my limited range of motion. It wasn't always comfortable but it made me feel better. I decided to do yoga every day and see where that took me. After six months, the range of motion in my neck and shoulders was almost back to normal. My energy and state of mind had also improved considerably. Six years after the accident, my sense of smell surprisingly returned and food tastes good again. I am now a Kripalu Yoga teacher and Phoenix Rising Yoga therapist. My range of motion and energy have never been better, and I love my life more than I ever thought possible.

—Anne Harris

EXPERIENCE: YOGA AT YOUR DESK

Here's a routine for the neck and shoulders that's a great work break. It can be done sitting or standing.

1. Sit or stand tall. Take a deep breath in. As you exhale, let the chin slowly drop toward the chest, stretching out the back of the neck.

2. Inhale the head back to the starting position and then lift the chin, looking up toward the ceiling. Keep the neck elongated and do not let the neck collapse and head drop back. Repeat this up and down movement several times, inhaling the chin up and exhaling it down. End by bringing the head back to center.

3. Take a deep breath in. As you exhale, lower the right ear toward the right shoulder, feeling the stretch on the left side of the neck. Inhale the head back to center. As you exhale, lower the left ear toward the left shoulder, feeling the stretch on the right side of the neck. Repeat this side-to-side motion several times, coordinating breath and movement. End by returning back to center.

4. Tuck the chin slightly and extend through the crown to elongate the neck. Take a deep breath in. As you exhale, rotate the head to look over the right shoulder, keeping the chin parallel to the floor and feeling the stretch to the neck muscles. The shoulders continue to face forward and the trunk does not rotate. Inhale back to center. As you exhale, turn the head to look over the left shoulder. Repeat this twisting motion several times, exhaling as you twist and inhaling back to center. End by bringing the head back to center and taking a moment to feel and relax the muscles of the neck.

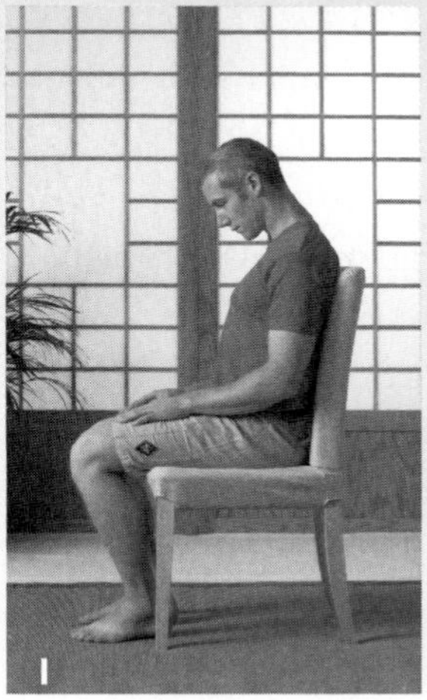

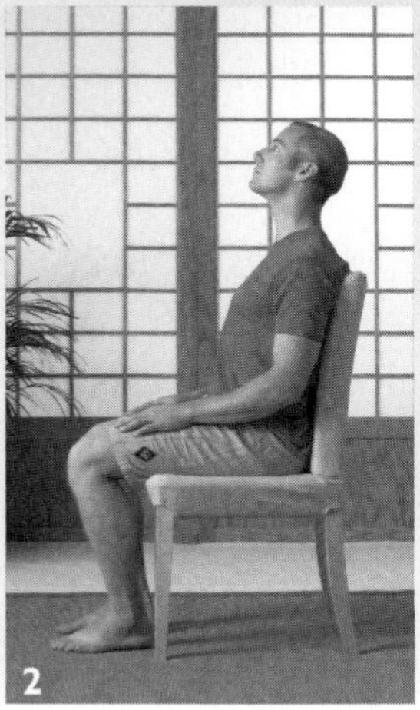

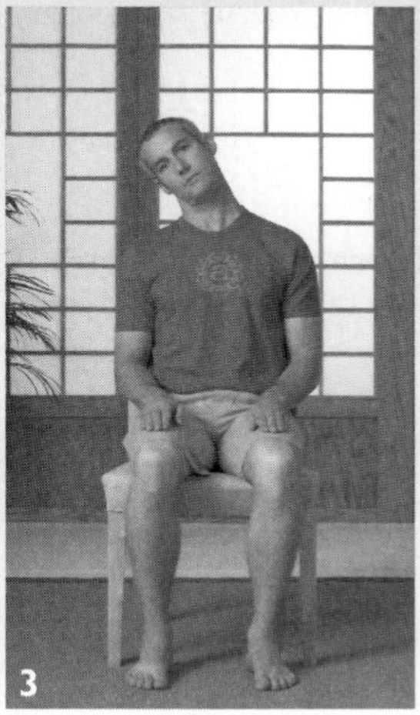

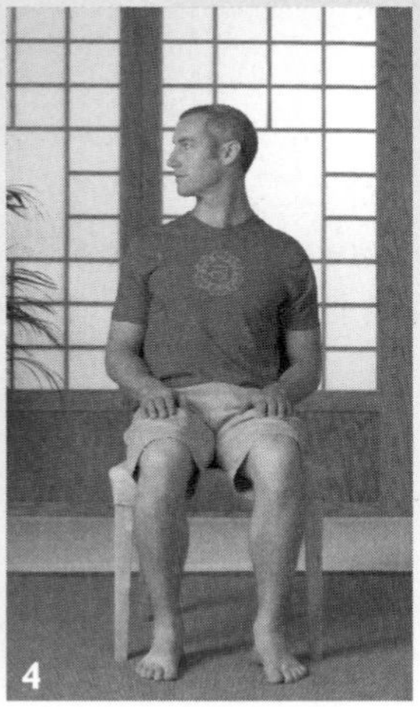

5. Take a deep breath in as you lift the shoulders up toward the ears. Hold the breath for several seconds, lifting the shoulders high, and then exhale with an audible sigh, allowing the shoulders to drop back down. Repeat several times.

6. Begin to circle the shoulders, rolling them forward, up, back, and down. Repeat several times, keeping the breath moving and letting the circles gradually grow wider. Pause and begin to circle the shoulders in the opposite direction, starting small and letting the circles gradually grow larger.

7. End by returning to an erect sitting or standing position. Let the tops of the shoulders drop away from the ears and the shoulder blades move down and back. Tuck the chin slightly and extend through the crown to elongate the neck. Rest for a minute or two in Mountain or Sitting Mountain, letting the breath flow freely.

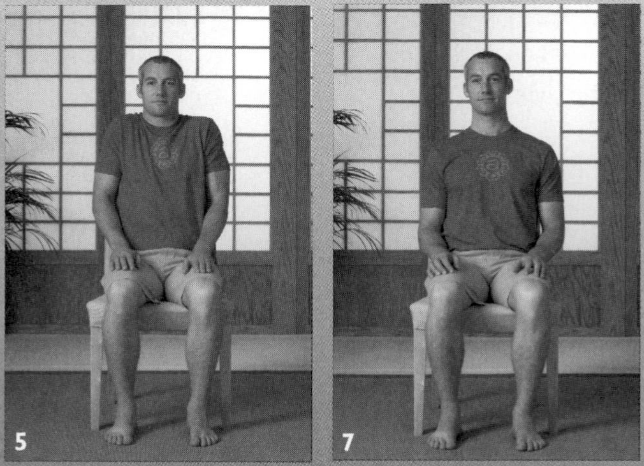

Working with the Abdomen

The abs are actually four different muscles. The *rectus abdominus* is the muscle closest to the surface, extending up the front of the body from the pubic bone to the sternum. A toned rectus abdominus will give you "six-pack" or "washboard" abs, but only if you are fortunate to have the genes that produce the "thin skin" look. When the rectus abdominus contracts, it draws the sternum toward the pubic bone to flex the trunk and helps you sit up or lie back. The *internal* and *external obliques* are a paired set of muscles that attach to the pelvic crest and ribs. The obliques help flex the trunk and rotate the spine. As the obliques are toned, the waistline gets smaller. The *transverse abdominus* is a deep muscle that wraps around the torso like a corset and attaches to the spine. A toned transverse abdominus stabilizes the spine, aids in elimination, and flattens the belly.

The abdominal muscles play numerous roles critical to health. They assist in respiration, protect the vital organs, keep the spine erect and aligned, protect the low back, and allow for the full and free movement of the torso and limbs. A healthy abdomen is strong, flexible, and responsive. Strength is required to fulfill its structural purpose of supporting the spine and torso through a broad range of movements. Flexibility is needed for fluid and graceful movement that originates from the body's center of gravity just below the navel. A healthy abdomen is also responsive to the needs of the moment. In moments of stillness and relaxation, the belly is soft and the breath can flow freely. When needed to initiate or brace movement, the abdomen contracts to support movement and quickly returns to a relaxed state without residual tension.

When working with the abdomen, it is necessary to do a series of different exercises that stretch and strengthen its complex of muscles. Resist the common tendency to overdo a single movement, often sit-ups or crunches, both of which are frequently criticized for straining the low back and neck. When not coupled with other exercises that strengthen the back and other muscles of the torso in a balanced fashion, intensive abdominal strengthening can shorten the muscles and pull the pelvis out of alignment.

Kripalu Yoga does not aspire to produce "abs of steel," a phrase that all too often refers to a buffed set of abdominal muscles that are chronically tight. Along with being the structural center of the body, the belly is also the body's feeling center. A relaxed belly helps you stay connected to your emotions, whereas chronic abdominal tension is a form of body armoring that blocks the ability to feel.

Back in 1997, I developed symptoms I now know as multiple sclerosis. For most of my life, I set demanding standards for myself and struggled to live up to them. Having MS destroyed the illusion that I was ever as in charge of my life as I thought. In the face of things beyond my control, yoga keeps me steady and mitigates the effects of stress, which really aggravates MS.

Leading MS researchers and physicians agree exercise is an underutilized strategy in the treatment of MS. Through some mechanism not yet understood, exercise rewires the brain and restores function. Because it is a comprehensive approach to well-being, yoga is widely regarded as one of the best forms of exercise for people with MS, a view confirmed by recent studies.

In addition to keeping me healthy, Kripalu Yoga has given me tools to help others. Working one-on-one with people with MS, many of whom were disabled and homebound, led a chapter of the National MS Society to sponsor my specialized classes. Now I've branched out to help people with all sorts of health challenges, from children with autism to people with heart problems to seniors who are regaining mobility after knee and hip replacements.

EXPERIENCE: MASSAGING THE LOW BACK

If your low back is sensitive, pause between abdominal strengtheners, or any exercises done on the back, and do this nurturing movement that massages the muscles of the low back and helps keep the lumbar vertebrae aligned.

1. Lie on your back and bring the knees into the chest. Reach the arms around the knees, interlacing the fingers. Allow the knees to be spread and supported in the crooks of the arms. If comfortable, touch the sides of the big toes together.

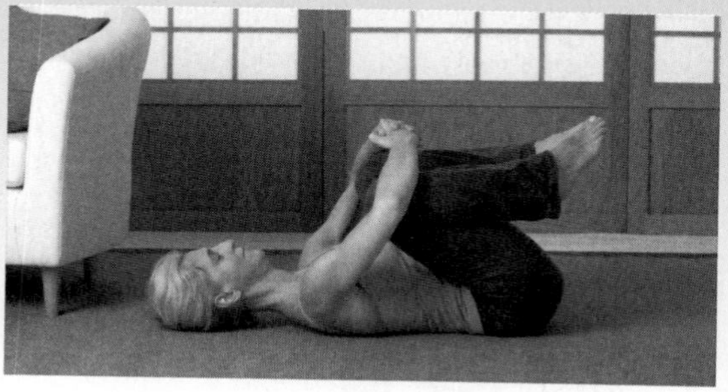

2. Slowly rock the right elbow and knee down a few inches toward the floor, and then back to center and rock the left elbow and knee a few inches toward the floor. Rock from side to side, gently massaging the muscles of the low back.

3. When your low back feels relaxed, move on to your next stretch or strengthener.

The message I give to each student is to honor what's happening in your body, know that there is no right way to be other than the way you are, and treat yourself with compassionate self-awareness. Grateful I am to have discovered yoga.

—Karen O'Donnell Clarke

Working with the Low Back

Half of all adults suffer bouts of low back pain in any given year. Despite its frequency, most low back pain is preventable. Between 70 and 90 percent of cases are caused by muscle or connective tissue strain, often stemming from weakness in the numerous muscles of the torso that attach to the vertebrae. In the past, bed rest was often prescribed as a treatment for acute back pain. Current research has shown that a targeted exercise program is the best treatment and defense against recurrence.

Contrary to conventional wisdom, low back pain is generally not a result of inflexibility. Exercises that strengthen and build endurance are more effective than stretching because they stabilize the spine, whereas increasing range of motion alone can be counterproductive. Unfortunately, no single exercise will do the job. Use a variety of exercises to gradually strengthen the muscles of the back, abdomen, hips, flanks, and chest. Exercises done from a neutral spine position—one in which the extremes of spinal flexion are avoided—are the safest because they maximize stability and minimize the risk of vertebral compression. To avoid strain, combine movements that strengthen with gentle movements that soothe and nurture.

BIRTHRIGHT

Despite illness of body or mind,
in spite of blinding despair or
habitual belief, who you are
is whole. Let nothing keep you
separate from the truth. The soul,
illumined from within, longs to
be known for what it is. Undying,
untouched by fire or the storms of
life, there is a place inside where
stillness and abiding peace reside.
You can ride the breath to go there.
Despite doubt or hopeless turns of
mind, you are not broken. Spirit
surrounds, embraces, fills you from
the inside out. Release everything
that isn't your true nature. What's
left, the fullness, light, and shadow,
claim all that as your birthright.

Both forward and backward bending can be a source of low back strain. However, if properly practiced, both movements are beneficial. In backbends, work to open the chest and arch the less flexible middle and upper spine. Avoid overstretching the low back, which arches back much more easily. Master the belly downs, especially Serpent and Sphinx, which use the floor to stabilize the low spine, and the Parabola, a standing backbend that teaches you how to properly bend backward. If you progress to deeper backbends such as the Camel and Wheel, listen to your body both during and after practice to make sure you are not overdoing it. Overstretching the low back is a frequent cause of lingering back pain for yoga enthusiasts. Although your low back may not hurt while doing the posture, skip the deeper backbends for a day or two and notice if the pain dissipates.

Begin your practice of forward bends from a standing position, which allows for a greater range of movement in the hips than sitting forward bends. Start with postures like Standing Angle or Pyramid with the legs spread wide, and avoid "toe touches" if your low back is sensitive. As you come forward, keep the knees slightly bent to release the hamstrings and avoid strain. Take care to keep the spine elongated by hinging forward from the hips, versus bending from the waist and rounding the lumbar spine. Support your weight by placing your hands on your thighs, shins, or the floor. As you move on to sitting forward bends, make sure to fully rotate the hip joints and resist the temptation to force yourself forward, another common way to overstretch the low back.

Ten years ago, the word balance *was not in my vocabulary. Working as a government affairs executive, I found myself*

YOGA AND CHRONIC PAIN

Interestingly enough, individuals suffering from chronic pain have been shown to benefit from using yoga and meditation practices that *increase* rather than dull sensitivity. Practice teaches them that pain is more than a physical sensation; it is a sensory experience steeped in emotion. Over time they learn to tease apart the sensation from its emotional overlay and to relax the associated muscle tension that aggravates pain. Although the physical sensations continue, many feel differently about them, and a high percentage find their pain becomes more bearable and much more manageable. Research continues to investigate whether regular practice may actually alter the neural pathways in ways that make pain more tolerable.

scrambling on a daily basis just to get by. I loved the work, but the time pressure, travel, and politics were taking a big toll. At this time, I had a lower back problem that my doctors were having difficulty treating. A friend told me about Kripalu Yoga, and I started taking classes with a local teacher. As I increased my yoga practice to three classes per week, my back pain stopped. Yoga opened my eyes in so many ways that changes just started happening. I saw there was so much more to me and life than being flat-out busy all the time. I came to realize that the lack of balance in my lifestyle was due to a lack of deeper meaning in my life.

—Sandy Weis

Along with muscular weakness, stress and emotional difficulties are believed to be significant factors in the onset of back pain. Deep breathing and relaxation techniques are proven ways to manage stress. A basic Kripalu Yoga practice includes all the elements recommended to prevent back pain. If you have a history of back problems, seek out a yoga therapist who can help you learn basic practices that help and do not hurt your low back.

Working with the Hips

The hip is a deep ball-and-socket joint structured to be strong and stable during standing, walking, and running. The upper leg bone, or *femur,* fits into the pelvis to form the hip joint.

EXPERIENCE: STRENGTHENING WITHOUT STRAIN

When your low back is sensitive, it is a challenge to strengthen the back muscles without straining them and compounding your problem. Belly down postures strengthen the paraspinal muscles that run up and down either side of the spine. In between a sequence of postures like the Serpent, Half Locust, and Boat, take a few moments to rest and do the following movements. Each gently releases sacrum and low back tension, helping to avoid strain.

1. Lie on your belly with your head turned to one side. Overlap the fingers to form a small pillow for your temple. Bend the legs at the knees and bring the shins perpendicular to the floor.

2. Wave the feet gently from side to side like windshield wipers. Feel the sensations of stretch and release in the sacrum and low back.

3. Then circle the feet, with the legs moving like the hands of a clock. The heels pass close by the buttocks and then farther away. Reverse direction of the circles.

4. Bring the feet back to center, and windshield wiper the feet in opposite directions, with the lower legs crossing one way and then the other.

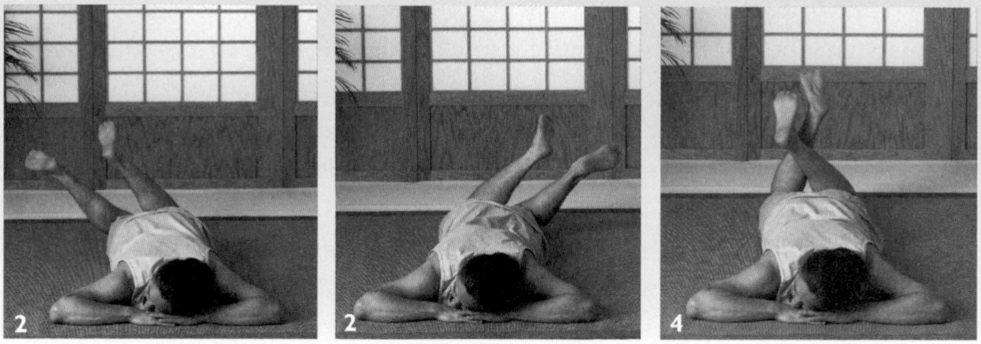

The femur is the longest and heaviest bone in the human body, and the hip is surrounded by a thick webbing of muscle and connective tissue that attaches the torso to the legs. Because of its heavy structure, it is not uncommon for the range of motion in the hips and legs to become limited by prolonged sitting and a sedentary lifestyle. When the muscles and connective tissues surrounding the hips are short and inflexible, they tend to pull the pelvis out of alignment, which causes muscle tension and pain in the hips or low back. Yoga is highly effective at restoring mobility in the hips. As with other conditions, it is wise to rule out any serious injuries such as arthritis, torn cartilage, or strained ligaments before beginning a practice.

A basic yoga routine such as the Sun or Moon Series will stretch and strengthen the muscles supporting the hip joint. If your hips are tight, it is advisable to work out the tension with gentle stretches done on the floor, where the hip is not required to bear significant weight. Slow and steady movements, repeated numerous times, are best. Begin with Inverted Frog as presented on page 207, then explore Happy Baby and Figure Four before Squat and Frog. As your hips open, you can move deeper into standing postures like Standing Squat, Goddess, Warrior, and Side Warrior that articulate the hip joint while stretching and strengthening the surrounding musculature.

Many yoga teachers feel that the pelvis and hips are places where repressed emotions and unresolved traumas are stored in the body. Because muscle tension and pain in the hips may have an emotional component of which you are unaware, be especially present to feeling as you open the hips.

I have always loved sports and vigorous activities like rock climbing, whitewater kayaking, backpacking, and backcountry skiing. In 1994, all this was suddenly taken away from me. I aggravated an old athletic injury to my left hip. The joint became severely arthritic, and within a year my once fluid and flexible body became twisted and hardened in a fruitless effort to escape the pain. Unable to walk more than a few steps, the wild places I loved became a distant memory. The life-energy that raced through me in torrents, like water in a mountain stream, slowed to a mere trickle. It took nine years of imprisonment in my body for me to realize that my only real option was hip-replacement surgery.

The surgery took all of one hour and twenty minutes. I was fifty-nine years old and my injured left side was considerably atrophied from years of compensation and neglect. Yoga practice flooded my starved tissues with life force, hastening not just my physical healing but also a return to normalcy in other facets of my life. I could actually feel how the yoga was untwisting and unwinding the frozen knot my body had become. As my body became softer and more malleable through the yoga, so did my mind. I found myself becoming the playful and enthusiastic person I had been before my ordeal began. It was only a matter of time before I was able to wholeheartedly shout from a mountaintop: "Free at last! Free at last! Praise God Almighty—I am free at last!"

—Dan Gryte

EXPERIENCE: OPENING THE HIPS WITH INVERTED FROG

The following series gently but effectively opens the hips and prepares you for deeper hip stretches.

1. Lie on your back with the knees drawn into the chest. Place the hands on the kneecaps.

2. Let the knees move out to the sides and begin to make small circles. Allow the movement to come from the hips, but steer the knees with the hands, lending the coordination of your hands to the less developed neural pathways of the hips. Moving slowly and smoothly, gradually allow the circles to grow wider.

3. Pause and begin to circle the knees in the opposite direction, starting small and letting the circles gradually grow wider. You will notice that this movement uses a totally different set of muscles. End by coming back to center.

4. Let the knees fall out to the sides, opening the hips and stretching the groin. Slide the hands down to hold the shins, and press the knees gently away to straighten the arms and deepen the stretch. This is Inverted Frog Pose. Breathe deeply as you hold.

5. Bring the knees back to center, and stretch the legs out into Corpse Pose. Take a deep breath in, and on the exhale let the whole body sink into the support of the floor.

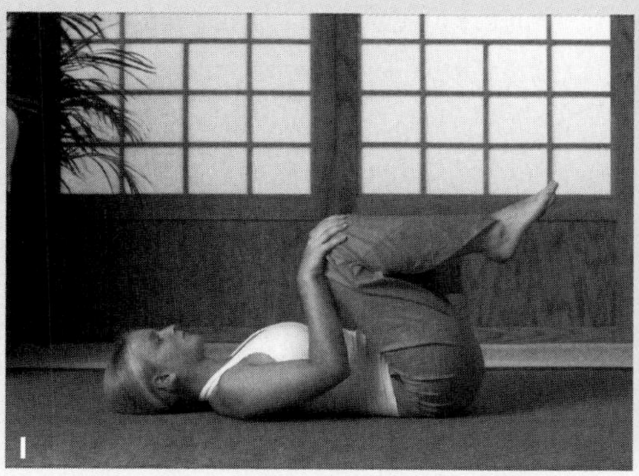

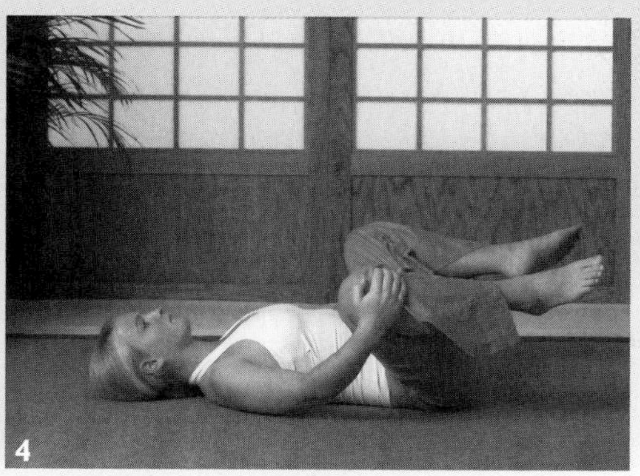

Working with the Knees

Many people come to yoga as a fitness alternative to running or other forms of high-impact aerobics that can cause or aggravate knee problems. Although it may look like a simple hinge, the knee is a complex joint that relies on an impressive combination of muscles, ligaments, tendons, and cushioning cartilage for stability. Strengthening the muscles and connective tissues that surround the knee, especially the thigh muscle or quadriceps, is the recommended way to stabilize the knee joint. Those with knee injuries may benefit from supplementing their yoga with strength training exercises aimed at the quadriceps.

Movements that tend to torque the knee, encouraging the knee joint to twist or move side to side, are to be avoided. So is hyperextending the knees, which happens to some people's joints when they lock their knees. While it is fine to keep the knees slightly bent while performing the standing postures, remember to press the feet into the floor to engage the muscles of the legs that support the knee joint. The Tree, Crane, and other one-legged standing poses are great ways to strengthen the legs. While doing them, press the four corners of the standing foot firmly into the floor while tightly contracting the quadriceps of the standing leg.

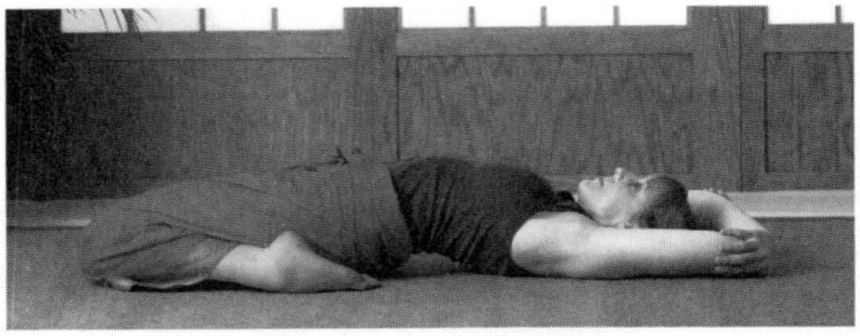

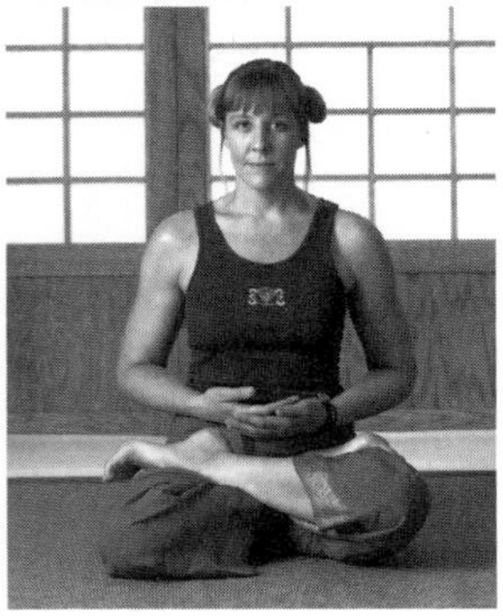

Hurdler's Stretch (Supta Vajrasana) and the Lotus are both classic yoga postures that present a real risk of knee injury.

This book does not provide instructions for the Full Lotus Pose, which is seen by many as a symbol of adeptness in yoga. Many newcomers to yoga injure their knees, in particular the delicate meniscus cartilage, by straining to get into Lotus before they have developed the requisite hip flexibility. Lotus Pose is not for everyone, and deep states of meditation can be attained without it.

> *I was diagnosed with arthritis and depression in the spring of 1998. Just walking made my bones ache inside and out. I was on pain pills, antidepressants, and arthritis medication. A friend told me that her Kripalu Yoga class was really good, so I decided to give it a try. I loved the combination of a workout coupled with breath and relaxation. My yoga teacher taught me a special series for my joints, and I began practicing it on my own at home and also added meditation. By fall, my spirits had lifted and I no longer needed any pain or arthritis medication. Yoga helped me feel playful and happy to be alive again.*
>
> —Karrie Vanderwarker

CAUTIONS AND CONTRAINDICATIONS

- *Glaucoma, detached retina, conjunctivitis, or other eye disorders*: Do not practice inverted postures because they increase eye pressure and can cause injury. This includes any posture in which the head is placed below the heart.
- *Back pain*: While yoga is a good treatment for many back problems, back pain can be a symptom of a wide variety of health conditions. Consult a physician rather than assuming that yoga will help. Do not practice Shoulderstand or Headstand if you have problems with the cervical vertebrae. Forward bends and twists can aggravate certain disk conditions and low back problems. In the case of spinal hypermobilty, avoid practices that increase flexibility without strengthening the spinal muscles.
- *Arthritis*: Don't strain the joints with extreme articulation or weight bearing, such as holding one-legged balancing postures. Gently articulate the joints without weight bearing pressure and avoid postures that cause pain.
- *Heart disease*: Some heart abnormalities require little restraint, while others involve significant restrictions. Seek professional advice. In general, avoid overly vigorous exercising, practices that significantly increase abdominal cavity pressure, and practices involving breath retention.
- *Cancer or tumors*: Depending on the type and locations, contraindications vary widely. Some cancers involve no restriction. Others demand extreme caution. Get medical advice.
- *HIV or other conditions that inhibit the immune response*: Avoid excessive physical or mental strain. Practice gently, emphasizing a flowing breath and easy stretching.
- *Digestive disorders, including colitis, hernia, gallstones, kidney stones, and ulcers*: Avoid postures that apply strong pressure to the belly.
- *Epilepsy*: Extended Yoga Nidra or sitting meditation, and intensive breathing exercises are contraindicated because they can trigger seizures. Short periods of relaxation are appropriate.
- *Severe mental disorders*: In the case of illnesses such as schizophrenia or bipolar disorder, relaxation, meditation, and intensive breathing practices should be done only in concert with professional treatment.
- *Other medical conditions*: Inversions are also contraindicated for those with unmedicated or severe high blood pressure, those recovering from a stroke, or anyone with an acute urinary tract infection, ear inflammation, common cold, or sinus problem. Those with low blood pressure should be careful in getting up after inversions or relaxation, as dizziness can result.

It's Not Just a Body

BY SENIOR TEACHER SUDHA CAROLYN LUNDEEN

Life is full of surprises. As an oncology nurse at a large Boston hospital in 1985, joining the Kripalu staff was the farthest thing from my mind. But I had been diagnosed with breast cancer the year before, and that catalyzed a willingness to make some major changes in my life. I had also been studying and practicing complementary healing modalities, such as Therapeutic Touch, to help patients recover from the rigors of cancer treatments and was impressed with the results. When I began my own treatments, I explored additional ways to help me deal with the side effects. I looked for practitioners who knew the value of treating more than just my body. Eventually, I took a deep breath and set out for Kripalu Center and what I thought would be a two-month stay.

Living at Kripalu, my eyes and my body discovered the new world of healing and nurturing possibilities I was looking for. In yoga classes, I found that I was not only strengthening my body, I was also learning how to relax and be present to the sensations and feelings that came up. The compassionate mindfulness I practiced on my mat began to integrate into other areas of my life. As I peeled away layers of fear, I started unlocking doors to previously unknown parts of myself. My yoga and meditation practice became the ground from which I could overhaul some old and limiting belief systems. Living this healthy lifestyle, I felt great. My six-month medical checkups said I was doing great too.

My story would be so much simpler if I could close on that high note. Little did I know that another shocker was on its way. But this time, when I needed more cancer treatments, I had the tools of my practices and wonderful community support to help me face the challenges and uncertainties. As anyone who has been there can attest, navigating a major health challenge is no small feat. For me, these challenges were mixed with a heavy dose of grace. By facing death, I opened to life. I am well again. And I know that life offers no guarantees. This is true for all of us, of course, but with a life-threatening diagnosis that truth becomes more compelling.

As a yoga teacher, workshop leader, and lifestyle coach for the past twenty years, I have worked with hundreds of people facing serious health conditions. When asked what has been most powerful in my healing journey, I can say there are a number of key practices and principles. It's important to breathe and stay present in your body.

It's equally important to treat yourself with compassion, not more aggression, and to quiet the inner critic. Don't give in to the temptation everyone feels to roll over and give up. Go to your edge. Remember that you are something more than your body, and learn to savor the good moments. There is no one right way when it comes to healing. Your journey will be different than anyone else's, and that's okay. These can sound like platitudes, but put into practice, they work. They make a difference. They helped me get my life back.

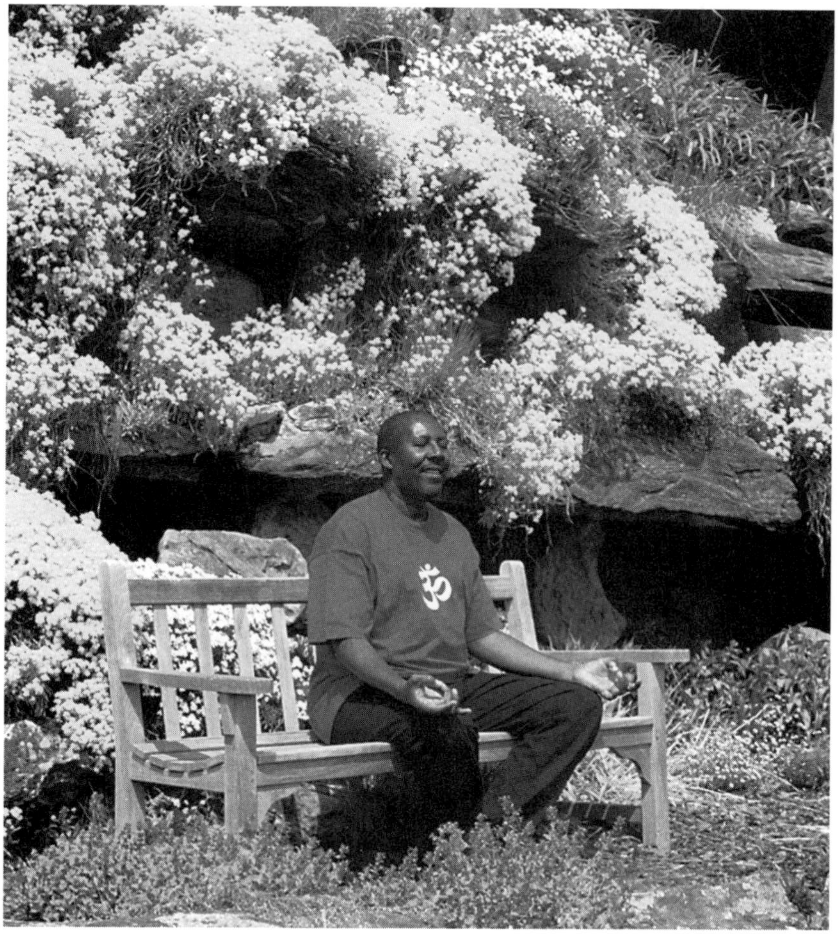

4. PSYCHOLOGICAL AND SPIRITUAL GROWTH

CHAPTER ELEVEN

DEEPENING YOUR PRACTICE

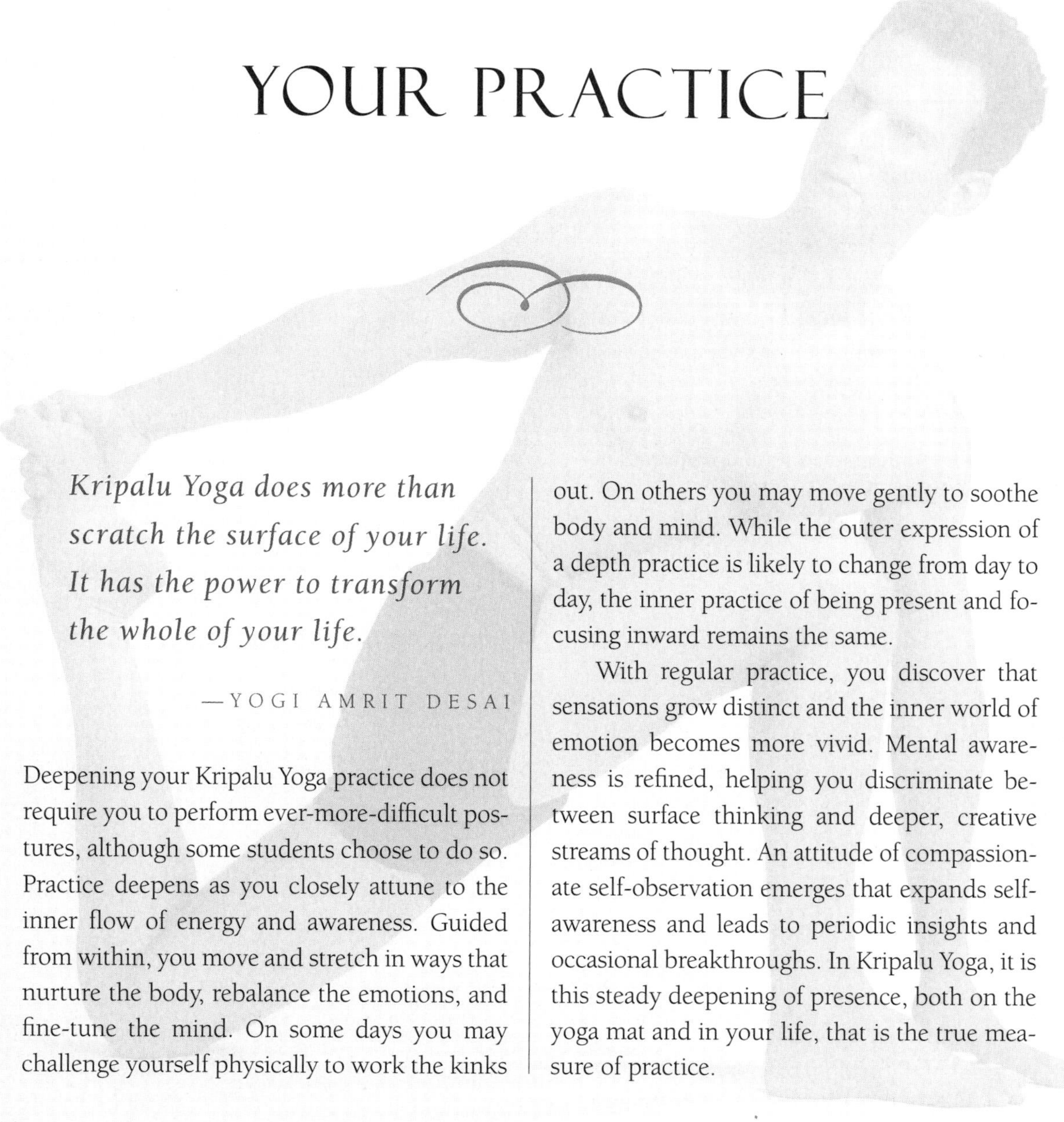

Kripalu Yoga does more than scratch the surface of your life. It has the power to transform the whole of your life.

—YOGI AMRIT DESAI

Deepening your Kripalu Yoga practice does not require you to perform ever-more-difficult postures, although some students choose to do so. Practice deepens as you closely attune to the inner flow of energy and awareness. Guided from within, you move and stretch in ways that nurture the body, rebalance the emotions, and fine-tune the mind. On some days you may challenge yourself physically to work the kinks out. On others you may move gently to soothe body and mind. While the outer expression of a depth practice is likely to change from day to day, the inner practice of being present and focusing inward remains the same.

With regular practice, you discover that sensations grow distinct and the inner world of emotion becomes more vivid. Mental awareness is refined, helping you discriminate between surface thinking and deeper, creative streams of thought. An attitude of compassionate self-observation emerges that expands self-awareness and leads to periodic insights and occasional breakthroughs. In Kripalu Yoga, it is this steady deepening of presence, both on the yoga mat and in your life, that is the true measure of practice.

Catalyst for Transformation

With contemporary yoga so focused on the physical, and postures woven into glitzy media images, it is easy to forget that traditional yoga was an esoteric tradition designed to initiate a profound process of personal transformation. Despite a few significant departures from the traditional approach, most notably the move away from the guru/disciple paradigm, Kripalu's experience is that yoga's potency has not been lost. Anyone able to maintain a consistent practice, ashram insiders and program guests alike, can attest to Kripalu Yoga's ability to catalyze psychological and spiritual growth.

> *My hairdresser knew I was a yoga teacher and asked me where he could learn more about yoga. I asked him, "Jeff, are you happy with your life right now?" He said he was. So I told him, "Then don't get into yoga. Your whole life will change." As much as I was kidding him, that's also the truth.*
>
> —Kathleen Grace Koch

The transformative process is best understood as an amalgam of three components: healing, growth, and spiritual awakening. Many of us come to yoga to address health concerns or to find a refuge from exhausting and hectic lives. We are in need of *healing,* the process of returning to normal functioning after trauma or injury. While the clearest example of healing is physical, as when a wound or broken bone mends, parallel types of healing occur on emotional and mental levels.

Those of us who stick with practice are pleased to discover that it stimulates a steady stream of insights that help us change in positive ways. This is *growth,* a gradual unfolding into a full expression of our human potential. Growth is not just steady, incremental progress. It also includes exciting quantum leaps brought on by peak experiences. Setbacks also provide grist for the mill of growth, as major lessons are learned from failures and the difficult tempering of character that results when we stand in the fires of loss and crisis.

An experience of *spiritual awakening* is different from healing and growth. It's a sudden shift in your sense of self that occurs when you touch the core of your being, the essential you that is already whole and complete, that doesn't need to change or get better in any way. This is the "true Self" that yoga depicts as infinite, eternal, and joyous. Because each of us is oblivious of material that has been pushed out of conscious awareness, it is normal to encounter surprises and confront more than a few pitfalls along the way to regaining our essential wholeness. The universality of this experience led Swami Kripalu to describe the transformative process as a "journey from the known to the unknown."

Everyone proceeds down the path of transformation in his or her own unique way. Your experience will depend on the specifics of your life history and current circumstances. Rather than a linear progression, it's a spiraling path forward in which you are constantly healing, growing, and awakening to deeper levels.

> *After my mother suffered a stroke at age eighty-seven, her health quickly declined. She made a conscious decision not to have a feeding tube and to refuse all treatment. The weeks that followed were heart wrenching. In that time, I learned something significant about my yoga practice. Over the years, my ability to do postures had not become what I might have liked. But my practice did give me a deeper awareness and understanding of life. It helped me become more accepting, more in touch with the fact that things change, and that nothing is permanent. In my mother's last days, I was able to practice the true spirit of yoga, bringing my attention to what was happening in each moment, being totally present in our interactions, drinking her in until the day she slipped away. In that hospital room, I saw that yoga had helped me grow.*
>
> —Elaine Sears

Awake in This Body

Traditional yoga sought nothing less than *mukti*, liberation. *Mukti* is a word rooted in the Hindu worldview that sees life as an endless cycle of birth, death, and rebirth that is shot through with suffering. Some yoga schools espouse the ideal of *videha mukti*, a liberation that requires the demise of the body and mind. Others believe in the possibility of *jivan mukti*, a living liberation.

LIFE COMES CALLING

Life itself expands me
when I let it. I point
to my known edge and
say, "That's it. I can't
go past there. That's
my limit!" But of
course life comes
calling as it always
does, not respecting
borders, asking me to
stretch again, and then
still more, until I can't
even recognize who
I am. You know
how it is—challenge,
tragedy, grief or ecstasy;
where I am right now
just can't stay static—
the pull toward growth
and evolution is too
strong. When I let go,
when I allow life in,
I grow before I even
notice what is happening.

Transformation in Kripalu Yoga leads to the experience of being *fully human*, *fully divine*, and *fully alive*. To be *fully human* is to be grounded in the everyday realities of life: inhabiting a body, relating authentically to others, responding to life's challenges directly and honestly. As you learn to accept yourself despite shortcomings, the wind is taken out of the sail of self-deception and denial. There is freedom and joy in just being you—no more and no less. Extending this acceptance to others enables you to embrace their humanity too, and the quality of your communications and relationships improves. A crack appears in the thick wall of separation from self and others that lies at the root of human suffering.

To be *fully divine* is to be in touch with the indwelling spirit. You have probably had moments of experiencing an aspect of yourself that is unblemished by life, perpetually fresh and brimming with energy. A depth Kripalu Yoga practice brings you into direct contact with spirit as the energetic source of body and mind. Rather than denying or negating the human experience, this kind of spirituality connects you to the world and allows you to reap a deep sense of fulfillment from the everyday tasks of life. It is important to understand that the word *divinity* is not meant to imply a particular deity, adherence to any creed, or even the existence of a supreme being. It is simply a recognition that a transpersonal dimension exists within everyone that goes beyond the limits of the mind.

Embracing your humanity and divinity, you are whole. There is a vitality that comes from being whole, a zest for life and a feeling of being *fully alive*. Taking good care of your body becomes a matter of honoring its clear signals. Open to a free exchange of energy with others, you can express yourself with less inhibition and listen with greater empathy. More and more, you live in a state where your body is relaxed, your heart is open, and your mind is clear.

I believe that what I experience in Kripalu Yoga is my natural state of being. When I get back in touch with that state, I both connect with my higher self and regain my humanity.

—Paula Linda Reed

Three Stage Approach

The three stages of Kripalu Yoga are a way to embark on your journey of transformation that integrates the wisdom of East and West. Western methods tend to focus on the physical and psychological changes you can see and feel—strengthening the body, opening the heart, and clearing the mind. Eastern yoga traditions emphasize the subtle energetic quickening that underlies these changes as a critical part of the equation. Kripalu Yoga integrates these views. Each stage includes yoga techniques that awaken energy to a higher level of activity, together with awareness focusing techniques that foster healing and growth.

If you are practicing the Sun and Moon

Series, you are already established in the first stage of Kripalu Yoga. The purpose of stage one practice is to stretch and strengthen the whole body, stimulating an increase in physical vitality. Postures are performed with the eyes open and awareness focused on alignment. While stretching and strengthening, it is common to encounter tight areas in which you habitually hold tension. These are the gross tensions that inhibit energy flow. Remaining present in the body, and cultivating an attitude of compassionate self-acceptance, you release tension by choosing to relax into the posture and fully feel sensation. As energy begins to stream through areas where its flow had been blocked, slow motion micromovements, audible sighs, and other natural sounds emerge to help the body let go. As stage one practice matures, a strong flow of prana is activated throughout the body and your mental powers of concentration begin to develop.

Stage one is often called *willful practice* to distinguish it from the later stages that emphasize *surrender*. In this context, *willful* means *volitional* or *directed by the mind*. It does not mean *forceful* or *effortful*. Willful practice is yoga's way to rejuvenate the physical body. It corresponds to the traditional stage of practice called *pranaprabalya* or *intensifying the life force*.

Focusing Inward

In the second stage of Kripalu Yoga, you learn how to systematically deepen your inner experience. Postures are held for longer periods of time, sometimes up to several minutes, with the body relaxed and mind focused on the heightened flow of sensation, emotion, and thought. Your gaze grows soft, or you close the eyes, to facilitate states of introversion and introspection in which the mind becomes absorbed in the inner world of your body and external distractions fade from awareness. Micromovements take you beyond the rigid parameters of the postures and into variations that release subtle tensions that go unnoticed in the basic form of the postures.

When coupled with breath and relaxation, prolonged holding causes buried emotion and other unconscious material to surface in awareness where it can be felt, seen, and let go. Two focusing techniques are introduced in stage two to support this inner work. Both build upon the Practice of Being Present—breathe, relax, feel, watch, and allow. *Riding the Wave* is Kripalu Yoga's approach to emotional release. As you hold the posture, focusing on areas of sensation that naturally draw your attention, energy builds in the body and the mind gradually shifts into a highly concentrated state. As deep-seated tensions surface, a powerful wave of sensation begins to rise. Staying present in your body and relaxing into the holding, you allow the wave to rise, crest, and dissipate. Riding the Wave is a highly effective way to regain your capacity to feel fully and is discussed in more detail in chapter 18.

The second focusing technique is *Witness*

Consciousness, which helps you sustain meditative awareness despite the steady stream of thoughts parading through the mind. Witness Consciousness builds upon the practice of watching—restraining the mind's tendency to grasp what is pleasant and push away what is painful—and produces a flowing state of equanimity and choiceless awareness that enables you to remain intimate with what is going on inside of you. (See chapter 20.)

Stage two is a shifting balance of will and surrender. As layer after layer of tension is released by willful practice, energy frees up. Surrendering to this awakened energy—experienced as urges, feelings, and intuitions—allows the energy to open the heart and clear the mind. During stage two, you may want to expand your routine beyond postures to include breathing exercises that flood the body with prana, or periods of sitting meditation that relax and refine the mind. It corresponds to the traditional stage of practice called *prana-furana*, or *releasing the life force*.

Meditation-in-Motion

Meditation-in-Motion is the hallmark of the third stage of Kripalu Yoga. With body and mind deeply relaxed, the body moves spontaneously as guided from within. During this experience, you drop everything learned from external sources and focus exclusively on allowing energy to awaken and express. You may have sensed the potential for spontaneous movement in athletes and dancers who seem to transcend technique, moving with a grace that staggers the mind. These individuals have instinctively learned how to allow their movements to originate from a place beyond mind. In the privacy of your yoga practice, you can do this too.

Prana awakening makes body wisdom accessible in your yoga practice. It allows you

THREE STAGES OF KRIPALU YOGA

Stage One	Stage Two	Stage Three
Practice of being present	Hold the posture	Invite prana to awaken
Ocean Sounding Breath	Ride the Wave of Sensation	
Yoga postures	Witness Consciousness	Release mind's control
Alignment principles	Posture variations	
Micromovements	Pranayama	Meditation-in-Motion
Deep relaxation	Sitting meditation	

Extraordinary Living

BY SENIOR TEACHER STEPHEN COPE

Kripalu Center is situated just across the street from Tanglewood, the summer home of the Boston Symphony Orchestra. From early on in my tenure at Kripalu, I found myself wandering across the street, sometimes every night, to watch conductor Seiji Ozawa's artistry and hear the genius of musicians like Yo-Yo Ma, Peter Serkin, and Kathleen Battle. What a treat!

Gradually, I began to notice something interesting—something that linked my daytime yoga practice with my nighttime revels at Tanglewood. These artists routinely entered into profound states of concentration. I recognized these states because they were precisely the same states cultivated in yoga and meditation—the same states I was cultivating in my own practice. What a surprise! I also noticed that the concentrated states into which the musicians entered affected not only themselves, but the audience as well. There was a profound "field effect" that extended to the thousands of people participating through listening.

All contemplative paths cultivate the mind's natural capacity to focus awareness. Yoga and meditation systematically expand and deepen this ability. In highly concentrated states, attention becomes one-pointed. External, distracting sensory input is completely tuned out. As the mind penetrates the object of its attention, the very architecture of the mental process is transformed. The stream of thought becomes laserlike, narrowed but highly organized. All extraordinary human endeavors involve this same quality of concentration. Ralph Waldo Emerson said, "What makes a man great is concentration of effort." "Winners focus, losers scatter," says Steven Covey, author of the acclaimed *Seven Habits of Highly Effective People.*

Yogis have another way of saying this that better conveys the spirit lying behind most extraordinary achievements: When you bring all of your energy and commitment to the table, God shows up. When you fully commit to one path, to one endeavor, then the Universe somehow responds. Mysterious doors open. We discover powers we did not know we had. Unseen beings come to our aid. We experience unboundedness—a mystical connection with the whole field of mind and matter—and act not from the individual personality but a state of unified mind.

I believe everyone has the capacity for extraordinary living. All that is required is that we bring our focus, skill, and energy together to serve one purpose. If we do, it can lead to astonishing powers of body, mind, and spirit—powers that are not "ours" in any sense of the word, but which we simply channel into worthy endeavors. My current focus is directing Kripalu Center's new Institute for Extraordinary Living, which is exploring what helps ordinary people, myself included, awaken their latent talent for goodness and greatness.

to respond directly to the body's signals without filtering them through the mind. Awakened energy naturally guides you into *kriyas,* intuitive actions that purify body and mind at an accelerated rate. As you learn to surrender into this experience, deep-seated tensions are released through postures, movements, breath patterns, and sounds. As energy flow intensifies, this process builds momentum as spontaneous actions free you of emotional armoring and psychological defenses. Stage three practice is a form of moving meditation accompanied by an experience of inner absorption. It corresponds to the traditional stage of practice called *pranotthana,* or the *rising of the life force.*

The Music of Transformation

The three stages of Kripalu Yoga orchestrate a grand movement within your being, transporting you from inner dissonance to states of harmony and oneness. This inner symphony is played not once, but each and every time you practice. The music of transformation is never stale or repetitive. It is evocative and enchanting, always inviting you to step free of blocks and limitations to experience the fullness of who you are. The following chapters provide a map of the journey—and yoga's role in it. The first step is exploring Kripalu Yoga's teachings on prana.

C H A P T E R   T W E L V E

PRANA, THE LIFE FORCE

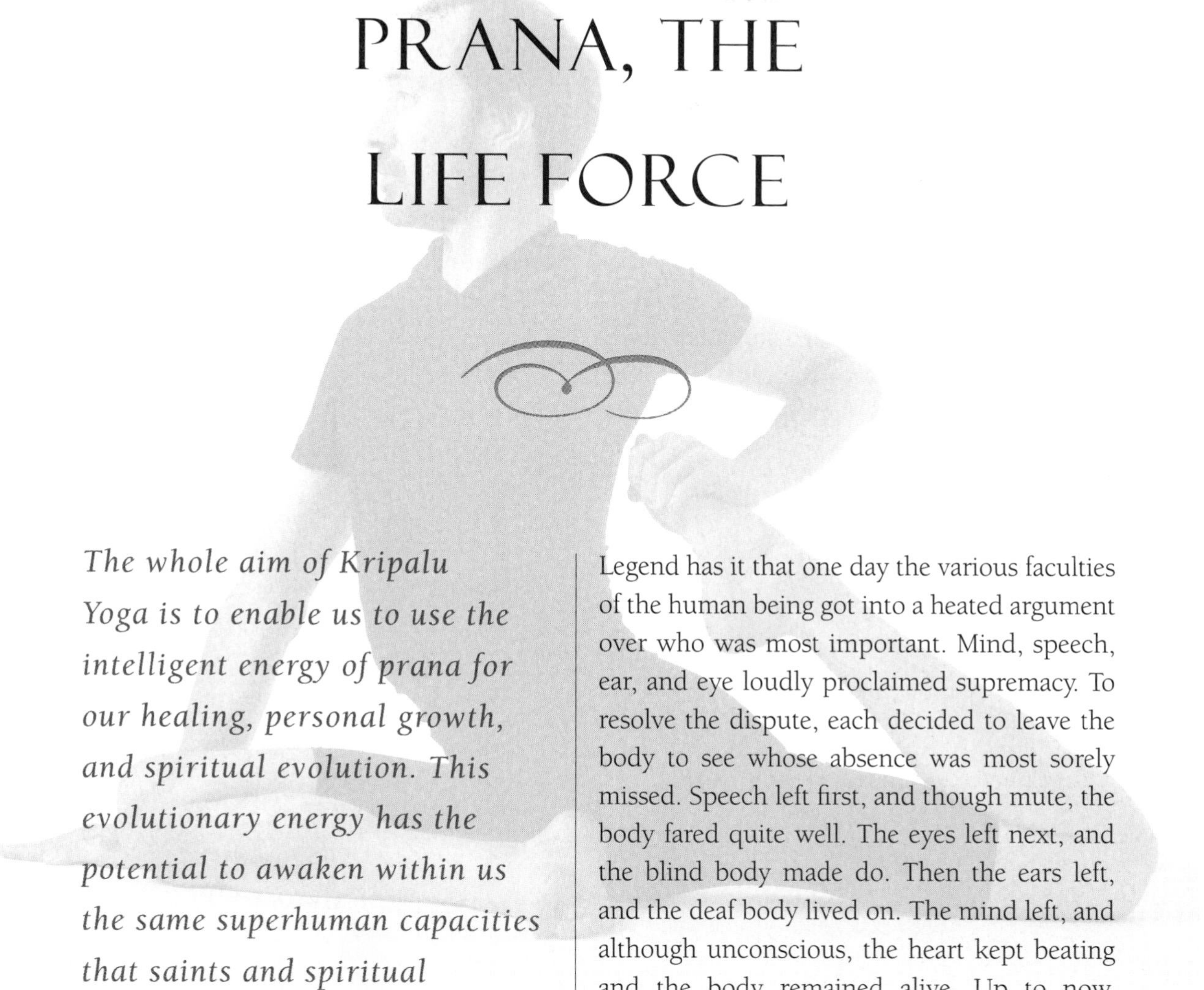

The whole aim of Kripalu Yoga is to enable us to use the intelligent energy of prana for our healing, personal growth, and spiritual evolution. This evolutionary energy has the potential to awaken within us the same superhuman capacities that saints and spiritual masters have experienced down through the ages.

—YOGI AMRIT DESAI

Legend has it that one day the various faculties of the human being got into a heated argument over who was most important. Mind, speech, ear, and eye loudly proclaimed supremacy. To resolve the dispute, each decided to leave the body to see whose absence was most sorely missed. Speech left first, and though mute, the body fared quite well. The eyes left next, and the blind body made do. Then the ears left, and the deaf body lived on. The mind left, and although unconscious, the heart kept beating and the body remained alive. Up to now, prana, the life force, had been sitting quietly in the background. As prana slowly got up to leave, the flow of breath ceased and the ground beneath the other faculties began to shake and heave. Mind, speech, ear, and eye fell to their knees and begged prana to stay, proclaiming for all to hear that it was indeed supreme.

The Discovery of Prana

In deep meditation, the sages of ancient India perceived that the physical body is the outermost expression of a subtle energy field. Focusing their concentrated attention inward, they observed that the field was composed of an intricate network of pathways and vortexes through which a luminous energy flowed. They named this energy *prana* and carefully mapped its flow through a system of pathways and centers they called the *subtle body*. When prana flows freely, the sages observed that a person enjoys radiant health and clarity of mind. When the flow of prana is obstructed by physical, emotional, or mental tensions, health is compromised and awareness dulled. While meditating, the sages found that prana would prompt their bodies to move and breathe in ways that released tensions and restored its free flow. The system of postures, breathing exercises, and meditation techniques that we know as yoga had its origins in the systematic study of prana by these Indian sages over thousands of years. The traditional name used to refer to their discoveries is *Prana Vidya,* which means *knowledge of the life force*.

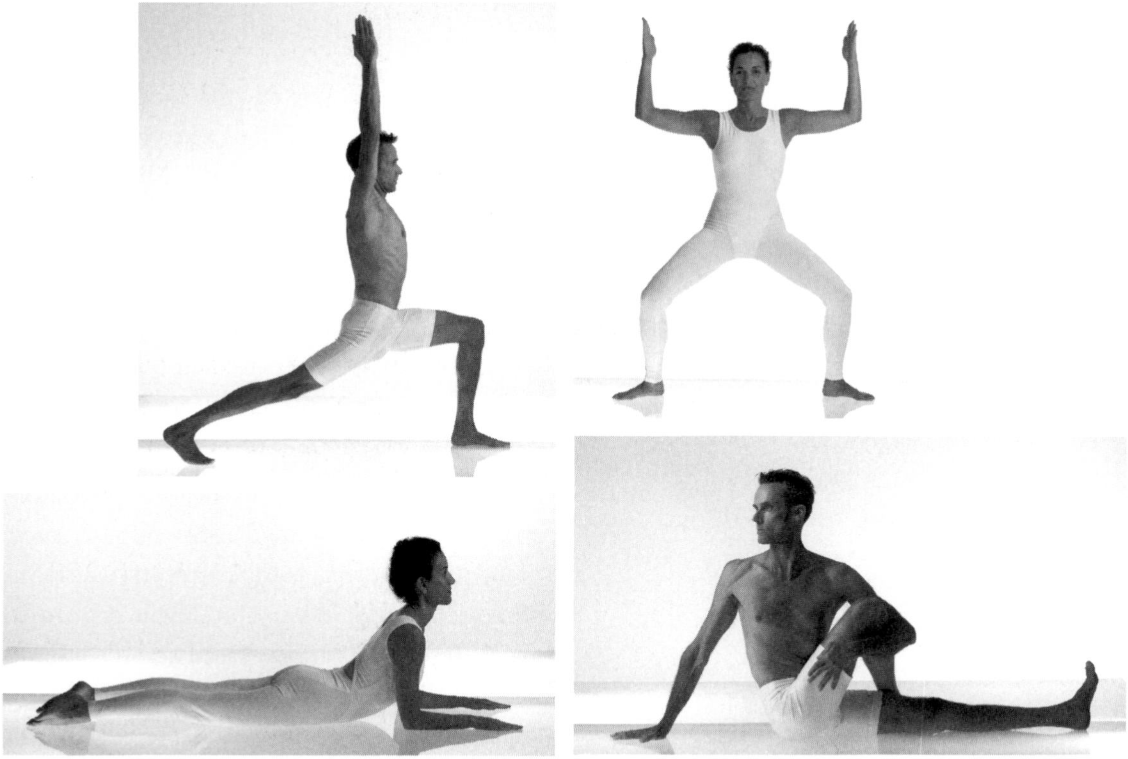

The coupling of conscious breathing and yoga postures is designed to charge the system with life force and encourage its free flow through body and mind. To the ancient yogis, the unimpeded free flow of life force through the body defined health.

What Is Prana?

The Sanskrit word *prana* means *primary energy* even though it is most often translated as *life force* or simply *breath*. Although intimately tied to the flow of breath, prana is not air or oxygen. Prana is the source energy that fuels the biological, emotional, and mental faculties. Just as electricity can be used to generate heat, light, and sound, prana enables you to see, hear, feel, taste, and think.

> *Prana is to the body what gasoline is to a car, electricity to a lightbulb, wind to a windmill.*
>
> —Amy Weintraub

Prana manifests on two different levels—spiritual and biological—and flows into your system differently from each. *Spirit prana* is the subtle energy that emanates from the soul to quicken the body and illumine the mind. Similar to the sun radiating light and heat, the indwelling spirit radiates spirit prana, which has the dual qualities of energy and awareness. It is this inner flow of prana from the spiritual dimension to the physical body that activates the breathing process and distinguishes a living person from a corpse.

Prana also surrounds us in the natural world. *Biological prana* is taken into the system through the air you breathe, the food you eat, the water you drink, and the sunshine that strikes the surface of your skin. A constant inflow of prana is required to sustain life. Spirit prana fuels the breathing process, which operates like the flywheel of an engine to bring additional biological prana into the system, where it is stored in the energy centers of the subtle body. From there, prana is distributed to various nerve plexuses to carry out the many functions that keep body and mind functioning properly. We expend prana in sustaining the basic metabolic processes of life, and also in physical, mental, and emotional activity. With an abundance of prana, we feel confident and able to meet life's challenges head-on. When reserves of prana are low, our well-being is compromised and life seems overwhelming. Absorbing prana is not merely a passive process; your state of mind plays an important role. Feelings of safety, happiness, fulfillment, joy, contentment, and love make you more receptive.

> *Prana, or the vital force, springs forth from the individual spirit or* Atman. *It brings the microcosm of the human body into being, and sets both body and mind in motion. From the inexhaustible reservoir of nature, the human body draws additional prana to carry out its activities throughout the span of a lifetime.*
>
> —Swami Rajarshi Muni

We are used to thinking of energy as an inanimate and neutral force, but prana is intelligent and evolutionary. Prana's intelligence is reflected in the intricate workings of the involuntary nervous system that sustains the internal homeostasis essential to life. It is prana that beats your heart in a steady rhythm, circulates your blood, makes you hungry, digests your food, eliminates your wastes, prompts you to stretch as you get out of bed in the morning, and makes you yawn off to sleep at night. When you have been standing for hours, prana makes you want to sit down and rest your legs. When you have been sitting too long, prana makes you want to stand up and

DISCOVERING THE SUBTLE BODY

Traditional yoga teaches that the *atman* or *true self* is encased in five bodies or *koshas*, a word meaning *sheath*. The innermost sheath is the *anandamaya kosha* (*bliss sheath*) or in Kripalu Yoga *spirit prana*. The second sheath is the *vijnanamaya kosha* (*wisdom sheath*) or *intuitive mind*, which also includes the higher emotional faculties associated with the heart. The third sheath is the *manomaya kosha* (*mind sheath*) or *thinking mind*, which includes the lower emotional faculties and instincts associated with the belly. The fourth is the *pranamaya kosha*, the flowing matrix of biological prana that underlies the function of our physical body. The outermost is the physical body or *annamaya kosha* (*sheath composed of food*). Contemporary yogis commonly refer to the four inner koshas as *the subtle body*.

THE FIVE BODIES

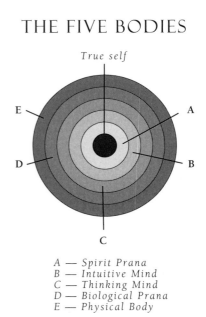

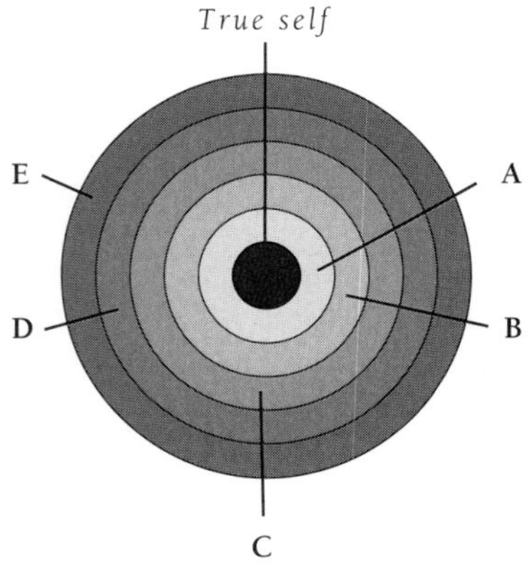

A — Spirit Prana
B — Intuitive Mind
C — Thinking Mind
D — Biological Prana
E — Physical Body

The practical importance of this model is that it places spiritual energy, rather than the material body, at the core of our being. Because it radiates out from the true self to vitalize the other bodies, spirit prana plays a crucial role in Kripalu Yoga practice. If you get still and trace either the breath or the mind's awareness back to its source, you will find spirit prana, which is the connecting link between all aspects of our being. Attuning to its inner flow frees the breath and brings the body, mind, and emotions into balance. In the state of dynamic equilibrium that results, health on all levels is uplifted and the indwelling spirit can be experienced.

move around. Because it is so close at hand, this wisdom of the body is easy to overlook.

> *The same supreme, universal wisdom that maintains the ecological balance of planet earth, and precisely guides the path of galaxies, is the wisdom of the body, guiding the life-giving functions that the body performs.*
>
> —Yogi Amrit Desai

> *Prana is the life force—the stuff of those million, zillion stars circling and exploding. Human beings receive it directly into the body through the air. We take it in in other ways as well—through live foods such as fresh fruits and vegetables, through fresh water, through living, breathing trees and vegetation, and, if we're open, through the love of other people and creatures. We probably take it in in more mysterious ways, too, I think—through music, and the sound of inspiring words and perhaps through beautiful sights.*
>
> —Stephen Cope

Prana is also the unseen source of our consciousness, imbuing our mental faculties with the quality of awareness that lies at the root of our capacity to perceive, reason, and act volitionally. Because prana functioning at the level of the mind has unique attributes and plays such an important role in life, yoga calls it by a different name—*citta*—to differentiate it from the wisdom of the body.

Other Cultures on Prana

Although the word *prana* originated in India, the concept of a life force linked to the breath is common to almost every traditional culture. Chinese sages called it *chi* and Japanese *ki*. Greeks called it *psyche,* and Romans *spiritus*. Polynesians used the term *mana* and Native Americans *orenda* and *wakan*. Africans called it *ashé* and Hebrews *ruach,* meaning *breath of life*. The healing methods developed by these traditional cultures also share a similar approach. Disease is believed to result when the flow of life force is blocked. Treatment is generally some noninvasive means to release blockages and allow the life force to again flow freely. Acupuncture, for example, is based on the flow of chi through a complex network of energy pathways called *meridians*. The exact placement of acupuncture needles is said to manipulate the flow of chi to promote health and healing.

Does Prana Exist?

While belief in a life force was central to traditional cultures, a host of scientists dating back to Sir Isaac Newton have tried to locate it, all without success. The past two decades have witnessed the meteoric growth in popularity of alternative health therapies, virtually all based on the principle that some vital force or bioenergetic field infuses organisms with the properties of life. While many of these therapies, including yoga and acupuncture, have been tested and proven effective, there is still no scientific proof as to what this life force is, or if it even exists.

Many scientists remain hostile to the notion. In an article in *Skeptical Briefs Newsletter,* Victor J. Stenger, Professor Emeritus of Physics and Astronomy at the University of Hawaii, comments: "Belief in the existence of a living force is primeval. . . . Despite complete scientific rejection, the concept of a special biological field within living things remains deeply engraved in human thinking. . . . This delusion has become so ubiquitous that it is appearing in books and journals that claim to practice scientific standards."

On the other hand, holistic physicians accept the life force as a practical reality. Andrew Weil, M.D., writes in *Spontaneous Healing:* "The energy that you feel in your body after [breathing exercises] is the energy that Chinese doctors call chi, their term for universal

The Importance of Playfulness

BY SENIOR TEACHER DEVARSHI STEVEN HARTMAN

I don't think yoga postures were meant to be static and stagnant. In the Kripalu approach, postures are tools to free up the flow of energy through the body. Micromovements are used to joyfully and safely explore a posture and discover creative ways to strengthen, open, and release. When I get in a pose, I like to ask myself, "What can I move? Can I spread my toes? Wiggle my tailbone? What happens when I shift my weight forward? When I shift my weight backward? Can I lift or lower my hips? Can I move my neck from side to side? How much space can I create in this pose that wasn't there before? Is there some part of me that can dance in this posture? What might a child do in this position? What is not flowing with energy?"

If I can allow myself to play, rhythmic movements and primal energies take on a life of their own. This kind of playful exploration opens a whole new realm of sensory experience. It reveals a wealth of information specific to my body. And I have found that it is almost impossible to enter into micromovements and hold my breath. Movement inspires breath, and breath gets the life force moving, even in areas where it may have slowed down to a trickle or ceased flowing altogether. It is this free flow of energy that revitalizes the body and brings forth a person's inner radiance and beauty.

EXPERIENCE: SLOW MOTION PRANA

Slow Motion Prana is a simple exercise taught by Swami Kripalu that can be used to verify the existence of prana. To be effective, it must be performed in ultra slow motion and with deep concentration.

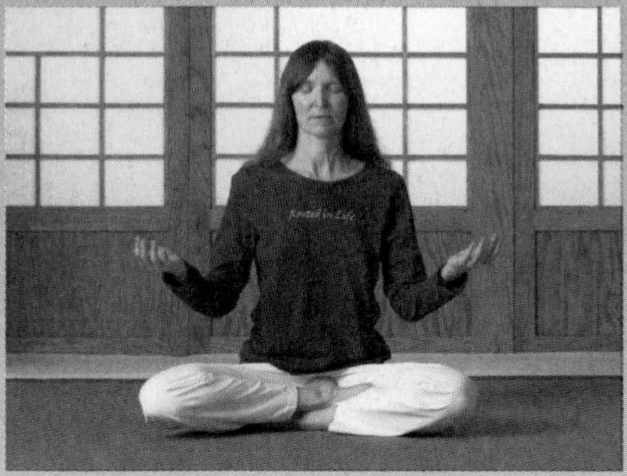

1. Sit comfortably on the floor or a straight-backed chair. Elongate your spine, close your eyes, and relax your body. Let go of any tension in your hands by gently shaking the hands, as if shaking water off the ends of your fingertips. Then vigorously rub the hands together as if you were trying to generate heat. Finally, bring your hands to rest palms up on your knees.

2. Consciously soften the belly and allow the breath to flow freely and deeply. Focus your awareness on the lower belly, a place where the body stores prana. As you breathe in and out, visualize the energy of prana gently pulsing brighter and brighter as luminous, liquid light. Breathe in this manner for several minutes.

3. Slowly lift your hands an inch or two off your knees. Visualize prana streaming down your arms and into your palms and fingers. Your fingertips may begin to feel especially sensitive or even vibrate with energy. Continue to breathe and concentrate on the energy flowing into your hands. Do not expect anything in particular to happen.

4. In extremely slow motion, allow your hands to begin to move upward, so slowly that your movement would be imperceptible to someone watching. Move so slowly that you can imagine the molecules of air rolling between your fingers as the hands lift.

5. At some point, allow the palms to turn toward each other and begin to slowly bring your hands closer together. As your hands approach, notice if you can feel an energy field between them. It may feel like your hands are two opposing poles of a magnet, or that you are holding a golden ball of energy. Slowly pulsing the hands toward and then away from each other may help you sense the edges of this field.

6. If you are not able to sense energy between the hands, as sometimes happens, let your hands come toward your face and notice if you can sense the energy field between your hands and face. There are also strong energy fields around the head and heart, and you can explore them too.

7. When you contact the energy, stay with this sense of subtle energy flowing through the hands. Take a few minutes to let the hands move in any way the energy wants to express.

8. Allow your hands to slowly return to their starting position on your knees. Remain sitting with your eyes closed to take in your experience, whatever it was. When you are ready, open your eyes, and stretch in any way that feels good.

life energy. Most people experience it as warmth or tingling or subtle vibration. With practice, you can learn to feel it more, move it about the body, and even transmit it to another person."

And in her book *Molecules of Emotion,* former National Institute of Health researcher Candace Pert suggests a biochemical basis for our experience of the life force: "It's my belief that this mysterious energy is actually the free flow of information carried by the biochemicals of emotion, the neuropeptides, and their receptors. When stored or blocked emotions are released through touch or other physical methods, there is a clearing of our internal pathways, which we experience as energy."

While the scientific debate rages on, spiritual practitioners work with the life force on a daily basis as they have for millennia, feeling its flow through their body and enjoying its beneficial effects.

> *Whatever yoga one may practice, directly or indirectly, one must worship the life force.*
>
> —Swami Kripalu

CHAPTER THIRTEEN

PATHWAYS OF ENERGY

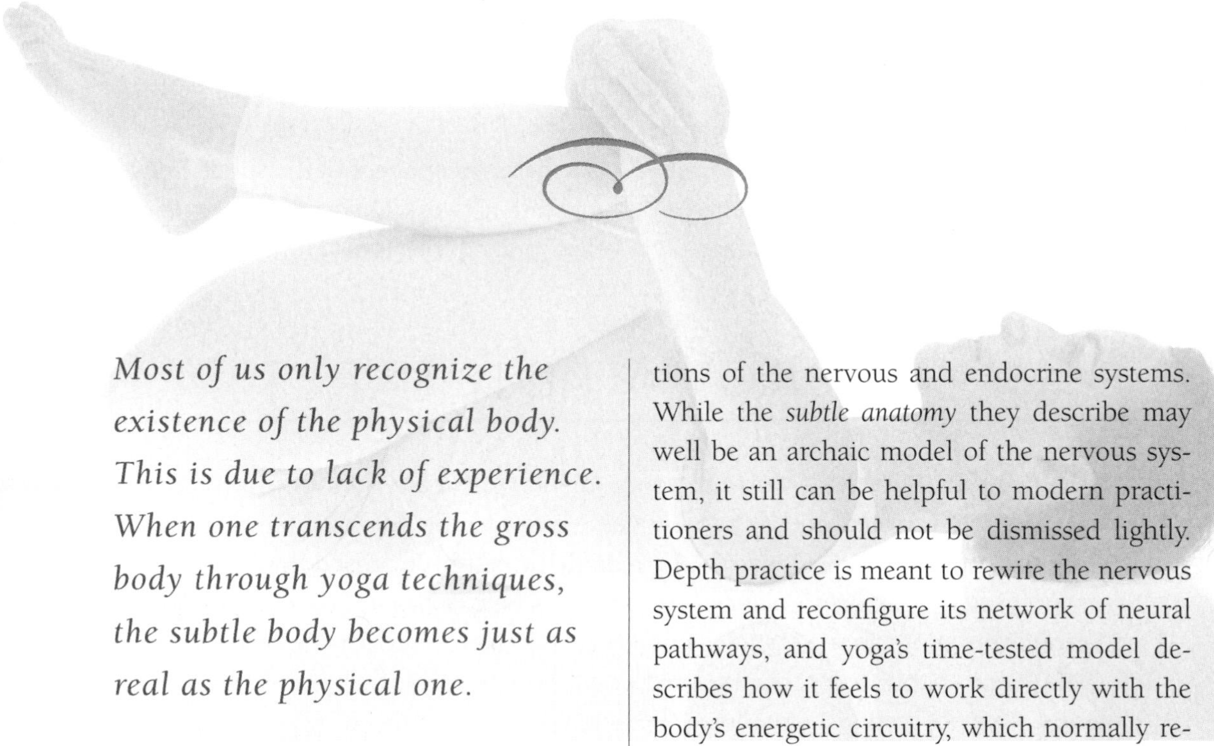

Most of us only recognize the existence of the physical body. This is due to lack of experience. When one transcends the gross body through yoga techniques, the subtle body becomes just as real as the physical one.

—SWAMI RAJARSHI MUNI

By rousing prana to high levels of activity, gifted yoga adepts are able to perceive the *subtle body* in considerable detail. Although based on subjective experience, their accounts over millennia are largely consistent and correspond in many ways to contemporary depictions of the nervous and endocrine systems. While the *subtle anatomy* they describe may well be an archaic model of the nervous system, it still can be helpful to modern practitioners and should not be dismissed lightly. Depth practice is meant to rewire the nervous system and reconfigure its network of neural pathways, and yoga's time-tested model describes how it feels to work directly with the body's energetic circuitry, which normally remains unconscious and outside of our control.

It is important to be clear at the outset that individuals vary widely in their ability to sense subtle energy. A small number are born with a perceptual gift for this task, feeling its flow inside their own bodies and even seeing its working in others with a type of second sight. Although it is true that a consistent yoga practice will sensitize you to the movement of subtle energy, it is not necessary to feel this inner flow to deepen your practice, realize all the desirable benefits yoga has to offer, or even become a yoga adept. Many practitioners start out as skeptics and over time become "energy believers" through their personal experience.

Yoga emphasizes the subtle body for two reasons. The first is that a consistent practice is intended to build an energetic matrix for higher functioning. Heightened prana flow is the invisible engine of the transformative process, catalyzing the positive physical, emotional, and mental changes that everyone can experience. The second is that the subtle body is malleable and can be shaped by the right mix of body position, breath, attention, and intention. A conceptual model of energy flow helps engage the mind in posture practice and empowers techniques such as visualization. The Kripalu Yoga approach is to hold the model lightly, using it as a guide to deepen your own inner experience.

Three Principal Pathways

The basic component of the subtle body is an intricate network of *nadis* or energy pathways that branch off into ever-smaller channels

ENERGY MEDICINE

A hot topic in today's world of complementary and alternative health modalities, energy medicine is the new name given to the age-old approach of activating the healing capacity of the body by restoring strong flow to energies that have grown weak or imbalanced. Practitioners believe that a field of electromagnetic and other more subtle energies provides an infrastructure for the physical body. Drawing from acupuncture, qigong, and yoga, energy medicine treatments include massage; tapping, tracing, or swirling the hand along identified energy pathways; postures or movements designed for specific energetic effects; and visualization and other techniques that focus the mind.

Since its inception, Kripalu Center has recognized the principles of energy medicine, offering an array of touch therapies including massage, shiatsu, polarity, reflexology, and many other forms of hands-on healing through its Healing Arts department. Applied by a skilled therapist, all these modalities restore optimal energy flow and integrate the physical, emotional, mental, and energy "bodies" to help you relax and heal.

much like the circulatory system. The Kripalu tradition describes 3 principal pathways, 14 major branches, 72,000 lesser branches, and 350,000 minute channels. This staggering number of pathways reflects the capacity of human beings for profound self-awareness when the flow of prana through the subtle body is not obstructed.

The *sushumna nadi,* or *central channel,* is the chief pathway, running from the perineum to the crown of the head through the center of the spinal column. The *pingala nadi,* or *solar pathway,* parallels the spine on the right side. The *ida nadi,* or *lunar pathway,* parallels the spine on the left side. The Kripalu tradition describes the solar and lunar pathways as connecting the nostrils to the *kanda,* or bulb, the egg-shaped origin point of all the energy pathways located slightly below the navel. When we breathe, taking in oxygen to sustain the physical body, yoga teaches that we also absorb prana to sustain the subtle body. As the air passes over the upper ends of the solar and lunar pathways located at the back of the nostrils, they charge the subtle body with prana. Other traditions depict the solar and lunar pathways as winding their way up the spine to join at the point between the eyebrows.

Yoga's ability to shift consciousness is rooted in its ability to influence prana flow and alter the functioning of the nervous system. Anatomically, the solar pathway corresponds to the sympathetic branch of the autonomic

THE THREE PRINCIPAL PATHWAYS

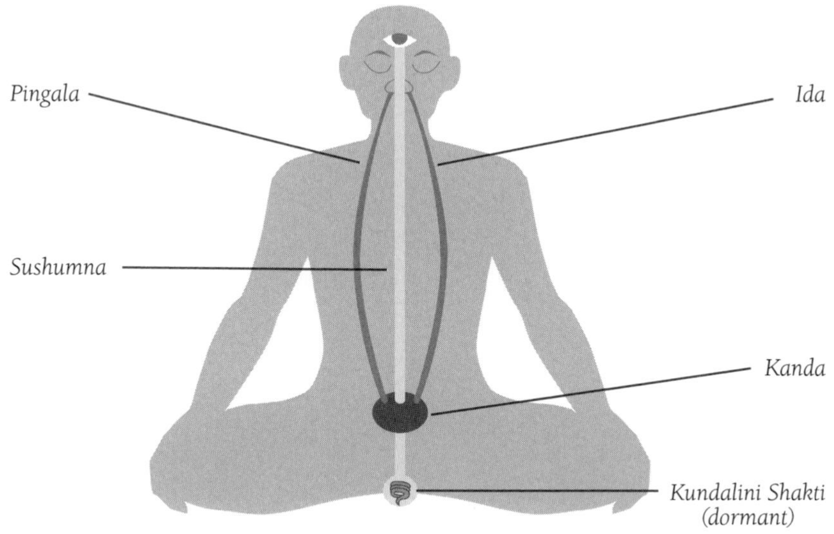

Subtle body with dormant Kundalini

nervous system, which is responsible for arousing the body to action. The lunar pathway corresponds to the parasympathetic branch, which calms the body. When prana flows smoothly and evenly through the solar and lunar pathways, the mind is integrated, free of agitation, and able to focus. Although a rarity in our world, yoga considers this our normal state of healthy functioning. Simple yoga techniques to produce inner balance include rocking, rolling, swinging, and side-stretching movements that repeatedly stimulate one side of the body, and then the other. Scissoring, twisting, and cross-crawl movements that cross over the midline of the body are another type of integrating movement pattern.

When prana flows through the central channel, the activity of the solar and lunar pathways is greatly diminished. The entire nervous system grows quiet, and awareness becomes internalized. This is the mechanism of introversion, which makes deep states of meditation and non-dual awareness accessible. The most common technique to stimulate energy to flow through the central channel is to direct the attention to the spot between the eyebrows, or visualize energy flowing from root to crown, often in combination with various breathing exercises.

Seven Energy Centers

The subtle body's network of energy pathways includes various *chakras*, or energy centers. The word *chakra* means *wheel* and describes a luminous vortex of swirling prana. Chakras occur at locations in the subtle body where

THE CHAKRA SYSTEM *(with awakened Kundalini)*

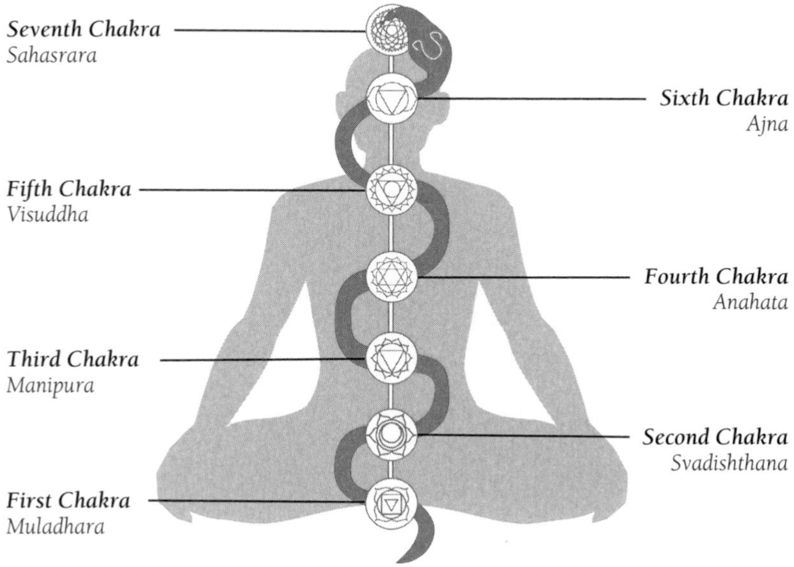

multiple energy pathways intersect. Yoga schools vary in the number of energy centers considered important, but almost all describe seven chakras arranged vertically along the spine and lesser centers in the palms and feet. The seven chakras are said to vibrate at different frequencies, appear as different colors, and influence various nerve plexuses, glands, and organ systems.

Contemporary spiritual teachers often attribute psychological attributes to the seven chakras, such as:

- Survival instinct and fear
- Pleasure and sexual desire
- Power and anger
- Love and empathy
- Knowledge and communication
- Wisdom and intuition
- Transpersonal awareness

Although this perspective has appeal, it is a recent adaptation. The approach of yoga has always been to increase the flow of energy to the centers through practice and supportive lifestyle, allowing the psychological issues to resolve themselves through the expansion in self-awareness that results.

Physicians are the discoverers of the physiological functions. Yogis are the discoverers of the chakras.

—Swami Kripalu

I was practicing one morning with a deep inward focus. As I released Standing Yoga Mudra, I let my arms slowly return around in front of me. I noticed a strong sense that my arms were floating and I let them hang in the air for a few moments, exerting no effort whatsoever to keep them up. It was then that I noticed the energy field all around my body. It was like standing in a pool with water swirling around me. From my lower belly streamed a spiral of energy extending farther than I could reach. There was another spiral flowing from my abdomen, another small pool of energy around my heart and strong streams of energy coming from my throat. After a few minutes spent entranced by these spiral streams, I thought to myself, "Oh my God, these are the chakras!" Afterward, I went outside and was taken aback. I could feel every person's emotions, energies, their very essence. I could also feel the grass, trees, and bushes. The plant life was so calm, nurturing, and accepting. Tears streamed down my face. This heightened state stayed with me for the next two hours. I didn't want the rapture to end, but alas, it passed.

—Yvette Bulger

Seven Major Energy Centers

Energy Center	Location	Element	Color	Physical Correlate
Muladhara, or Root Center	Perineum	Earth	Blood red	Excretory system, coccygeal plexus, gonads
Svadishthana, or Base of the Self Center	Genitals	Water	Bright red	Reproductive system, lumbo-sacral plexus, ovaries, prostate
Manipura, or Jewel Fortress Center	Navel	Fire	Green	Digestive system, epigastric or solar plexus, adrenal glands
Anahata, or Unstruck Sound Center	Chest	Air	Golden	Respiratory system cardiac plexus, thymus gland
Visuddha, or Pure Speech Center	Throat	Ether	Smoky gray	Pharyngeal plexus, thyroid and parathyroid glands
Ajna, or Command Center	Forehead	Subtle Energy	White	Cerebral cortex, cavernous plexus, pineal and pituitary glands
Sahasrara, or Thousand-Petaled Center	Crown	Spirit	Luminous light	Beyond physical form

EXPERIENCE: SINKING INTO THE SUBTLE BODY

The following technique induces a state of introversion and absorption called *pratyahara* which means *drawing inward.* In that state, the flow of energy through the subtle body can be perceived. This experience is best done with soft and soothing background music, which aids introversion and is also used to time the experience. It requires a minimum of thirty minutes but can be done for as long as one hour. It is an extension of deep relaxation (Yoga Nidra).

1. After turning on your music, make yourself comfortable in Corpse Pose. Take a few long deep breaths. Then consciously relax the body, letting it sink into the support of the floor.

2. Begin to let the breath flow freely. Don't force the breath in, or push it out. Let the breath flow freely and naturally, consciously releasing any tensions that inhibit or restrict its natural flow. Let the pace of the breath be set from within, finding your own rhythm which will change and shift over the course of the experience.

3. Connect your in-breaths and out-breaths by letting inhalations and exhalations flow smoothly one into the next. This circular breathing pattern minimizes the nervous system flutter that occurs as the breath shifts phases, which is also where the mind tends to wander off into distraction.

4. As you are learning this breath, just do your best to stay with it. Expect some initial agitation and resistance. Breathing in this way will gradually produce a profound state of inner absorption. To get there, you will play the edge between sleep and wakefulness. It is fine to drift off and lose the breath; but when you become aware of the music, come back to a free-flowing, circular breath.

5. Rest your attention on the flow of breath and the felt sense of the body. As the body deeply relaxes, let the mind remain conscious and aware. As your attention is drawn inward, relax completely while remaining totally awake and aware. Gradually become absorbed in the world of inner awareness.

6. Deep absorption is often accompanied by a heightened sensitivity to subtle energy flow. Rest in this realm of subtle energy, noticing any sensations of warmth, tingling, or flowing currents of energy. Explore the feeling, contours, and boundaries of your subtle body.

7. When the music ends, let go of the breath and take a few minutes to rest and integrate your experience, whatever it was. Get up slowly, gently stretching the body back to normal awareness.

Energy Blocks

The flow of prana through the pathways and centers of the subtle body varies among individuals. In a typical person, the flow of prana is obstructed by three major tangles of knotted pathways in the belly, throat, and head called *granthis*. Granthis can be likened to the ball of hair and dirt that clogs a bathroom drain. They slow the flow of prana to a trickle, dulling the vitality of tissues and causing a buildup of waste products and other impurities. The flow of prana can also be blocked by localized obstructions at various vital points on the body called *marmans*. From the vantage point of the subtle body, a primary purpose of yoga practice is to untangle these knots and free up the flow of prana. The revitalization of the body and mind that results is called *shuddhi,* or purification, the topic of chapter 14.

The Serpent Power

An intriguing component of the subtle body is the *Kundalini Shakti,* or *serpent power,* a reservoir of concentrated primal energy symbolized as a coiled snake that lies sleeping at the base of the spine. *Prana* and *Kundalini Shakti* are not synonymous terms. When flowing through the lesser pathways that correspond to the autonomic nervous system and the peripheral nerves, the life energy of the subtle body is called *prana*. When flowing through the central channel or spinal cord, the force it exerts on consciousness is magnified to such an extent that it is referred to by an altogether different name.

A depth practice of Kripalu Yoga is designed to activate prana and encourage its free flow through all the pathways of the subtle body. This uplifts health and stimulates a natural process of psychological and spiritual growth. A consistent practice steadily removes energy blocks and, over time, opens the central channel to a manageable amount of Kundalini energy. Kripalu Yoga is a safe practice, one suitable for those living active lives, and a reliable way to access deep states of meditation.

When quickly roused to full activity by the intensive techniques of Kundalini Yoga, prana coalesces at the core of the body and forcibly awakens what Swami Kripalu called the *evolutionary force.* The central channel opens wide and a powerful energy surges from root to crown. With repeated practice, this energy flow purifies and pierces each chakra, causing it to blossom into vivid aliveness. As Kundalini courses through the central channel, dramatic shifts in perceptual awareness occur. Traditional yoga texts state that the awakened Kundalini Shakti bestows psychic powers and liberates the yogi from the cycles of birth and death.

Intriguing in theory, and often wrongly associated with techniques to bestow extraordinary sexual powers, Kundalini Yoga is a path fraught with difficulties. Swami Kripalu described the force it awakens as "uncontrollable and terrifying," one that renders the

SWAMI KRIPALU ON KUNDALINI YOGA

What makes Kundalini Yoga unique is that it awakens the evolutionary force in its complete, uncontrollable, and terrifying form. Most aspirants cannot withstand its intensity. Even the best do not practice this yoga for long. In other forms of yoga, the mind remains tranquil all day. In Kundalini Yoga, the awakened energy surges powerfully through the system and the mind becomes unsteady. Disease and hallucinations are always standing nearby, and an aspirant's self-control can be lost at any moment. Traveling this path, I have come close to death five times. Through the grace of God and guru, I somehow survived and can say that to pass these difficulties is not easy.

In both Kundalini Yoga and Kripalu Yoga, it is necessary to awaken the evolutionary force. Without this, it is not possible to develop spiritually. In Kripalu Yoga, the evolutionary force is awakened in its partial and tolerable form. The physical health and mental stability of those following the path of Kripalu Yoga is protected. This is the most advantageous practice for a person living an active life in society. The sincere practitioner of Kripalu Yoga awakens prana, which is the only doorway to Kundalini Yoga, and it becomes possible to enter that path without special initiation.

mind unsteady and prone to hallucinations and madness. The rapid purification it engenders is cathartic and often damaging to physical health. The traditional teachings are clear that Kundalini Yoga requires an unusually gifted aspirant, a cloistered lifestyle, and personal guidance from an adept teacher.

Kripalu Yoga can serve as a bridge to this more intensive form of practice. Depth Kripalu Yoga practitioners experience the reality of the subtle body, but usually in more basic ways than traditional yoga's highly stylized network of nadis and chakras. The subtle body is like a magnet, with strong poles at the body's core and head. In early stages of practice, energy often can be felt pulsing at the core. As practice continues, it may radiate outward from the core to the periphery of the body. In depth practice, the energetic connection between the two poles is strengthened, gradually opening the belly, heart,

EXPERIENCE: ALTERNATE NOSTRIL BREATHING

Traditionally called *Nadi Shodhana,* which means *energy pathway purification,* this technique clears the energy channels and balances awareness. Begin with just a few minutes of practice, letting the breath flow through alternate nostrils in a relaxed and easy manner, free of any tension or strain. Gradually lengthen to twelve minutes. If your arm becomes tired, support the elbow with the opposite hand.

It may take some time for your system to adjust to breathing in and out of only one nostril. If you find yourself straining, release the practice and breathe normally for a few moments before resuming. After becoming accustomed to the technique, most people find it soothing. Don't do alternate nostril breathing if your nose is stuffy from a cold or sinus infection.

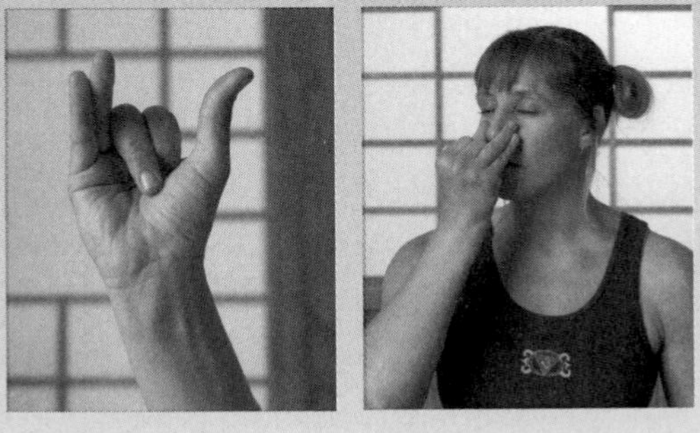

To come into Vishnu Mudra, bend the index and middle fingers to touch the palm. This hand position allows you to close one nostril with the thumb and the other with the combination of the ring and little finger.

1. Sit comfortably on the floor or a straight-backed chair with your hands resting palms up on the knees. Elongate your spine, close your eyes, and relax your body. Consciously soften the belly and allow the breath to flow freely and deeply.

2. Bring your dominant hand into *Vishnu Mudra* as shown above and exhale through both nostrils. Close the right nostril and slowly inhale through your left nostril.

3. As soon as you finish inhaling, close the left nostril and exhale through your right nostril. At the end of the exhalation, inhale through the right nostril—the same nostril through which you just exhaled.

4. Close the right nostril and exhale through the left. At the end of the exhalation, inhale through the left nostril—the same nostril through which you just exhaled.

5. Continue to breathe in this pattern, keeping the body relaxed and letting the breath flow freely and easily.

6. As the meditative quality of your experience deepens, the breath will become slow, deep, and flowing.

7. To complete your practice, exhale through the left nostril and return the hands to your knees or lap. Sit quietly for several moments to feel the effects.

8. If you want to deepen your practice, gradually progress from twelve to eighteen to twenty-four minutes of Nadi Shodhana. After six months of practice, you can begin to transition into the practice of Anuloma Viloma pranayama, a form of alternate nostril breathing that involves holding the breath in after each inhalation. Begin with a short pause between inhalation and exhalation. Then begin to gradually lengthen the pause, relaxing body and mind as you hold. Don't strain or struggle to hold the breath longer than is natural. Over time you will find your breath moving toward a 1–4–2 ratio. This means that if you breathe in for a count of three, you will hold to a count to twelve, and exhale for a count of six. Striving to attain this ratio can create tension in the body and mind. Instead, let your practice naturally evolve in its own meditative rhythm, using the ratio as a tool to be more attentive to your natural breath pattern. Never strain when working with the breath, which can stress the nervous system, and do not hold the breath in excess of this ratio.

and throat. Increased energy flow along the central channel integrates the animal, human, and divine aspects of our being. Kripalu Yoga is one way to activate prana and do the inner work needed to prepare the body, mind, and nervous system for an unforced and natural awakening of the evolutionary force.

The Science of Pranayama

Although the word *pranayama* is usually translated to mean *breathing exercise,* it is actually a sophisticated method of using the breath to direct the flow of prana. Its goal is to charge the subtle body with prana, clear it of obstructions, and by so doing bring the mind into a state of focused equilibrium. At a basic level of practice, sustaining a rhythmic breath stimulates the flow of prana, and postures direct its flow through various parts of the body. In deeper practice, more vigorous breathing exercises are employed to flood the subtle body with prana, and various forms of alternate nostril breathing are used to direct its flow through desired energy pathways.

The yoga tradition explains the ability of alternate nostril breathing to clear the subtle

Where Your Attention Goes

BY SENIOR TEACHER REBEKKAH KRONLAGE

My life was in upheaval when I visited Kripalu for the first time in 1986. I was ending a relationship, insecure in my work, and my mind was wild as a tornado. In a program called *Body Alive*, we explored yoga, pranayama, and meditation in a context of learning to be present with ourselves and our energy. Over the course of one week, my mind went from being crazy to being focused and at times even blissful and content. Like so many of my friends, the power of that experience led me to join the Kripalu staff and embark on a whole new life.

It was in that program that I was introduced to the principle "Where your attention goes, energy flows." This was such a core teaching for me, and one that has stood by me over many years. I trained in bodywork and energy healing, served guests for many years as a healing arts therapist, and eventually taught the professional bodywork program. Kripalu Bodywork is more than massage; it's a yogic approach that develops one's sensitivity to subtle energy—whether you call it spirit, God, or healing presence. Focusing attention on love and compassion invokes this divine energy and shifts the energy field between giver and receiver. Something connects and the intelligence of the energy flows in a way that both people receive the healing.

A few years back, I began directing the Kripalu Yoga Teacher Training program using the same approach I did in Kripalu Bodywork: ground the body, get present, stay with the breath, focus inward, and allow your intuitive self to come forth. I think this is the heart of the three stages of practice. For me, discipline is important because once I start paying attention, concentration of mind eventually results. I applied these principles to energize my life and make space for everything I want to create, not in a rigid way but by being open and receptive to the intelligence of divine energy. I've found they are applicable to everything: writing a story, creating a garden, or being intimate with a loved one. Where your attention goes, energy flows.

body of obstructions quite simply. In the same way that you might clean a clogged pipe by flushing water through it one way, and then the other, breathing through alternate nostrils clears the energy channels. The ability of alternate nostril breathing to bring the mind into equilibrium can also be explained, although not so simply. Scientists know that the breath of a healthy person oscillates from one nostril to another in a regular rhythm due to the swelling of the right then the left respiratory turbinates located in the sinus cavities. Although the mechanism that causes this is understood, medical science is not aware of why this occurs.

Yoga teaches that breathing through the right nostril causes prana to flow through the solar pathway, activating the sympathetic nervous system. Breathing through the left nostril similarly activates the lunar pathway and parasympathetic nervous system. The natural oscillation of the breath is one way the body maintains a healthy state of balance. Alternate nostril breathing makes use of this natural mechanism. By equalizing the flow of prana in the two pathways, it brings the two branches of the autonomic nervous system into a precise balance. In a similar fashion, the activity of the two hemispheres of the cerebral cortex is equalized, bringing the central nervous system into balance. With the entire nervous system in a state of equilibrium, a yoga practitioner finds it easier to enter deep meditation.

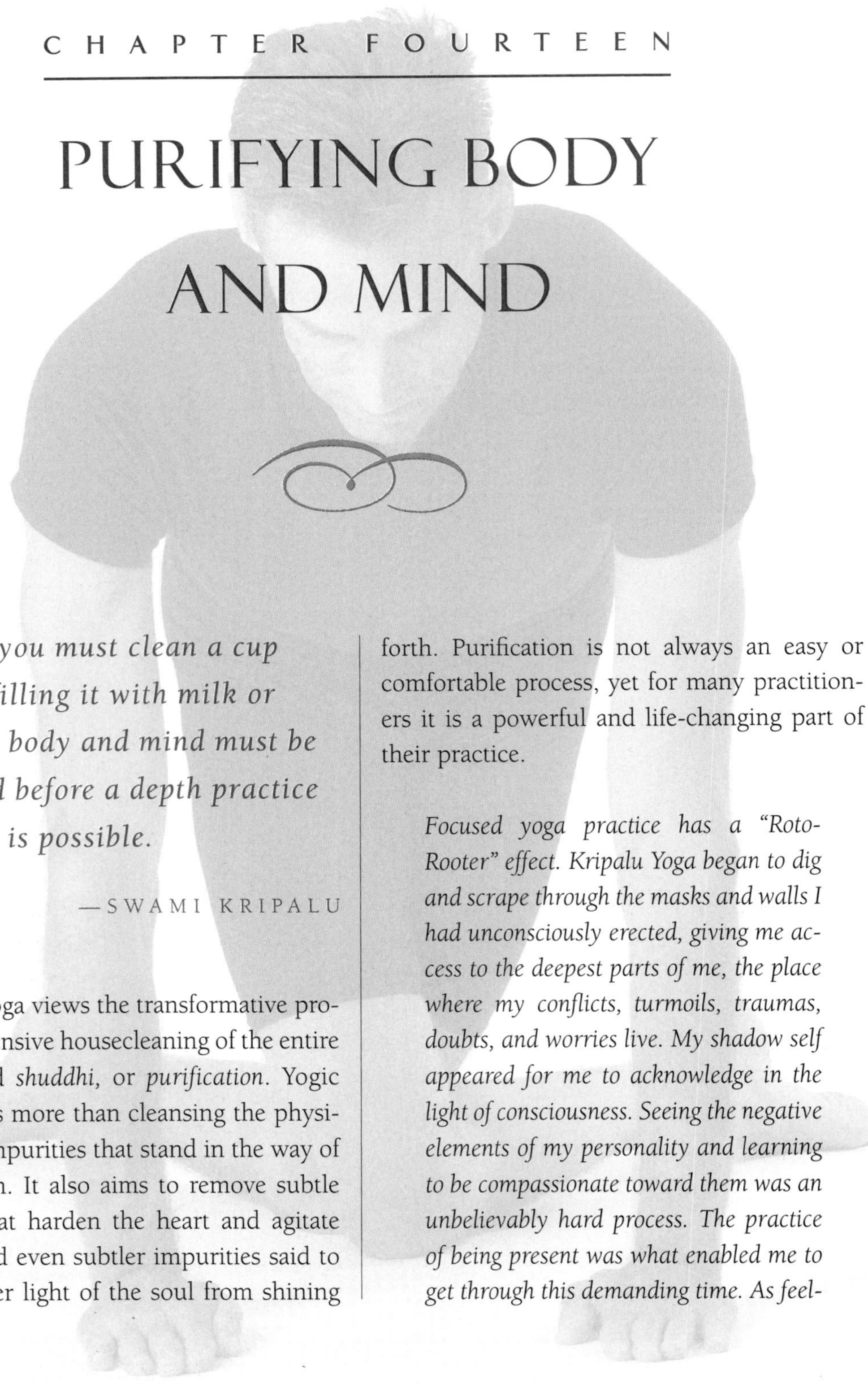

CHAPTER FOURTEEN

PURIFYING BODY AND MIND

Just as you must clean a cup before filling it with milk or tea, the body and mind must be purified before a depth practice of yoga is possible.

—SWAMI KRIPALU

Traditional yoga views the transformative process as an intensive housecleaning of the entire system called *shuddhi,* or *purification.* Yogic purification is more than cleansing the physical body of impurities that stand in the way of vibrant health. It also aims to remove subtle impurities that harden the heart and agitate the mind, and even subtler impurities said to keep the inner light of the soul from shining forth. Purification is not always an easy or comfortable process, yet for many practitioners it is a powerful and life-changing part of their practice.

> *Focused yoga practice has a "Roto-Rooter" effect. Kripalu Yoga began to dig and scrape through the masks and walls I had unconsciously erected, giving me access to the deepest parts of me, the place where my conflicts, turmoils, traumas, doubts, and worries live. My shadow self appeared for me to acknowledge in the light of consciousness. Seeing the negative elements of my personality and learning to be compassionate toward them was an unbelievably hard process. The practice of being present was what enabled me to get through this demanding time. As feel-*

ings and thoughts arose, I developed the inner strength to ride them out, listen inside, and learn from myself. I thought about, cried about, and finally came to terms with the part of my personality that had always caused me the most trouble. I grew able to see that part of myself without blinking. As my mind and personality were remolded, I was able to change my behavior. I know without a doubt that my Kripalu Yoga practice has strengthened the very fabric of my personality and soul, allowing me to withstand the pressures of life as a whole and grounded person.

—Leslie Oster

The purification process starts on a tangible level with the physical body. Many individuals find themselves trapped in a sedentary lifestyle. Eating too much, exercising too little, smoking, and abusing alcohol and drugs all cause the body to produce more wastes than it can eliminate. As wastes accumulate in the tissues and cells, the body becomes heavily laden with what yoga calls *mala* and holistic healing modalities refer to as *toxins*. Instead of feeling light and clear, an impure body feels heavy and stagnant.

Regular exercise and moderate eating allow the body to begin eliminating its backlog of waste products. Yoga enhances this natural process by increasing blood circulation throughout the entire body and stimulating organ function. Physical impurities that sap vitality are flushed from the tissues to enter the bloodstream and be eliminated, primarily by the liver and kidneys. What traditional yoga calls *bhuta shuddhi*, or *purification of the gross elements*, contemporary practitioners refer to as *healing*.

Transformation came to me via an encounter with breast cancer. Diagnosed, I underwent a year of caustic treatment. By the end, I was exhausted and depleted. Looking in the mirror, the light had gone out of my eyes. I felt chemotherapy had taken my soul from me. I began Kripalu Yoga and my eyes steadily regained their light. For the first time, I began to feel at home in my body. I have infinite respect for Kripalu Yoga's power to heal.

—Ava Wolf

Meditation and other contemplative practices stimulate a parallel process on a psychological level. Traditional yoga teaches that subtle impurities called *vikshepa* cloud and agitate the mind. This includes anything that prevents awareness from flowing freely through the emotional and mental faculties. Emotional impurities include buried trauma, repressed feelings associated with undigested experiences, and everyday emotional baggage that dulls sensitivity and acts as a barrier to full feeling. Mental impurities include preconceptions, rigid and compartmentalized thinking, inaccurate belief systems, and other conditioning that filters perception and distorts reality.

JUICE FASTING FOR PURIFICATION

All spiritual traditions have used fasting to purify body and mind. The word *fasting* conjures up a total abstention from food, but it describes a variety of approaches that help the body eliminate toxins and give the digestive system time to rest. The purification brought on by water fasting is too intense for most people. Periodic *juice fasting* is a gentler way to cleanse the body, which consists of drinking modest amounts of fruit and vegetable juices throughout the day. Cooked vegetable broth is also used to supply the body with needed potassium. Another approach to purification is a *mono-diet.* This is eating one type of food, such as fruit or brown rice, for a given period of time. Kripalu Center offers a regular schedule of supervised juice fasts and mono-diets that include yoga practice to support the purification process. Participants report that fasting not only revitalizes the body, it also provides an opportunity to recalibrate your relationship to food. An effective tool for cleansing and purification, fasting is not a strategy for weight loss. Fasting can serve as a stepping stone to conscious and moderate eating, a practice supportive of the gradual and long-term purification sought by depth yoga practitioners.

By relaxing and focusing the mind, meditation causes mental and emotional impurities to rise and enter the stream of consciousness. The mental faculties that allow us to feel fully and see clearly serve a similar purpose as the liver and kidneys. When unconscious material is held in the light of conscious awareness, it is released to pass through you, leaving your heart more open and mind clearer. Yoga regards psychological purification as an *unlearning* process, a stripping away of layer after layer of conditioning to reveal our essential wholeness. The purified mind is steady, creative, and surprisingly simple. Its faculties are responsive to the moment and free from the scars of past disappointments, resentments, and wounds. Today's yogis consider *sattva shuddhi,* or *purification of the subtle elements,* to be a process of psychological growth.

Yoga teaches that our core problem is that we have forgotten who and what we really are. This *avidya,* or spiritual ignorance, is the most subtle impurity. Convinced that we are defined by our bodies, beliefs, personalities, preferences, possessions, careers, and nationalities, we live estranged from an authentic sense of self and cut off from a vital spiritual connection. Purification consists of *vidya*—the direct experience of spirit. What yoga calls *chitta shuddhi,* or *purification of the self-sense,* contemporary practitioners refer to as *spiritual awakening.*

Healing Crisis

When the body is sluggish and the world is viewed through a thick filter of emotional baggage and mental clutter, it is impossible to see reality clearly and respond appropriately. This is why approaches to healing and growth that do not work to purify body and mind prove superficial. It is important to know, however, that the kind of purification brought on by intensive yoga practice can be a challenging proposition. Imagine the morning after a party where you ate a lot, drank too much, and didn't get much sleep. Physical purification sometimes feels like that. When the pace of purification is rapid, it can lead to a *healing crisis* and temporary reduction in function. Common experiences include headaches, nausea, colds, fevers, or areas of soreness that suddenly come and go. As the crisis passes, vitality rises to a new level.

The most potent forms of purification are emotional and mental. Purification can cause powerful emotions to surface and break through unconscious barriers to feeling in the phenomenon called *catharsis.* Catharsis can dramatically cleanse an emotional system that has grown congested and dull. Although it leads to greater sensitivity and balance, fully feeling the mental content associated with catharsis often pushes you outside comfort zones and beyond perceived limits.

Mental purification can similarly lead to insights that reconfigure a mind grown cluttered and compartmentalized. Although increased clarity and creativity is the result, clearing the mind requires bearing the pain of confronting material that has been pushed out of conscious awareness, experiencing inner conflict, reliving past memories, and acknowledging unseen shortcomings.

Several years after I discovered Kripalu Yoga, I was doing postures one morning as I always did, when a wave of anger rose through me, moving from my feet to the top of my head. I felt explosive, like Mount St. Helens on the day before the big eruption. The thing that unnerved me was that the anger had no object, and no story attached to it. I was just angry—I was anger, personified. I came out of the posture I'd been holding and stormed into our guest room, where I flung myself onto the bed and began to beat it with my fists. I buried my head in a pile of pillows and screamed until I was hoarse. When the storm finally passed, I sat up and took stock of myself. I was exhausted, but actually felt lighter, like something old and long buried had been released. Gingerly, I went back to my yoga room and finished my postures.

For a period of several months, my

EXPERIENCE: SKULL SHINING BREATH

Skull Shining Breath, or *Kapalabhati pranayama,* is one of the *shat kriyas,* or six purifying actions, traditionally used to prepare the body for depth practice. Practiced before or after postures, it powerfully works the lungs, oxygenates the blood, and eliminates carbon dioxide and other impurities through the exhalation. It also clears the nasal passages, strengthens the diaphragm, and massages the vital organs.

Skull Shining Breath is a rhythmic series of exhalations through the nostrils, accomplished by contracting the muscles of the abdomen, which lifts the diaphragm. Each exhalation is followed by a passive inhalation of air through the nostrils, which happens naturally as the abdomen relaxes, which allows the diaphragm to lower. The time taken for the inhalation is slightly longer than the exhalation. As you become established in the practice, you will be able to maintain a smooth rhythm that starts slow and builds momentum over the course of a round. Skull Shining Breath may be done in a slow, medium, or fast rhythm and sounds a bit like a steam engine puffing along at different speeds.

Practice on an empty stomach. If you feel light-headed or short of breath, slow down the pace and make sure you are completely relaxing the abdomen, which is the key to a passive inhalation that takes in enough air. If the practice feels awkward or difficult at first, know that it is normal for it to take some practice to build strength and coordinate your breath with the movement of the abdomen.

This is an intensive breathing exercise which should not be practiced if you are menstruating, pregnant, have epilepsy, unmedicated high blood pressure, have recently undergone surgery, or have any other active injury or inflammation in the abdomen or chest. If after practicing you feel overly light-headed, anxious, or irritable, either decrease the number of exhalations or rounds or stop altogether and resume practice of Ocean Sounding and Sun Breath. If you start gently and work into the practice gradually, you are likely to find this an enjoyable and energizing addition to your daily yoga routine.

1. Sit comfortably on the floor or in a straight-backed chair. Elongate your spine, close your eyes, and relax your body.

2. Consciously soften the belly and allow the breath to flow freely. Come into a few minutes of Ocean Sounding Three-Part Breathing to warm up the lungs and breathing muscles.

3. Place your hands on your lower belly. Begin to slowly and rhythmically contract the muscles of the abdomen, expelling air through the nostrils. These are sharp exhalations, followed by passive inhalations. Allow the abdomen to relax between exhalations to facilitate an inhalation of adequate depth. Feel the abdominal contractions and movement of the diaphragm with the hands, noticing that only the abdomen moves

while the rest of the body remains stationary. When you have become acquainted with the movement of the belly, you can bring the hands onto the knees or lap.

4. Find your rhythm, and let its pace build slightly. After twenty expulsions, take in a deep breath. Hold the breath for a few seconds, then exhale slowly. Let go of any effort to control the breath and watch as it naturally rebalances.

5. After the breath has returned to normal, repeat steps 3 and 4 two more times for an initial practice of three rounds of twenty expulsions. You can add ten more expulsions per week until you are doing three rounds of fifty expulsions.

6. After you are established in that practice for some months, you can incorporate *Alternate Nostril Kapalabhati* into your practice. Toward the end of each round, bring your dominant hand into Vishnu Mudra. Close off one nostril with the thumb, and exhale sharply through the other. Inhale through both nostrils, and then close off the other nostril with the ring and pinky fingers and exhale sharply. Continue in this fashion, inhaling through both nostrils and exhaling through alternate nostrils. Take a deep breath in, hold the breath for a few seconds, and exhale slowly.

7. End by sitting in stillness, watching the natural flow of breath. Feel the effects, noticing if you can sense energy moving in your body.

yoga mat felt like a psychic battlefield. Every now and then, I'd move into a posture and find myself facing a painful childhood memory, or flooded with anger, grief, sadness, doubt, or despair. While I didn't exactly like what was happening, it felt necessary and even "right" in a way I couldn't put into words. Through trial and error, I always found a way to deal with whatever difficult memory or painful emotion arose. Mostly I breathed, cried, or beat the bed. Sometimes I went for a walk.

At times I questioned what was happening, but deep down I knew that I was clearing out old and toxic emotional baggage. Looking back, it is clear that I was dealing with the uncomfortable emotions I'd always shoved aside in the past.

—Danna Faulds

Anyone who goes through a fiery time of purification emerges on the other side knowing firsthand its value and benefit. While making a sincere effort to clean up your lifestyle is important, remember that purification is just one aspect of the transformative process. Taken to extremes, it can turn into a puritanical asceticism that dead-ends in dogmatic behavior, emotional deadness, and self-righteousness.

An Elegant Approach

BY SENIOR TEACHER DIANA DAMELIO

My experience training yoga teachers has taught me how important it is for new students to engage in a disciplined willful practice to "strengthen the container." This means developing a body and mind strong enough, both physically and emotionally, to contain a higher voltage of energy. Until this work is done, the capacity to be the witness remains out of reach, and with it the ability to sense the subtle body activity that distinguishes the deeper stages of Kripalu Yoga practice. As the witness develops, it invariably brings a student into a state of absorption and flow.

Students sometimes form the mistaken impression that once the container is strengthened, Kripalu Yoga is all about Meditation-in-Motion. My own practice almost always includes a mix of willful postures and flowing yoga. I use postures and pranayama to prepare my body and mind for sitting meditation, which is the real core of my practice. When outer movement ceases, an inner flow continues that is the gateway to depth meditation and non-dual states.

Every month or so, a new crop of fledgling yoga teachers arrives at Kripalu Center. Sometimes, I start out resistant to the intensity of leading a large retreat that combines life-changing personal transformation with learning how to teach yoga. But as I return to the discipline of my own practice, and watch the students individually progress on their journeys, my resistance fades and disappears. This simple and elegant approach really works, and I remember again what a gift it is to be able to share this yoga and become grateful, very grateful.

Because the challenges presented by purification are very real, Kripalu Yoga recommends slow and steady lifestyle changes and deepening your yoga practice at a modest pace.

> *The transformation that took place in my mind, body, and spirit in the year I started doing Kripalu Yoga was amazing. At first I tried to be the perfect yogi, thinking that being involved in yoga meant I should give up everything I shouldn't be doing. I found that all I really needed to do was be true to myself. Truth is, I really didn't want those cigarettes or need those drinks to cover my pain. I became able to trust my body and eat what it really calls for. I discovered that when I just stay with my yoga practice, everything else falls into place. Along the*

way, I learned to let go of my attempt to be perfect. I may not reach enlightenment, but I'm more concerned now with being present to life and all the people in my life. This has become my yoga.

—Kathleen Grace Koch

A significant number of earnest spiritual seekers take up the practice of yoga. Unfortunately, many stop because exactly the right thing happens. That thing is purification.

—Swami Kripalu

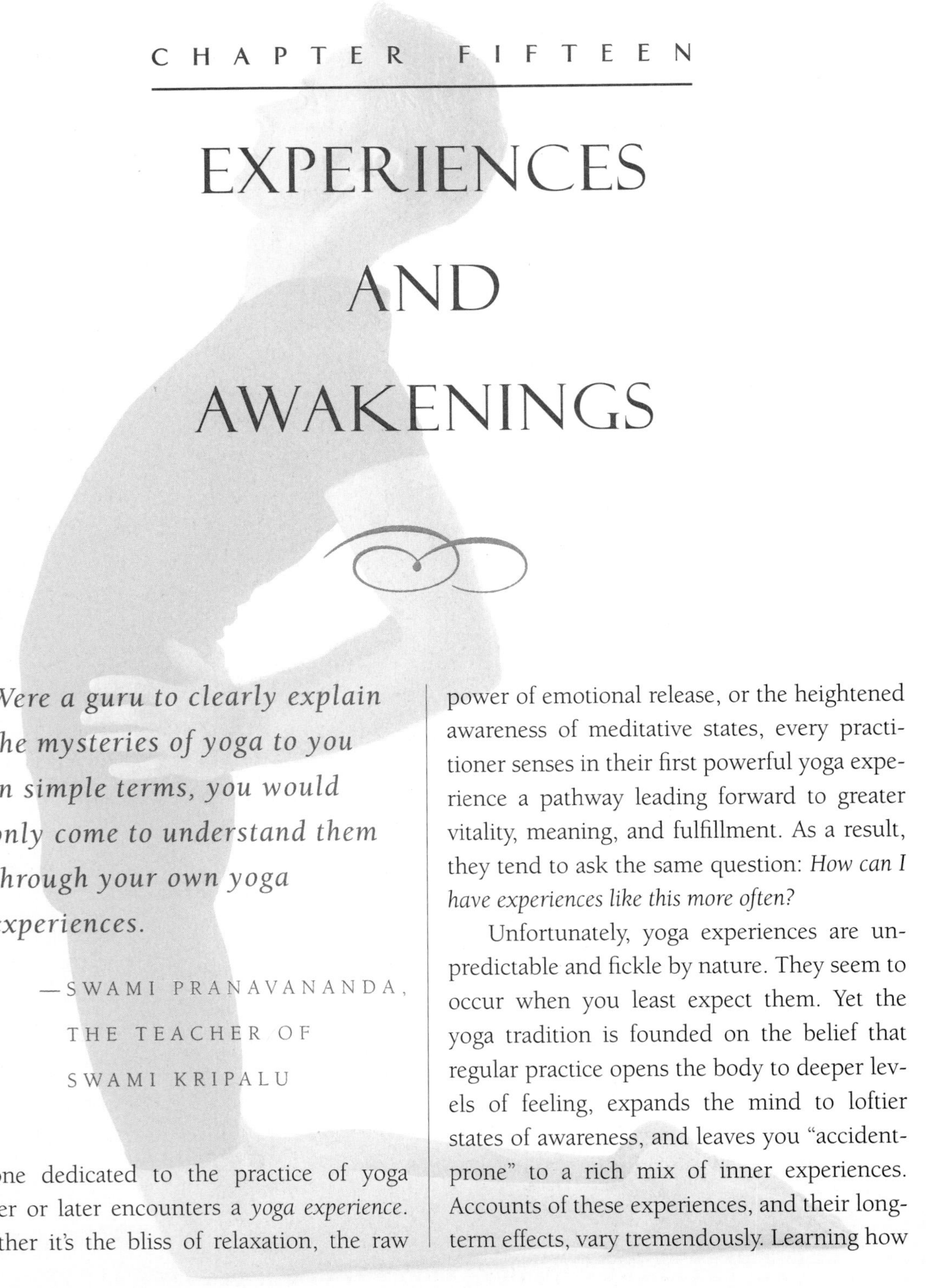

CHAPTER FIFTEEN

EXPERIENCES AND AWAKENINGS

Were a guru to clearly explain the mysteries of yoga to you in simple terms, you would only come to understand them through your own yoga experiences.

—SWAMI PRANAVANANDA, THE TEACHER OF SWAMI KRIPALU

Anyone dedicated to the practice of yoga sooner or later encounters a *yoga experience*. Whether it's the bliss of relaxation, the raw power of emotional release, or the heightened awareness of meditative states, every practitioner senses in their first powerful yoga experience a pathway leading forward to greater vitality, meaning, and fulfillment. As a result, they tend to ask the same question: *How can I have experiences like this more often?*

Unfortunately, yoga experiences are unpredictable and fickle by nature. They seem to occur when you least expect them. Yet the yoga tradition is founded on the belief that regular practice opens the body to deeper levels of feeling, expands the mind to loftier states of awareness, and leaves you "accident-prone" to a rich mix of inner experiences. Accounts of these experiences, and their long-term effects, vary tremendously. Learning how to open yourself to these experiences, and to let them touch and teach you, is one aspect of what takes your practice into the deeper realms that lie beyond body mechanics and physical fitness.

What Swami Kripalu described as a yoga experience is known in psychology as a *peak experience,* a term coined by one of the founders of humanistic psychology, Abraham Maslow. Peak experiences are moments of sudden joy and well-being that are often accompanied by heightened awareness, feelings of wonder and awe, and a notable lack of fear, anxiety, and doubt. Less often, they include a direct experience of "ultimate truth" or the unity of all things. Beyond their intrinsic value, Maslow believed peak experiences are catalysts for growth, releasing creative energies, transforming an individual's view of themselves and the world, increasing empathy, strengthening life purpose, and integrating the personality. After a lifetime of study, Maslow concluded that simply being aware of the potential to have a peak experience makes them more likely to occur. Yoga would agree, adding that our capacity for higher states can be consciously cultivated.

Deep yoga experiences are like flashes of lightning that illumine the landscape on a dark night. They momentarily crack open the psyche, revealing a glimpse of deeper truths and possibilities. Along with helping you stay inspired and motivated to practice, yoga experiences point the way toward the deeper awakenings and realizations yoga is designed to produce.

While being led in an experience of holding the Goddess Pose, I felt a wave of energy move up from my feet and through my whole body. A strange laugh started to come out of me, and within a split second I found myself sobbing uncontrollably. I decided to go with this experience and just witness what was happening. It was as if I went into a time continuum thirty years earlier. I saw myself as a ten-year-old, feeling my father's disapproval. I moved onto the floor and into Seated Angle Pose. I was so full of emotion that I could barely stay composed. An inner voice said to go deeper, and I became the little boy who was told that he would never be good enough, never ever quite right. I curled into a fetal position to take in the fullness of the moment. That experience shined the light on a part of me that felt unlovable and set me on my way to coming to terms with my father's inability to love me for who I am.

—Guy Matthews

What Causes Yoga Experiences?

Swami Kripalu taught that yoga experiences are signposts on the path of self-development, indicators that progress is being made in the underlying tasks of purification and growth. Although they often seem to arise out of the blue, yoga experiences result from a combination of three factors:

- A focused and introverted mind
- A heightened sensitivity to feeling
- An increased flow of life force

Although they may seem extraordinary, yoga experiences are actually the ordinary fruit of a committed practice, both on or off the mat. Avoid the pitfall of practicing with an unconscious belief that a depth practice requires the development of otherworldly faculties beyond your reach.

> *I was taking Yoga Teachers Training at Kripalu and doing yoga every day. At the beginning of a morning session, I was struck with a painful pressure in my right ear and felt dizzy. I tried to do some simple warm-ups and found myself submerged with feelings and emotions. A torrent of tears burst forth, and the pain spread to my jaw and neck. I started Ocean Sounding Breath to calm down and deal with the pain, but the dizziness only grew worse. I felt an outside pressure pressing in on my body. My right arm pinned itself against my side, hand tightly clenched. The thought of a stroke flashed through my mind and I grew frightened. The pressure continued to increase, changing into rumbling and shaking. It felt like an energetic tornado working its way down my arm. When it reached my clenched fingers, it slowly forced my hand open. Reaching my fingertips the energy shot out my now straightened fingers as if they were fire hoses. Twice more that morning the energetic tornado kicked up again in my legs and hips. These times I was not afraid and kept saying to myself, "Let it go, let it go." The difference in how I felt before and after these experiences astounded me. It was as if I had taken off an ugly, tight, heavy coat that I didn't even know I was wearing. I am still in awe over the transformative power of this experience.*
>
> —Yvette Bulger

What Is an Awakening?

It can be life changing to sob away profound grief, recover a part of yourself split off in childhood, glimpse with great acuity the beauty of creation, or break through to an exalted mind state. As compelling and revelatory as yoga experiences like these may be, however, they differ from the more fundamental *awakenings* that emerge from a deep practice of Kripalu Yoga. No matter how profound, experiences come and go. Although they may leave you changed in positive ways, they are a transient phenomenon. Yoga experiences tend to be extremely personal; they arise from a constellation of energetic patterning and psychological conditioning unique to you. In the midst of a moving experience, it often seems you could never forget the chain of events that unfolded, or the insights sparked as a result. A year or two later, you may or may not remember it.

Holding Bridge Pose, I was breathing deeply. I felt all the energy in my body collect around my navel. I shifted my focus to my heart, and felt the energy move into my chest and a series of images flooded into my mind, showing me that everything is life force, pulsating, malleable, flowing, interconnected. I thought, "This is God," and was completely awed. Releasing the pose, I slowly sank into relaxation, wanting to cry because what I experienced was so beautiful. I again felt sensations rise from belly to chest to throat, where they were constricted and I wanted to cry. I received another flood of images, this time from childhood, showing me incidents when I didn't say how I truly felt, relationships with old boyfriends where I didn't express my needs, all the times where I wish I had expressed myself, but didn't.

—Kim Kuhns

The word *awakening* suggests that you have sleeping capacities that can be roused to wakefulness. It asserts that you can open to whole new ways of being. Where an experience comes and goes, an awakening brings some essential aspect of you into full aliveness. After a little time to adjust to a fuller experience of yourself and life, the once latent ability feels entirely natural. It might be hard to remember that you were ever any other way. Yet reflecting back, you know for sure that a fundamental shift in your being has occurred. As developmental theorist Ken Wilber writes, there is a big difference between *states* and *traits*. Rather than temporary *states*, the object of spiritual practice is to embody higher qualities in all aspects of your life as stable character *traits*.

Spiritual teachers and practitioners use the word *awakening* differently. At times, it is used to describe a powerful experience that shifts the trajectory of a person's life, often setting him or her on a path of conscious growth. It is also used to refer to enlightenment, an ultimate state beyond separation and struggle. The awakenings sought in Kripalu Yoga may sound more modest: the vitality of the body, the ability to feel sensation and emotion fully, and the capacity of the mind to see reality clearly. But not only are these the awakenings that produce yoga experiences, they are also the capacities that help you progress along the path of transformation.

Awakenings of all kinds tend to be heralded and solidified by yoga experiences. There are gradual awakenings in which a latent ability gently sprouts and flowers over an extended period of time, accompanied by numerous experiences. There are sudden awakenings in which a single experience gives birth to a whole new way of being. It is not unusual for a person new to yoga to have a number of deep experiences over a short period of time as encrusted barriers fall away and basic sensitivities come alive. The dramatic nature of these initial experiences is usually more a result of the thickness of the filters that fall away than the depth of awakening that occurs. As practice begins to foster sustained growth, the rate of these experiences often slows down. After being dazzled by the fireworks, it can feel like nothing is happening and a temptation arises to discontinue a practice that has plateaued and is no longer producing results. If practice is continued, the slower and steadier cycles of long-term growth become apparent.

> *The value of any spiritual discipline can be measured by the degree to which it is capable of transforming one's personality.*
>
> —Swami Rajarshi Muni

Powerful experiences can sometimes produce a negative side effect by raising expectations about what should—or should not—be happening during your time on the mat. Expectations create tension and can be a barrier to the openness required to experience yourself in new ways. Resist the tendency to fixate on transient experiences. Also remember that doorways into deeper practice often swing open unexpectedly. It is not unusual for practice to feel mechanical at one moment, and in the next suddenly shift from distraction to sharp focus or deep absorption. With time you learn that the best anyone can do is suit up, show up, and let grace take care of the results.

SYNAPSE IN THE MIND OF GOD

In deep blue, dawn blue,
translucent blue, I lose
myself. I am a synapse
in the luminescent mind
of God. My heartmind
opens wide as I slide
inside the light, sensing
the link from the center
of my being to the inner
core of everything.

I am one pearl on a string
of pearls extending nowhere,
everywhere; bare awareness
filled with breath. Energy
pulses, toes to crown, or
down from throat to loins,
and I am tingling, so alive
I ache, eons or one breath
away from consummation.

CHAPTER SIXTEEN

BUILDING CHARACTER

> *You can straighten out the tail of a dog, but the moment you let it go, it snaps back into its original shape. That is why yoga places such importance on character building principles.*
>
> —SWAMI KRIPALU

Elite athletes do the impossible when *in the zone*. Artists enter *flow states* that heighten creative powers. Top executives learn to function at *peak performance*. Patients with life-threatening conditions heal themselves with prayer and visualization. All signs indicate that humans possess extraordinary capacities that are largely untapped, but can ordinary people really learn to access these deeper potentials?

For thousands of years, yoga and other contemplative traditions have sought to awaken humankind's sleeping capacity for extraordinary living. In addition to a set of practices integrating body and mind, these systems include a philosophy that encourages adherents to embark on a path of conscious self-development. Looking below the surface, one discovers that all these traditions emphasize ethics, linking what psychologists call *moral development* to extraordinary functioning. Why is this so?

Yoga teaches that humans are by nature caring and ethical beings. This is not a Pollyanna view that overlooks our capacity to do wrong. It is a statement that we cannot be at peace as long as we act in ways that go against what we know is right. Each time we ignore our moral compass, we create mental and emotional dissonance. In the short run, this disturbs our happiness. In the long run, it renders the mind unsteady and sabotages our powers of concentration. The contemplative traditions speak with one voice in saying that it is impossible to progress very far along a path of growth without developing a genuine concern for others. Only when the foundation of an ethical life is laid can practice deepen and bring extraordinary capacities to life.

The Four Aims of Life

Yoga teaches that humans are born with four primary drives. Exerting a steady pull of desire, each drive gives rise to what yoga calls a *noble aim of life*. The first aim is to acquire a steady supply of the material goods needed to keep body and soul together. Although referred to as *artha,* a word meaning *wealth,* this does not imply the hoarding of riches. It acknowledges our basic needs for food, shelter, and security.

We all long for something more than survival, and the second aim of life is *kama,* or *pleasure*. The good life is pleasant and comfortable. Yoga is often seen as founded upon asceticism and self-denial, but it actually acknowledges the need for pleasure and views the task of achieving it as noble.

The third aim of life is *dharma*. A word with no English equivalent, *dharma* has two distinct meanings. The down-to-earth definition of *dharma* is *an ethical and virtuous way of life*. It takes discipline to follow the rules of your society and be willing to look at situations from the perspective of others. Adherence brings self-esteem and the respect of your peers, both of which are required for success in life. The next level of dharma goes beyond what developmental psychologists call conventional or rule-bound thinking. *Dharma* also means *living in harmony with the divine order of the cosmos*. This is a call to attune to the subtleties of the circumstances at hand and act appropriately to the moment, drawing on intuitive knowing and the genuine concern for the welfare of others acquired in the first-level practice of dharma.

The fourth and final aim of life is *moksha,* or spiritual freedom, which arises from a drive to go beyond our mortal and limited sense of self. According to yoga, true fulfillment requires more than wealth, pleasure, status, and self-expression. It requires knowing that we are something more than body and mind, which can only come from personally experiencing our unlimited spiritual nature. In today's yoga world, moksha is most often called *self-realization*.

Dharma Is Pivotal

Satisfying the four aims of life while honoring the ethical precepts of dharma is a challenging task. It requires us to acquire practical skills, gain knowledge, expand our capacity

EXPERIENCE: ARE YOU GROWING?

H. C. Berner, an American student of Swami Kripalu, posed the following questions to help ascertain if you are progressing along the yoga path of growth:

- Are you taking better care of yourself and your body?
- Are you expressing your creative energies more freely?
- Are you increasingly successful in your work and personal life?
- Are your relationships with others improving?
- Are you more in touch with your true nature?

Answering "yes" to these questions indicates that you are pursuing all four aims of life.

for self-expression, hone discernment, practice restraint, and ultimately transform our conception of who and what we are. If measured by the four aims, success in life requires comprehensive self-development. The key to applying these principles to your life is understanding what dharma is—and isn't.

Where contemporary society views ethics as relative and subjective, the Indian sages taught that certain ethical principles are universal and apply regardless of time, place, or circumstance. They called these principles *yama* and *niyama*. *Yama* means *restraint* or *behavior to avoid*. *Niyama* means *observance* or *conduct to cultivate*. With five yamas and five niyamas, it is easy to think of yama and niyama as the Ten Commandments of yoga. Rather than a right/wrong morality rooted in obedience to a judging God, they affirm the positive qualities that reside in the heart and soul of every individual. Instead of assigning blame or guilt, yoga aims to awaken inner sensitivities and reveal the virtuous character lying dormant within everyone. Yoga lore portrays our lost virtue as a golden statue buried underground for centuries. Exhumed, it requires cleaning, but encrusted layers of dirt have not corrupted its beauty. This attitude that yoga's ethical precepts mirror every individual's innate goodness waiting to be revealed is very different from the "thou shalt not" approach many of us grew up with.

> *The success achieved by men and women in various fields is founded upon the practice of the principles contained in yama and niyama. I can confidently state that anyone who ignores yama and niyama is clearly stunting his own growth and development.*
>
> — Swami Kripalu

Yama or Restraints

AHIMSA: NONVIOLENCE

When one practices nonviolence, one refrains from causing distress in thought, word, or deed to any living creature. Nonviolence is the root of all other ethical precepts.

SATYA: TRUTH

Truth destroys the walls between hearts, transforming strangers and even enemies into loved ones. Truth is speaking that which promotes the welfare of all beings, and which is not adulterated with untruth. To practice truth, we should decrease our practice of untruth.

ASTEYA: NON-STEALING

When we obtain what we desire by honest means, our mind remains at peace and free of fear. Non-stealing is not desiring anyone's wealth by thought, word, or deed, and not taking anyone's possessions, no matter how small, without their permission.

APARIGRAHA: NONATTACHMENT

A person practicing nonattachment cultivates a voluntary simplicity and discharges his or her duties in life while remaining free of obsessive desires. Any action performed for the love of God or welfare of humanity is a form of nonattachment.

BRAHMACHARYA: MODERATION

Brahmacharya literally means *movement toward the Lord* and its practice involves moderation in all sense pleasures. If you want to bring forth harmonious music from your body and mind, you will have to walk the path of moderation.

While holding high ethical principles, the Indian sages recognized that genuine virtue requires something more than following the letter of the law. A person of great integrity has embodied these principles to the extent that his or her actions naturally spring from them.

Yoga Versus Morality

Yoga and *morality* are not synonymous terms. Morality is concerned with issues of right and wrong. Yoga is a comprehensive path of self-development that fosters moral development. Rather than aspiring to be a "good person,"

Niyama or Observances

SAUCHA: PURITY

Purity involves cultivating a healthy body through habits such as proper diet, bathing, and regular exercise. It also includes cultivating a wholesome mind through positive thinking, good company, prayer, and meditation. Virtuous conduct is the chief characteristic of mental purity, since one can act virtuously only when his or her mind is pure.

SANTOSHA: CONTENTMENT

Contentment is joyfully accepting whatever life provides and not wanting more than is at hand. Contentment renders the mind steady and is a source of true happiness. A content person is able to bear the experience of mental distress.

TAPAS: AUSTERITY

Tapas means *to generate light or heat.* It refers to the psychic energy generated by the voluntary practice of disciplines that purify the body and mind and generate spiritual radiance. Just as fire purifies gold, austerity purifies the seeker.

SWADHYAYA: STUDY OF SELF AND SCRIPTURES

One practices swadhyaya to get to know one's true Self. The highest form of swadhyaya is a continual process of self-observation and inquiry into the true nature of self and psyche, but it also includes reflecting upon scriptures and inspirational reading. Study integrates knowledge and action.

ISHVARA-PRANIDHANA: SURRENDER TO THE DIVINE

In order to find peace and experience our inborn divinity, we must surrender to a higher principle. *Ishvara-pranidhana* means to dedicate one's every thought, word, and deed to the Divine with total faith.

yoga advises you to stay connected to your individual needs, which are the source of your drive and energy. Channeling this energy to meet the four aims of life, you will discover that your own happiness and well-being require you to become a better person. When you encounter a person of great spiritual maturity, like Swami Kripalu, it may appear that he or she is scrupulously moral. On closer inspection, you discover that they are deeply integrated in their being. Their personal needs are no longer in conflict with the world around them, which brings them a measure of peace and freedom. As one is maturing toward this state, the dynamic tension involved in meeting competing needs produces what Swami Kripalu referred to as *character building.*

> *A few years ago I had a series of difficult experiences, including some challenging relationship issues within my family. To cap things off, my dog was hit by a car and killed. I came back to my Kripalu Yoga practice and found that I understood the teachings more deeply. I was able to put myself back together again, using postures to ground me in my body. Breathing helped me to keep letting the emotions flow through and not build up inside me. Gradually I gained strength and regained the ability to feel. I began practicing the yamas and niyamas—seeing myself as a human who makes mistakes just like everyone else, accepting all that had happened in my family. Over time, I began to feel the Divine inside of me, and it filled me up again, helping me find my true being and real purpose in life.*
>
> —Jennifer Alexander

Self-Observation Without Judgment

When you boil yoga down to its essence, you discover that all its practices are designed to provide the key ingredient needed for character building, what Swami Kripalu called *self-observation without judgment.* At other times he used the phrase *self-observation with love.* Although self-observation begins with self-acceptance, an attitude praised by many psychologists, it eventually goes considerably deeper.

Self-judgment is the force that causes material to be pushed out of awareness and gives birth to the inauthentic personas we unconsciously adopt to meet our needs in a less than straightforward manner. Unless we can refrain from self-judgment, layers of fearful thinking, defensive posturing, and primitive urges like rage, lust, greed, and envy remain buried in the unconscious. Self-love is the essential tool needed to disarm the mind's self-protective mechanisms. In shedding light on those parts of the psyche that have been repressed, we can access the tremendous energy locked in the unconscious and use it to fuel a transformative process that jettisons masks and conditioning to reveal our authentic character.

Learning how to cultivate a non-reactive awareness is the essential skill. When you can feel powerful emotions arise in the body, or see distracting thoughts and conditioned responses arise in your mind, without losing yourself in them, you grow able to learn from your direct experience of making your way through life. Yoga practice has an important role to play here, helping you stay connected to your inner experience. When practiced with compassionate self-observation, yoga not only quiets the inner critic. It sets the stage for

Why Character Matters

BY SENIOR TEACHER DINABANDHU GARRETT SARLEY

I began my practice of yoga when I was eighteen. For several years, I was consumed with making rapid progress in postures, pranayama, and meditation. I tracked the hours spent in practice each day and took great pride in my growing flexibility and calm. While I read about the need for character development, it seemed tangential to my main practice. Somehow I assumed that along the way to enlightenment I would just naturally become pure of heart and develop self-control.

After a few years of this approach, I began to hit a ceiling in the results I was getting from practice. I could now touch my toes, but I was no less insecure or competitive. Many of the unconscious patterns of behavior I had before yoga remained intact, and fulfillment remained beyond my reach. Slowly the realization dawned on me that the quality of my relationships with others was a better indicator of my success in yoga than my flexibility. If I really desired the unity consciousness that is yoga, I had to embody it in all of my life.

Practically speaking, this meant finding ways to see and uproot habitual ways of interacting with others that were creating conflict and separation. I began to carefully observe my actions in daily life. At that time, I honestly believed that I had basically developed good character, that I only occasionally lied, was hurtful, engaged in addictive behaviors, etc., and when I did it was minor and didn't really matter. I quickly discovered that I was constantly shading the truth to look good, hiding my failures to avoid embarrassment, and unintentionally hurting people because I was so focused on meeting my own needs. Where yoga practitioners are guided to be indifferent to pleasure or pain, and success or failure, I could not escape the fact that I was a veritable storehouse of preferences and desires.

Yoga is a path beyond separation, a way to return to the truth of our connectedness with all beings and all things. Seen through this lens, character development started to make a lot more sense. If we look at yama and niyama in this light, we see that each of them prevents a tear in the fabric of connectedness and union. When I lie, I separate myself from truth and everything else. When I give in to greed, I retreat into my most disconnected sense of self that can never get enough. And when I adhere to yama and niyama, I protect my connection to my essential self, the one that is always safe and at peace.

When we come into a posture properly, most of us report a feeling of "rightness." By aligning our bodies as nature intended, we somehow come home to our selves. In much the same way, when we practice the tenets of yama and niyama, our spirit remembers who we are. We feel good about ourselves and grow a little more alive. There is no morality at play here, just the natural intelligence of the universe working patiently to restore a tear in the fabric of one reality. Doing this again and again removes fear, creates confidence, and generates a nobility of Self that brings happiness, security, and fulfillment within our reach. For anyone on the path to yoga, character really does matter. Not someone else's, but your own.

character building and extraordinary functioning.

Tools for Growth

Coupled with compassionate self-observation, yama and niyama become powerful tools for growth. Practice begins with yama, the restraints designed to bring the instinctual urges of the body into balance and harmonize social relationships. The peace of mind that results makes it possible to practice niyama, the conscious cultivation of positive qualities. Wholesome traits are nurtured. Faults are simply witnessed and allowed to wither. Remember that self-observation is intended to expand your ability to see yourself objectively, which includes both your positive and not-so-positive qualities. At first your shortcomings and negative traits are likely to loom large and stand out in high relief. Gradually it becomes possible to see your positive qualities too.

It is natural to feel overwhelmed at the prospect of tackling all ten restraints and observances at once. Swami Kripalu recommended choosing one to practice intensively for a time, saying that by firmly grasping any one of its flowers you can lift the entire garland of yama and niyama.

> *Do not wrestle with a fault that you want to remove. Wrestling increases the disturbance of the mind and allows the excited fault to lift you up and slam you to the ground. Unable to pull yourself up to fight again, you will eventually give up the fight forever. The best way to remove a fault is to practice its opposite virtue, which decreases mental restlessness. By applying this principle, a person can gradually eradicate his or her bad character traits and formulate the best possible personality. This process, however, inevitably requires patience, enthusiasm, tolerance, and ardent perseverance.*
>
> —Swami Kripalu

CHAPTER SEVENTEEN

OPENING THE HEART

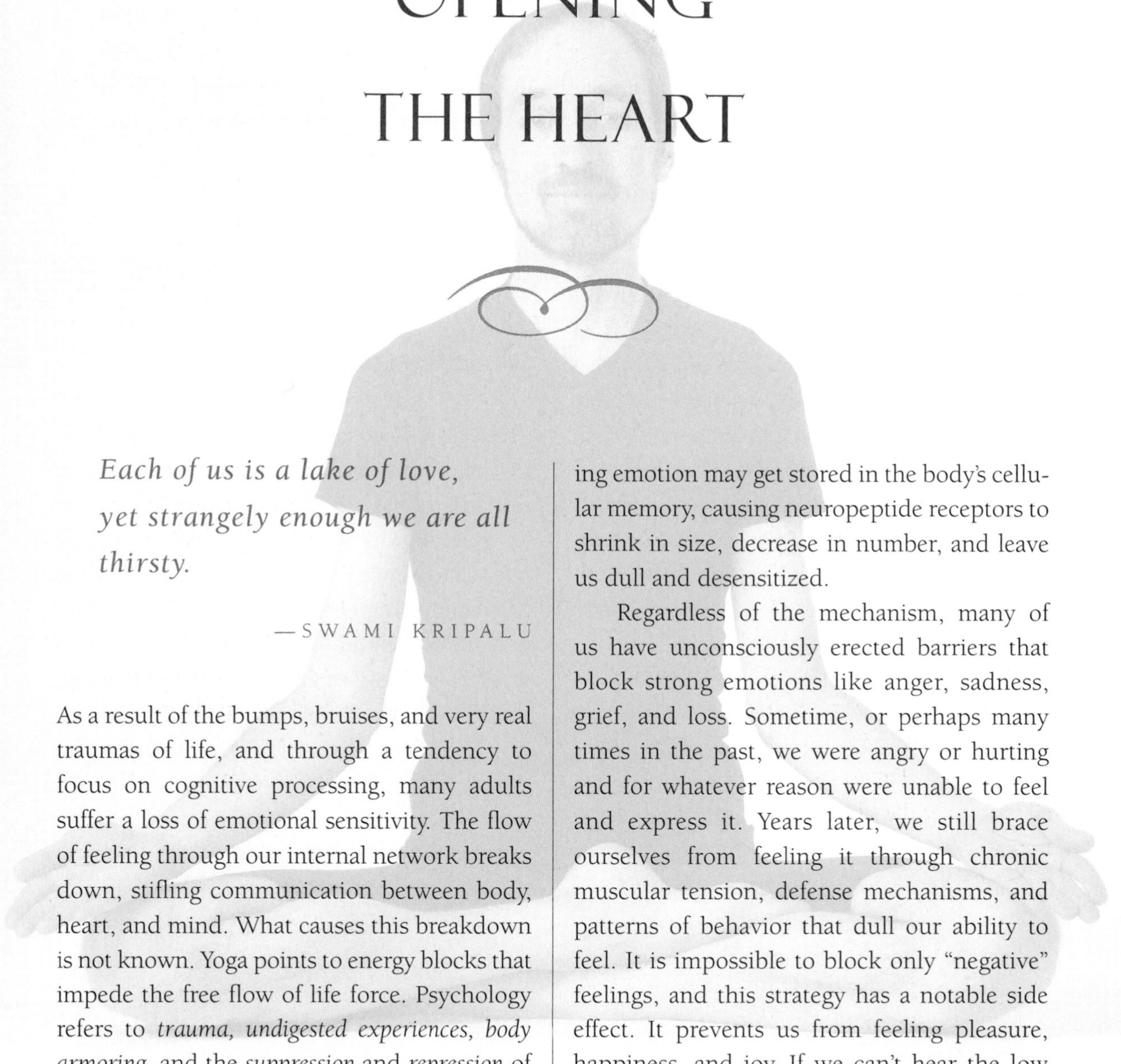

> *Each of us is a lake of love,*
> *yet strangely enough we are all*
> *thirsty.*
>
> —SWAMI KRIPALU

As a result of the bumps, bruises, and very real traumas of life, and through a tendency to focus on cognitive processing, many adults suffer a loss of emotional sensitivity. The flow of feeling through our internal network breaks down, stifling communication between body, heart, and mind. What causes this breakdown is not known. Yoga points to energy blocks that impede the free flow of life force. Psychology refers to *trauma, undigested experiences, body armoring,* and the *suppression* and *repression* of feeling. Neuroscience posits that overwhelming emotion may get stored in the body's cellular memory, causing neuropeptide receptors to shrink in size, decrease in number, and leave us dull and desensitized.

Regardless of the mechanism, many of us have unconsciously erected barriers that block strong emotions like anger, sadness, grief, and loss. Sometime, or perhaps many times in the past, we were angry or hurting and for whatever reason were unable to feel and express it. Years later, we still brace ourselves from feeling it through chronic muscular tension, defense mechanisms, and patterns of behavior that dull our ability to feel. It is impossible to block only "negative" feelings, and this strategy has a notable side effect. It prevents us from feeling pleasure, happiness, and joy. If we can't hear the low notes, we can't hear the high notes either.

Inhabiting a narrow band of feeling not only limits us individually, it restricts our ability to connect with other people. When severe, it can leave us isolated, lonely, and unable to create and sustain intimacy.

To make matters worse, there is a strong tendency for this state of affairs to spiral in the wrong direction. Suppression is like holding a beach ball under water. As the beach ball grows in size, more and more effort is required to hold things in place. Pressure builds within the psyche and we become reactive, carrying around an emotional charge and apt to fly off the handle by responding to situations with too much intensity. Bottling up emotion also agitates the mind, and we lose clarity. Acutely aware of the pressure, we are often in the dark on what is causing it, or how to alleviate it. All this makes the prospect of opening up to feeling even more threatening, so we clamp down harder still. The path to opening the heart starts with reversing this process and regaining the ability to feel.

> *The past four years have been the most challenging of my life as I have made my way through the pain of separation, divorce, deception, and betrayal. Anger, bitterness, negativity, self-pity, unutterably deep sorrow and grief, overwhelming devastation and despair are just a few of the emotions that ran through me. Without Kripalu Yoga, I'm sure I would not be where I am today. Instead of repressing my feelings, yoga gave me a way to release those feelings safely—to process them through my body. Time and again, I felt emotions rising to the surface while practicing postures. I breathe and stay in the moment and soon the emotion subsides. I always leave my yoga practice uplifted and inspired to "take the high road" in my actions. Kripalu Yoga has a very cleansing and purifying effect, and helped to make this very difficult time more bearable.*
>
> —Mary Yoke

What Are Feelings?

The term *feelings* covers a lot of real estate. Feelings are the colors, textures, and tones of your response to the world around you. When you are in touch with your feelings, life is vivid and real. Cut off from your feelings, life occurs as dry, hollow, humdrum, and meaningless. You may find it helpful to distinguish between two types of feelings that arise during yoga practice, *sensation* and *emotion*. Sensation is the raw physical experience of being in a body that pulses with life and is equipped with five senses. It includes the ability to sense the body's position in space, feel movement, and identify differences in warmth and cold, tension and relaxation, heaviness and lightness. It also includes the visual images, sounds, textures, tastes, and smells associated with the outside world. Mediated by the cerebellum and brain stem, sensations are basic messages essential for our safety and survival.

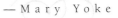

THE MOLECULES OF EMOTION

The pioneering work of neuroscientist Candace B. Pert, PhD, suggests that emotions are part of a biochemical information network linking body and brain. The body has a "chemical nervous system" that operates through the flow of neuropeptides, information-carrying molecules produced all over the body that link with specific receptor sites in the brain. Pert believes that emotion is the felt sense of this exchange of information. As she describes in her book *Molecules of Emotion:*

Every second a massive information exchange is occurring in your body. Imagine each of these messenger systems possessing a specific tone, humming a signature tune, rising and falling, waxing and waning, binding and unbinding, and if we could hear this body music with our ears, then the sum of these sounds would be the music that we call the emotions.

My research has shown me that when emotions are expressed—which is to say that the biochemicals that are the substrate of emotion are flowing freely—all systems are united and made whole. When emotions are repressed, denied, not allowed to be whatever they may be, our network pathways get blocked, stopping the flow of vital feel-good unifying chemicals that run both our biology and our behavior.

What Are Emotions?

Emotions, on the other hand, are richer, meaning-laden feelings that seem to occur at the interface of body and mind. While the biological basis of emotion is not yet fully understood, it is clear that emotions are processed by different parts of the brain—the amygdala, hypothalamus, and limbic system—known to play important roles in decision-making and memory.

Emotions convey a wide range of important messages. The flow of emotion is not an occasional occurrence, as suggested by the phrase *getting emotional*. The emotional system is working all the time to sustain a familiar *emotional tone* that governs mood, colors thought, and helps us act appropriately. A consistently angry or sad person has often grown so accustomed to their emotional tone that they are unconscious of how it impacts their behavior and their reception by others.

> *Kripalu Yoga makes more room inside of me, and I've discovered that there is so much to explore. It's not always pleasant, but I've become emotionally and spiritually stronger. I used to be reserved and guarded and let the past rule the future. Now I can express myself more freely and love more openly.*
>
> —Suzanne Swang

Emotions are complex and sometimes confusing. It is not uncommon to flip-flop between opposing emotions in response to a situation. You may be happy that you got a promotion at work, but sad that a hard-working colleague was passed over. You may feel genuine warmth for a loved one, yet be enraged at how they are treating you. You may be elated to have accomplished a major goal in life, but feel overwhelmed by yet another hurdle looming on the horizon. To further complicate matters, your emotional and cognitive response to a situation may conflict. Thoughts and feelings can diverge in different directions, leaving you confused and needing time to sort things out.

Kripalu Yoga teaches you how to hear and honor the full range of emotional messages flowing through you. By listening closely, most practitioners discover that their body is far from a mindless brute. Dancing for joy, or sobbing with sadness, the body is highly sensitive and profoundly wise. It is the seat of an attribute as old as the hills but only now being recognized as important: emotional intelligence.

> *Kripalu Yoga so fundamentally altered the way I see myself and the world around me that years later I am still moved to tears writing these words. Thanks to Kripalu Yoga, I was able to reinhabit my body and release a lifetime of accumulated tension and psychic pain. As I practiced with awareness, the adult I had become was able to make space for the forlorn little girl I had once been. As I experienced my own suffering and welcomed it into the light of consciousness, my sweet, true Self emerged and compassion gradually awakened in me; compassion for myself—both as a child and as an adult—and by extension for all others who suffer as well. In this mysterious and graceful way, Kripalu Yoga opened my heart, teaching me what it is to love and be loved. For that great gift, I will always be immensely grateful.*
>
> —Suzanne Selby Grenager

Regaining Sensitivity

Kripalu Yoga offers a way to safely reclaim your ability to feel. It is based on a simple but powerful truth: you do not need to do anything to

ARE TRAUMATIC EMOTIONS STORED IN THE BODY?

Yoga and traditional healing systems have taught for millennia that repressed emotion can be stored in the tissues of the body, dull vitality, and even cause illness. In the 1920s, controverisal psychiatrist Wilhelm Reich introduced a similar idea to Western medicine. Reich believed the body responds to external threats by contracting muscles in areas that feel threatened. Initially, this state of contraction reduces vulnerability and dulls pain. When chronic, Reich called it *body armoring* because it had the parallel effect of limiting the capacity to relax and feel pleasure. Reich's work formed the basis for a number of body-centered therapies that utilize movement and breathing to release body armoring and repressed emotion. Contemporary "body psychotherapies" such as Phoenix Rising Yoga Therapy and Core Energetics help clients contact and release buried emotion. Candace Pert, whose research suggests that emotional memory is stored in neuropeptide receptor sites throughout the body, calls herself a *molecular Reichian*.

change or fix your emotions. You just need to stay present in your body and ride the waves of whatever feelings arise during practice. Sensations and emotions are messages conveyed in the language of feeling. You can learn to receive the message and let it go. With each message received, you grow in self-awareness and a layer of tension melts away.

During practice, uncomfortable or even painful emotions should not be rejected. Instead of evidence that you are *doing it wrong*, their presence is a strong indication that you are *doing it right*. There is simply no way to free yourself of an emotional burden without feeling the weight, bit by bit, of what you have been carrying. Buried emotion rises from the subconscious and unconscious to be fully felt, pass through you, and leave you lighter and wiser. When you really catch on to this, strong, painful, and even neurotic emotions become your light in the darkness. Watch them enter your consciousness. Feel them in your body. Breathe into them. Notice as the sensations shift and change. When held in the light of awareness, what was feared as an obstacle often befriends you and reveals a profound secret.

Yoga and Depression

BY SENIOR TEACHER AMY WEINTRAUB

For many years, I had a shaky sense of my own worth and suffered from depression. Empty and numb, I often woke up feeling like there was a layer of cotton batting between my brain and my cranium. Despite medication and psychotherapy, I felt doomed to an unsatisfying life, no matter how much I loved and was loved, no matter what I achieved. I recovered from depression through my practice of yoga, which balanced the biochemistry of my brain, stimulated my endocrine system, created a state of healing relaxation, and dissolved the beliefs I carried from childhood that made me feel unworthy of love.

Depression is a deadly disease—it's the fourth leading cause of death worldwide and by 2020 is expected to rise to number two. Recent studies have shown yoga techniques create an immediate biochemical state that feels good, elevating the hormones prolactin and oxcytocin (the "cuddle hormone"); increasing glucose and oxygen, the building blocks for the neurotransmitters, including serotonin; balancing dopamine and norepinephrine; and reducing the stress hormone cortisol. Yoga also stimulates the parasympathetic nervous system so the body feels calm and relaxed. Many practitioners say their yoga practice has beneficial effects on their emotional well-being, their mental acuity, and in many cases alleviates the symptoms of depression.

When depressed, your shoulders may slump forward, closing the chest and rendering the breath shallow. This body posture tends to reinforce the state of low energy that characterizes depression. Yoga practice opens the chest, improves posture, deepens the breath, and increases the amount of energy traveling through your system.

When we practice yoga with sensitivity to our inner experience, we meet our depression at its source. We strip away the layers of tension that make us feel separate and release emotional blocks held in the body that prevent us from experiencing our wholeness. I hope that you will be encouraged by the news that I felt better after my very first yoga class. Within a year of beginning my yoga practice, I was free of antidepressant medication. In gratitude for my recovery, I am passionate about sharing the gifts I have received on my yoga mat with others who suffer.

For additional information, see Amy Weintraub's *Yoga for Depression: A Compassionate Guide to Relieve Suffering Through Yoga* (Broadway Books, 2004).

Being gentle with myself has never been easy—and that includes my yoga practice. One morning, I stepped forward into the Warrior. I had practiced this posture for five years and it hadn't opened for me at all. Most days I'd push myself past my edge and when my body didn't meet my rigid expectations, thoughts would start coming like "You've been doing this long enough that your thigh should be horizontal." This particular morning, I guess I got fed up with the crap I'd been giving myself. It was as if I said "No more!" to that critical voice inside me. I decided to just be with where I was in this pose instead of forcing past my limits. As soon as I eased up, something beautiful started to happen. I felt a deep sense of peace come over me. My heart glowed. I experienced a glorious feeling of interconnectedness. If I'd known self-acceptance would feel this good, I would have started a long time ago! I am continually reminded of this experience whenever I don't like where I am emotionally or physically. I still struggle from time to time, but having felt the love available to me just from being with my edge in the Warrior, I find it easier to back off and accept myself with compassion whenever I'm not meeting my expectations.

—Kristin Herbst

INSTRUCTIONS

Hold the silence like
a mother holds her child.
Hold your ground while
all around you structures
crumble into nothing.
Focus on the still point
in your center until you
are filled with light, until
Spirit speaks to you in
words you understand,
until the love in your
heart grows so strong
it must be shared.

Emotional Benefits of Yoga

There is an intrinsic value to feeling, not as a means to gain self-awareness or foster healing, but simply to be more alive. As the emotional system clears, it feels good just to feel.

As you open to feeling, it is likely that you will experience a gradual lessening of whatever emotional charge you are carrying. If your emotional "set point" has become stuck in one place, it may shift. If you are melancholy by nature, yoga won't necessarily turn you into a perpetually upbeat person. But practice will help you regain a buoyant emotional tone, one that rises and falls appropriately with the circumstances you are facing. Over time you will recover the ability to feel a wider range of

EXPERIENCE: BECOMING A WELL-WISHER OF ALL

The Kripalu Yoga tradition encourages practitioners to become a *well-wisher of all*. The following technique is a way to actualize this aspiration of opening your heart to others. Based on a prayer used by Swami Kripalu, it is also informed by the Buddhist practice of Metta or Loving-Kindness meditation.

1. Adjust your sitting posture to make your body comfortable. Press the sitz bones down and lift through the crown of your head to elongate the spine. Bring yourself fully present through the five steps of breathe, relax, feel, watch, and allow. Take a few long, deep breaths.

2. Now, bring your attention to yourself. Inwardly repeat the following prayer:

   May I be happy.
   May I be healthy.
   May I prosper in all ways.
   May I be free.

   If you notice any discomfort in wishing yourself well, just witness that with compassion.

3. Bring your attention to a person for whom you feel a natural love. Inwardly repeat the following prayer:

   May you be happy, as I wish to be happy.
   May you be healthy, as I wish to be healthy.
   May you prosper in all ways, as I wish to prosper.
   May you be free, as I wish to be free.

   Then repeat the prayer for a person with whom you have difficulty. If you notice any discomfort in wishing this person well, just notice that with compassion.

4. End by bringing your attention to all beings everywhere, and inwardly repeating the following prayer:

   May everyone be happy.
   May everyone be healthy.
   May everyone prosper.
   May everyone be free.

emotions, giving you a larger palette of colors from which to paint your experience of life.

People often push away uncomfortable feelings out of a fear that letting them in would render them an emotional basket case. By teaching you how to be with powerful emotions and not react in a knee-jerk fashion, Kripalu Yoga helps you do the inner work required to clear your system without becoming overwhelmed or dysfunctional. Current research reveals that the emotional brain and cognitive brain are partners, debunking the old notion that emotion-free reason is at the pinnacle of a decisive mind. This lines up with

A Man's Heart Opens

BY SENIOR TEACHER RICHARD FAULDS

I had been practicing Kripalu Yoga for several years, in part to get more in touch with my feelings. I knew that I was a sensitive person at heart, but I had somehow fallen out of touch with myself. As a result, I was often less than clear in my communications and somewhat awkward in relationships. At times I would have moments of deep feeling in workshops or while practicing yoga, but they would pass and I would resume my normal state. I felt something was eluding me but didn't know exactly what.

One day I was practicing yoga and out of nowhere had a clear vision of an electrical junction box situated right in the center of my chest. It was not just a vision; I could also feel it there. I stayed with the experience and gradually saw that the wires leading into the box had been disconnected so the current couldn't flow. This was perplexing. What did it mean?

The image and feeling stayed with me. On the next morning, I noticed that the wires had been neatly tied off with electrical tape and wire nuts. An immediate knowing flooded into my mind. This was the handiwork of my father, a consummate do-it-yourselfer. Outrage and then just flat-out rage filled me. How could he possibly have done this? Who would ever do something like this to anyone else, let alone their own son?

These feelings haunted me for several more days. They came unbidden into my mind whenever I lost focus on whatever else I happened to be doing. I stayed with the experience each morning as I practiced yoga. Somehow or other I got through the rage by once again noticing how neatly the wires had been treated. Clearly my father had done this job with great care. This must be how he thought a man's heart should be wired. He was just following the blueprint he had been given! Love for my father filled me and I wept. And then another thought came to me. Even though I am no match for my father with a pair of pliers, I could rewire the box myself. I could make a start right now by taking off the wire nuts and removing the electrical tape, which looked easy enough.

What happened next I will always remember with profound feeling. Without any conscious thought on my part, the wires came alive and slowly melded into one another perfectly, as if they had never been cut. The junction box dissolved and the center of my chest turned into a glowing, golden, exquisite, and perfectly functioning human heart. The effects of that experience rippled out into my entire life. Now, some years later, I would find it surprising not to be in touch with my own feelings. But back then, it was a revelation. I am happy to say that my father is still alive and we have grown close.

the consistent experience of Kripalu Yoga practitioners who discover that as the emotional faculties clear they become trustworthy sources of intuitive information about the world around them. A mature emotional connection is empowering. Instead of losing life hardiness, you actually gain strength.

Opening your heart to yourself and others is not without risk or challenge. Emotional release can be cathartic, and confronting the associated mental content difficult. In the presence of strong emotions, it is easy to fall into the trap of trying to understand or fix them. This is often motivated by the conscious or unconscious belief that understanding will make the uncomfortable feelings go away. Strong emotion can also lead you to act out by engaging in habitual or inappropriate behavior. Instead of pushing the feelings away, trying to understand them, or channeling them into compensatory behaviors, choose to feel them fully in your body. This is the simple, but not necessarily easy, key to overcoming all these challenges.

The full flowering of emotional health is larger than intrapersonal wellness. It is the capacity to live in a web of authentic and caring relationships. As your heart opens, your capacity for empathy expands and relationships take on more meaning. Close relationships allow you to be real and genuine, sharing whatever it is you are feeling. They are also a place where you can listen deeply, understand another's experience, and express true caring. When your heart is open, even casual interactions can be intimate and meaningful.

> *Kripalu Yoga taught me that yoga is about paying attention on the yoga mat and in life. With this learning, my life began to transform. I began to notice the abundance and grace already in my life, rather than everything I didn't have and thought I needed. As I deepened my practice, I found my heart opening, and more love coming in and flowing out—not just to my family, but to everyone I came in contact with.*
>
> —Jashoda Rona Edmunds

Love Is Your True Nature

Using the tools of yoga to strengthen your connection to your feeling self makes it possible to feel the love that is already there, even when shields and scars obscure it. By helping you regain sensitivity, Kripalu Yoga offers a pathway back to the treasure trove of love hidden in your own heart, and in the hearts of others.

> *Truly the wise proclaim that love is the only path, love is the only God, and love is the only scripture. Impress this verse upon your memory and repeat it constantly if you want to realize your dreams of growth.*
>
> —Swami Kripalu

CHAPTER EIGHTEEN

RIDING THE WAVE OF SENSATION

In everyone's body passions and strong emotions arise. Passions are expressions of intensely flowing life energy. Yogis know how to derive benefit from passions through the techniques of yoga.

—SWAMI KRIPALU

Many spiritual traditions consider strong emotion as an impediment to practice, an obstacle to attaining the peaceful state of mind you seek. Kripalu Yoga takes a different approach. It honors the wisdom that brings an emotion into awareness at a particular moment in time. It views emotion as an important message and potent form of transformative energy. Push away painful or uncomfortable feelings to get on with your practice, and you turn away an opportunity for growth. Rather than make matters better, it further distances you from yourself.

Three years ago, I was under a lot of stress and knew that something was desperately missing in my life. I stumbled upon an article about yoga. Something inside just clicked and I went to my first class and loved it. In the second class, something happened toward the end of class. The teacher was guiding us into the twist and said, "Breathe. Relax. Let go." I tried to hold back the tears but started to cry. We moved on to the other side and again the teacher instructed, "Breathe. Relax. Let go." I began to sob and the release that followed was powerful. That day the door to a new life opened for me. Breathe, Relax, Feel, Watch, and Allow. Ride the Wave. This simple yet powerful discipline is truly profound.

—Elysa DeMartini

Riding the Wave of Sensation is the technique that helps you take this different approach. It teaches you how to move toward sensation and become absorbed in the felt experience of strong emotion. This is not as easy as it sounds. We resist emotions like fear, anger, and sadness precisely because they are so painful to bear. Riding the Wave is not about delving into the thoughts or story line associated with the emotion. Rather than going into your head, it takes you into your body. You release trapped emotion by choosing to feel it fully, by going through the experience and not under, above, or around it. In the process of encountering strong emotions, it is natural for mental content to arise in the mind. Some thoughts, images, and story lines take you deeper into the process. Others are distractions that take you out of the process. The key is to stay anchored in the felt sense of your body. While mental content often arises that afterward proves meaningful and helpful, during the experience you stay present to sensation, which allows the wave to build and ultimately crest.

Years ago, when I was learning Kripalu Yoga, I was led in an experience of holding the Camel. We came into the pose progressively, with a variety of warm-ups, and I felt safe to explore. Coming into the full posture, I immediately began to have noticeable physical experiences. Parts of my body trembled. I continued to breathe and hold the posture, riding the waves of sensation streaming through my body. Suddenly, and with great clarity, I remembered an experience years before when I was flying through a thunderstorm with lightning flashing and the plane rising and falling in the turbulent air. Staying with the posture, I broke into a sweat, and then felt clammy and cold. My breath grew shallow and fast, and my hands shook. Noticing the physical sensations that accompanied holding the Camel I realized that this is what fear feels like in my body. *Now that I knew what I was feeling, now that it had a name, it was no longer fear—it was curiosity and excitement. In the safety of holding the Camel, I could explore fear, staying with it in a way I had never allowed myself to do before. Afterward I saw yoga in a very different way, knowing that it was a way to deeply connect with myself and release trapped feelings.*

—Rasmani Deborah Orth

How to Practice

Powerful feelings are experienced in wavelike movements of energy and sensation. As you learn to Ride the Wave, the process of emotional release becomes quite natural. You start by simply being attentive to the physical sensations that arise as you breathe, stretch, and relax. Often what proves to be the beginning of a wave of energy starts small and can easily be ignored. By being sensitive and self-aware, you gradually realize that your yoga mat floats on the surface of an ocean of feeling. If you open to feeling, there are always big or little waves to ride.

As you practice postures, the first step is to let your awareness rest on the areas of greatest sensation and "breathe into them." The flow of breath is intimately connected to the flow of emotion. Any effort to block feeling will be reflected in a minor or major restriction of diaphragmatic breathing. Conversely, breathing freely automatically opens the door to your inner world. The next step is to notice any areas of the body that are contracted or tense and consciously relax them. Muscular tension inhibits the flow of feeling. As you breathe, relax, and hold the posture, the wave rises and begins to build in intensity. You may have to repeatedly relax your belly, diaphragm, shoulders, face, and other areas that chronically tighten to hold back the flow of emotion. Just keep breathing and let the tension go.

As sensation and emotion flow, focus your attention there, actively feeling and becoming absorbed in the energy experience. Watch the sensations shift and change. There are lots of ways to express this in words—being with whatever is there for you, opening up to it, not pushing it away. All these phrases describe the same experience of not avoiding the in-your-body felt sense of powerful energy, sensation, and emotion moving through you. If you feel that spontaneous movements or sounds want to emerge to deepen your experience, let that happen while keeping your attention focused inward on sensation.

> *As my yoga class drew to a close, my mood shifted into sadness. Instead of pushing the feelings away, I relaxed and let my body feel. I acknowledged my grief and began to sob. As I allowed the waves of emotion to wash over me, I felt release. The tears were like rain, cooling the emotions that burned inside of me. I experienced a great feeling of peace.*
>
> — Lynne LaSpina

During this process, your mind may get activated and attempt to distract you in various ways. This is the time to hang in there with the experience, simply letting thoughts arise and pass away. Choose to stay focused and let the sensations build. Emotional release does not result from making fleeting contact with a powerful emotion in order to select the right mental label to describe how you feel afterward: "I now know that I am sad." It comes from fully experiencing how that sadness feels, where it shows up in your body, and

EXPERIENCE: HOLDING THE BRIDGE

The Bridge is a safe and powerful posture for prolonged holding. This experience is designed to familiarize you with how to Ride the Wave of Sensation. Before beginning, you may want to review Bridge posture (pages 157–158) and warm-up. Then explore holding the Bridge for three to five minutes as guided below.

1. As you begin, affirm your intention to hold the posture and experience the deep release possible through this technique.

2. Then take the time to start with several pelvic lifts, inhaling the hips up and exhaling them back down to the floor. When your body feels ready, press into the feet and lift the hips into an easy Bridge.

3. Come into Ocean Sounding Breath, letting the breath flow freely and deeply. Allow the diaphragm to move and the belly to balloon in and out. Sustain this deep and flowing circular breath for the entire period of holding. Breathe, relax, and feel.

4. Slowly feel your way into the full expression of the Bridge, consciously relaxing any contracted muscles that are not essential to holding the hips high. Isolate the muscles that are essential, and engage them fully. Tease out the effort from the let go, relaxing everything you can. Find the balance point where you can hold without strain.

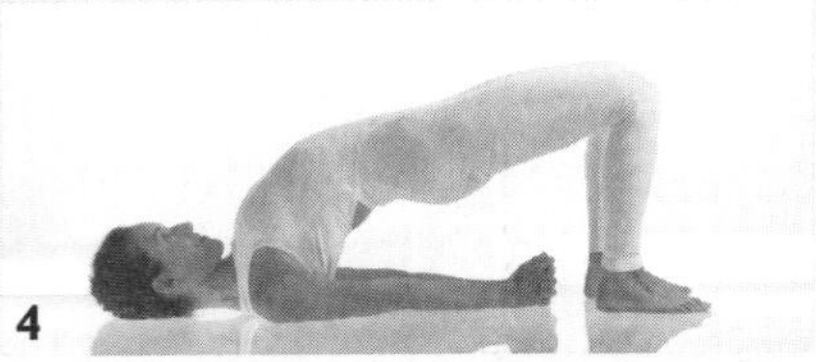

4

5. Focus your attention on areas of sensation, anchoring your mind in the body. Breathe, relax, feel, watch, and allow. Let the energy intensify as the wave begins to rise. If fear or distraction surfaces in the mind, let it go and come back to breath, energy, and sensation. Let any micromovements or sounds that naturally emerge from the holding process happen. Allow the wave to steadily build.

6. Watch the content of the mind without judgment, comparison, or trying to understand. Don't push away discomfort or grasp hold of pleasure. Keep awareness anchored in the body and focused on feeling. Invite physical tension to melt from the hips, pelvis, belly, and chest. Allow emotional and mental tension to surface from the depths of the mind. Let the energy build to a climax.

7. As the wave crests, allow the mind to become fully absorbed in the felt sense of the body. Let energy and awareness flow freely through you. When the wave dissipates, release the posture in slow motion.

8. Let the body rebalance by moving in any ways that feel good. Gradually come into Corpse Pose and integrate the experience with a few minutes of deep relaxation.

how it responds to your awareness. Release distracting thoughts and allow the experience to be whatever it is. After you have stayed with the experience for a while you may want it to "go away now" when in fact the wave is still actively rising. Don't expect anything to change, or try to make the tension dissolve. Just surrender to whatever is happening.

BEING HOME

Where can I soften
in this posture?
Where is the edge
between opening
and force, the line
between stretch and
too much effort?

The mind and body
serve up a feast of
feelings, each breath
another chance to
deepen and release.

The smallest motion,
or even just a quiet
sigh could be all that
I require to shift my
focus from the outer
to the inner realm,
a change from feeling
lost to being home.

As the wave crests, emotional release is often accompanied by the bliss of heightened energy flow. It is not unusual for awareness to pervade the body as you become totally absorbed in sensation. You, the separate experiencer, may momentarily disappear as the mind dissolves into the gap of pure awareness that exists between thoughts, connecting you with what lies beyond. Be courageous and let that happen, trusting the wave to carry you safely to shore when the time is right. After the wave has crested and sensation begins to subside, slowly release the posture. Stay with the feelings as you integrate the experience with stillness or gentle complementary movements. The wave is dissipating but it has not yet passed. This is when valuable "ahas," insights, and intuitive knowings often arise effortlessly in the mind. After the wave has passed, the critical mind may come in to disavow the experience or reassert old beliefs. Just remain present, watching even this without judgment.

While Riding the Wave often starts out as an uncomfortable or even threatening process, it soon becomes a natural one. The body has a wisdom all its own, and there is an organic intelligence and safety underlying what comes to the surface. No matter what you may think, there is a good reason for why you feel, what you feel, when you feel it. There were also good reasons in the past that led you to block whatever is now coming to the surface to be felt. Seeing why emotions were buried can

The Body Remembers

BY SENIOR TEACHER RASMANI DEBORAH ORTH

As a Gestalt psychologist, I became fascinated with the Riding the Wave technique I learned in Kripalu Yoga. Through applying it off the mat, I had one of the most powerful experiences of my life. I was at the beach with my partner on an early June vacation. Falling asleep on my stomach, the backs of my arms, legs, and even earlobes got badly sunburned. Determined that this would not ruin our vacation, I ignored the seriousness of the injury and went for a long evening walk on the beach. On the way back, I started feeling chilled and weak. I sat on a rock wall and felt my teeth begin to chatter. I had to lean on my partner to make it back to where we were staying.

My symptoms were so severe that my partner was beside herself with worry and wanted me to go to the emergency room. I wanted to be alone and ride this out. I sent her to get soda and popcorn, which was all I could imagine eating. When she left, I began the process of Riding the Wave: Breathe, Relax, Feel, Watch, and Allow. The sensations in my body were strong and a bit scary. I considered for a moment that I might be dying, but really didn't believe it. I began to talk to myself like I would to a scared child. "It's okay, you didn't do anything wrong. You didn't mean to fall asleep in the sun or walk so far that you couldn't get home."

I let the waves of sensation wash through me. There were the obvious sensations from too much sun, but the sensations began to move to different areas of my body. The arm I broke in the fifth grade, the knee that had been dislocated, my throat where I had mumps. I coached myself like I would talk to a child: "Just relax. It's okay. It's safe to be right where you are, even if it's scary. Just relax into what's happening."

I was truly frightened, but another part of me was intensely alive and curious. I was shivering uncontrollably and aware of pain in my jaw and neck. I remembered all the people around me who had died when I was small: my grandmother, my uncles John and Paul, my aunts Ella and Christina. At this point the experience had been going on for more than a half hour. I said to myself, "You aren't going to die," and the waves of sensation subsided so abruptly that I was shocked.

Seven people in my family died before my twelfth birthday and those experiences imprinted me with a deep fear of death. By Riding the Wave, I was able to access and release some portion of that fear. The message I took from that experience is that everything is carried in the body. When my partner returned with the soda and popcorn, I was able to eat and drink. For the rest of the vacation, I was physically slowed down, but on a deeper level felt blissful and grateful for an experience that helped me let go of so much I had held on to for so long.

allow you to view yourself in a new light, which can be a profound avenue for personal growth. But the process of Riding the Wave does not always produce such understanding. Sometimes a deep release may occur and your conscious mind may never know the details. Although it is odd that profound feeling can arise without a story line attached, this is not an uncommon experience for regular yoga practitioners.

C H A P T E R   N I N E T E E N

CLEARING THE MIND

Mind is the sole source of bondage or liberation.

—MAITRI UPANISHAD

An agitated mind squanders a tremendous amount of energy by running in circles, fighting with itself, and hankering after relief from its distracted state. A calm mind is a fount of creativity, cogent thinking, and productive action. Although the suffering born of agitation is apparent, it is not so easy to rid ourselves of mental unrest. Efforts to tame the mind often compound the problem by creating a backlash of further disturbance. Yoga teaches that there are different levels to the ocean of awareness called *mind*. Its choppy surface is the *thinking mind*, which is by nature unsteady and subject to distraction. With awareness confined there, our mental life is exhausting. Dropping below the surface, we discover the *intuitive mind*, which is naturally contemplative and creative. Rather than fighting to still the surface of the mind, yoga teaches us to explore its depths. It is only by deepening our awareness that we can find the inner peace we seek, and realize our potential to grow toward wholeness.

Growing up was full of contradictions. There were fun times in our household, but there were also instances where my parents were unsupportive, negative, and even abusive. Those times left me with low self-esteem, an inability to speak what was true for me, and difficulty receiving a simple compliment. I imagined those limitations would stay with me for life until I discovered Kripalu Yoga. Twelve years later, I can speak my truth, smile my smile, and even sing in front of other people.

—Rose Campisi

Thinking Mind and Ego

When you use the word *mind,* you are probably referring to the *thinking mind.* The distinguishing feature of the thinking mind is that it is extroverted, directing awareness outward through the five senses. Using sensory input to assemble a picture of the world, the thinking mind is constantly attending to changing stimuli. The primary purpose of the thinking mind is to take care of your safety and survival needs. It is always on the lookout for danger. If the coast is clear, it is scheming how to meet your need for food and comfort. Its nature is to scan for threats and opportunities.

The thinking mind loves to understand, which allows you to predict future events, avoid danger, and maximize comfort. In pursuit of understanding, the thinking mind is driven to sift, sort, label, and classify the data flowing in from the senses. Thought-bound and logical, the thinking mind is skillful in creatively organizing information in new ways. In other words, it cleverly manipulates data, but it is not very skilled at coming up with entirely new ideas. Because of its focus on survival and comfort, the thinking mind is inherently self-centered and fear-based.

Western psychology calls the self-image that forms around the thinking mind the *ego.* Yoga uses the term *ahankara,* which means *I-maker.* The ego is the executive of the thinking mind, making decisions based on its likes and dislikes, and seeing the world through the filter of its egocentric needs. Each of us has an ego, a basic identity as a person born on a certain date, with a unique life story and a particular set of values, attitudes, preferences, and beliefs. In Western psychology, the ego is considered the self-organizing principle of the psyche and the command center of the personality. Strengthening the ego is considered good because it allows you to be effective in the world and satisfy your needs and desires. A strong ego can also draw on conscience to restrain instinctual urges and function harmoniously within an ordered society.

Spiritual traditions tend to see the ego in a totally different light, as a *false self* that is incompatible with unity, inner peace, and selflessness. The ego fragments reality into pieces, dividing the world into categories like me, mine, and other. Using its powers of analysis, it then strives to manipulate external variables to satisfy its own ends. Founded on the view that each of us is inherently separate, supported by sense perceptions that suggest I am "in here" and there's a world "out there," the ego is forever blind to the spiritual unity underlying the material world. Tied to the restless thinking mind, the ego is always looking for the next threat, the next meal, or the next romance. It lacks the capacity to rest in the now and experience peace or fulfillment. For all these reasons, many spiritual traditions define the goal of practice as "killing the ego."

Identity Formation

Unlike some traditions, Kripalu Yoga views the egocentric self that originates in childhood as a natural and healthy aspect of identity formation. As we mature to face life's challenges, we all need to develop a sense of self that is positive, stable, and cohesive. Identity formation is a prodigious task, however, and one that must continue throughout the lifespan for us to remain healthy and vital.

Emerging from adolescence, the ego takes its place at the center of an understandably superficial identity that is molded from mental concepts of how we should look, behave, think, and feel. Unproven in life, and facing a momentous number of developmental challenges, most young adult identities are undergirded by a sense of fear and inadequacy. On the surface, they tend to be dominated by a superiority complex, a grandiose view of one's qualities and abilities, or an inferiority complex, a demeaning view of self. It is not unusual for them to sway back and forth between extremes, alternately playing the roles of hero and victim, and projecting blame or praise on others.

As we grow into full adulthood, we gain life experience and are confronted by situations that challenge simplistic notions of who we are and how life works. In response, we can choose to develop a more accurate and authentic sense of self. Alternatively, we can turn those opportunities away and resist further development. If we fail to shift and change in response to life's feedback, our entrenched identity becomes a *persona* and we begin to stagnate. A persona can accurately be called a *false self* because it is a mental abstraction, divorced from the reality of what is, and often cut off from a vital connection to the body. In Kripalu Yoga, the goal is not to kill the false self but rather to create the conditions that allow us to grow beyond it. To do this, we must learn to dive below the surface of the thinking mind and awaken the intuitive mind.

> *My practice mirrors back to me who I really am—centered, focused, whole, and complete.*
>
> —Angelena Craig

Buddhi: The Intuitive Mind

Beneath the thinking mind and ego lies the *intuitive mind,* sometimes called the *wisdom faculty*. Free from the distractions of the senses, the intuitive mind is steady and reflects the brilliance of the pure awareness from which it was formed. Rather than skimming across a conceptual surface of thought, the intuitive mind is contemplative by nature and able to penetrate to the essence of things and bestow depth knowing. Rather than fragmenting reality into pieces, the intuitive mind is always integrating disparate parts into a larger whole.

OUTSIDE THE THINKING MIND

I find sustenance outside
the thinking mind.
As the thought stream quiets,
awareness comes to focus on
a single point, then moves—
shooting through me like the
light from distant stars.
Focus follows energy, rides
like a feather on the breath,
flies to the source of ecstasy
and life force.
Focus carries me everywhere
and nowhere, flowing like
water in a fountain.
Is it any wonder I return,
morning after morning,
to the still point at
the heart of motion?

The intuitive mind is not thought-bound, nor does it operate on logic. It comprehends directly through *intuition,* the ability to know without conscious reasoning. Innately creative, the intuitive mind is the source of insight and generates entirely new ideas by what is often called *out of the box thinking.* In a mature psyche, the intuitive mind is an active partner of the thinking mind and provides a necessary counterbalance to the self-centeredness of ego. Where we tend to think of intuition as something that flashes on and off, the aim of yoga is to allow us to rest in intuitive knowing and benefit from the reliable flow of insights that results.

> *The perceptive/logical mind can, at most, help one obtain word-based, indirect knowledge of Spirit. But the basic ignorance of the real Self is not destroyed by such knowledge. On the other hand, knowledge obtained by direct contact with the intuitive mind destroys the hindrances that prevent one from realizing one's true nature as Spirit. That is why the intuitive mind plays a central role in yoga.*
>
> —Swami Rajarshi Muni

The Authentic Self

A significantly different sense of self emerges in a mature psyche with a highly functioning intuitive mind. This *authentic self* is founded on the acceptance of reality as it presents itself in the moment. It is integrated, drawing body, heart, thinking mind, and intuitive mind into wholeness. Where the false self is preoccupied with the endless stream of ideas, images, and concepts that flow across the screen of the thinking mind, the authentic self is able to see beyond the hypnotism of the thought stream. Attuned to a wider reality, it is less likely to fall into self-deception and delusional thinking. Activating the intuitive mind and establishing yourself in an identity that is less fear-based than the ego-centric self is a big step forward on the path of

Marrying Yoga and Meditation

BY SENIOR TEACHER SUDHIR JONATHAN FOUST

Raised a Quaker, I was steeped in a tradition that shunned external forms. No minister, no altar, and no one with any closer affiliation to spirit than anyone else. Our practice was silence and contemplation. Although this sounds spacious and enlightened, I felt frustrated from an early age. Quakers speak of the inner light, but all I noticed was a never-ending stream of thoughts. I craved a technique to awaken the still, small voice within that is core to Quaker tenets.

I was a student at a Quaker prep school when my mother introduced me to Transcendental Meditation. Experiencing that wonderful state of restful alertness that comes from mantra meditation, I felt that I had discovered the secret of the universe. After only a few weeks of practice, I was more happy, creative, and courageous than ever before. Sensing that meditation would be with me for the rest of my life, I committed to a regular practice.

The school gave me a key to the school library and a small but dedicated group of us meditated every day before dinner. This convinced me of the power of practicing with like-minded people. During college, I managed a thousand-acre farm with a fellow meditation junkie. Even during the intensity of spring planting, we'd throttle down the tractors to find a corner of the field in which to sit. I joined the Peace Corps and meditated with friends in intense heat, with sweat dripping off our elbows in West Africa. To sustain my practice, I meditated in planes, trains, cars, libraries, churches, dentists' offices, cathedrals, and on park benches. I used various techniques to make myself less conspicuous, such as pretending to be napping, pulling a hat low over my eyes, and even wearing sunglasses while holding a newspaper.

I moved into Kripalu Center in the early '80s to immerse myself in meditation and was surprised to find an entirely different set of practices. Instead of silent meditation, there was yoga, pranayama, and high-energy chanting and drumming. When we did meditate, the guru talked at us incessantly. Surrounded by yogis, I felt more alone in my personal practice than ever before. There was hardly any interest in what I considered meditation.

While continuing to sit, I began to explore the deeper potentials of the body through postures and pranayama. I learned that Kripalu Yoga views the body as a doorway to the present moment. Absorbed in sensation, I came in direct contact with the energetic here and now experience of being in my body. Because riding the waves of energy and emotion stimulated deep purification in me, I had to learn how to remain the objective observer of my inner process to stay with the practice. I saw that cultivating this ability to be the witness is how meditation fit into the Kripalu approach.

As time passed, a cadre of Kripalu residents began to seek out deeper instruction in sitting meditation. We started sneaking off to Buddhist retreat centers and our minds were blown away by their teachings on cultivating awareness. At the same time, hard-core meditators began slipping into Kripalu to drop deeply into their bodies and leave their minds far behind. I watched as two seemingly different spiritual traditions were woven together in a profound and wonderful way.

After three decades of practice and teaching, I believe each of us must find a personal practice that integrates body, mind, and spirit. Swami Kripalu taught that we are constantly balancing our energy (prana) and awareness (citta). That teaching rings true for me. Yoga awakens my energy and brings me deeply present in the body. Meditation helps me quiet the reactivity of my mind and pay steady attention to whatever is unfolding. It grounds me in equanimity and compassion, and allows me to release everything that is not really me. Instead of one or the other, it's the blend of awakened energy and witness consciousness that brings yoga and meditation into a dynamic and fulfilling relationship.

As a child I longed for the direct experience of the inner light. I think we all intuit the potential for a world filled with more peace, wisdom, and compassion. A regular practice of yoga and meditation is the best way I have found to realize my potential to live and love fully.

yoga. Instead of being driven by unconscious fears and desires, you glimpse your higher evolutionary potential and feel drawn to realize it.

Myths describe the end of the false self's clinging to "me" and "mine" as an epic struggle, for it does not give up the ghost gracefully. An inner revolution is required to reconfigure the psyche, stripping away fears and fantasies in a process of embracing reality. At first this is slow going, as the clouded thinking mind obscures the presence of the intuitive mind. When the light of the intuitive mind starts to shine forth, the pace of transformation picks up. Gradually the complex tangle of feelings, thoughts, and ideals that is the false self is consumed in the fire of moment-to-moment awareness. When the process comes to fruition, a shift occurs in the center of gravity of your identity. Where before you viewed yourself through the lens of thoughts and concepts, you now identify with the spacious awareness in which feelings and thoughts arise. Instead of bringing yourself fully present, the realization slowly dawns that you are presence itself.

> *The deepest structures of the mind are evoked in this process of seeing clearly—the intuitive awakened mind,* buddhi. *This is a mind, an awareness, a consciousness, that can move anywhere, that is not separate from anything in the whole field of mind and matter, that is not restricted by fear, clinging, holding on. This is the mind that can acknowledge, experience, and bear all of life. This is the mind and body that can be fully in the dance and, at the same time, be fully in the calm, abiding center.*
>
> —Stephen Cope

Story, Stuff, Shadow

In the midst of focused spiritual practice, it is helpful to have some idea of exactly what it is that you are clearing from your mind. What psychology calls *conditioning,* traditional yoga calls *ashaya* (impressions) or *samskara* (subtle activators). Experience has led the Kripalu Yoga community to develop some less academic but useful terms to describe the inner conditions that lead us to be mechanical and patterned, versus fresh to the present moment.

In the quest to break free of conditioning, you are likely to find yourself getting lost again and again in your *story*. In many ways, our egocentric identity is a complex and inconsistent narrative about who we are, who others are, what life is, and how it all fits together. We repeat this story in our heads constantly, update it continually, and in many ways steer our actions by its assumptions, plots, and themes. The only problem is that it's a story *about* who we are, and has embarrassingly little to do with the actual substance and being of us. As spiritual practice activates the intuitive mind, you will gain insight into your story. It is likely that your core strategies for getting needs met, your tactics to avoid suffering, and your well-worn ways to rationalize shortcomings and failures will become clear to you. While that is all to the good, it is important to understand that the point of spiritual practice is not to sort it all out, which is an impossible task. Practice helps you discover firsthand that you are not your story, which lessens your fascination and obsession with it.

Stuff is the word used to describe the uncomfortable thoughts and feelings that are part and parcel of everyone's practice—and life. The phrase *That's just your stuff coming up* is a way to suggest that you not be overly concerned with your temporary state. Remain present, breathe into your experience, feel what's there fully and see it clearly, but don't take it too seriously. Examined more closely, stuff is the highly personal residue that results from incomplete development. Given an opportunity, it will always arise in your awareness to help you complete the developmental process.

To make this more concrete, an important stage of early childhood development is described by psychologist Erik Erikson as *trust versus mistrust*. To the extent that you don't embody a basic trust in life, a fearful sense of mistrust will color your inner world and be projected onto your outer circumstances. In a very personal and nuanced way, this will arise as *stuff*, making your anxiety evident and giving you a chance to look deeper and choose differently. Staying with Erikson's developmental model, other elements of *stuff* include shame, doubt, guilt, inferiority, identity confusion, various blocks to intimacy, and despair. Because it helps you address and remedy many life issues, your stuff is a great friend decked out in a most convincing disguise.

Shadow is a very different phenomenon. Whenever you hold tightly to an identity, you block a whole range of feedback about the larger truth of who you are. If you see yourself as a "nice guy and team player," you will censor and literally not see all the ways in which you compete and jockey for status with those around you. In the fairy tale "The Emperor Has No Clothes," the king's vanity renders him totally blind to the obvious. This speaks of the danger of the shadow. If a friend or coworker tells you in a straightforward manner exactly how you are coming across, you will vehemently disagree and fight tooth and nail to disprove her. Why is this so? Because it runs exactly counter to who you think you are. The truth of what she is saying is obscured by your shadow.

Everyone casts a shadow, and peering into it is one of the most potent catalysts for transformation because it reveals material entirely outside your story. Doing so, you learn firsthand that who you are on a psychological level is an ever-changing flow of thoughts and feelings versus any fixed and rigid identity. Faced with this reality, the best anyone can do is be authentic and self-disclosing, casting as small a shadow as possible. And even after making that effort, blind spots will remain. Contemplative practices of all sorts are excellent tools to work with stuff and story. Seeing into your shadow is much more difficult and usually requires input from outside the conscious mind. Although this can include gifts of intuition and inner guidance, shadow work entails cultivating sensitivity, self-awareness, and especially a willingness to learn from the feedback that others and life provide.

> *Unfortunately there can be no doubt that man is, on the whole, less good than he imagines himself to be. Everyone carries a shadow, and the less it is embodied in the individual's conscious life, the blacker and denser it is. If a weakness is conscious, one always has a chance to correct it. But if it is repressed and isolated from consciousness, it never gets corrected.*
>
> —Carl Jung

The Better Part of Valor

Where many spiritual traditions encourage practitioners to take on the ego in full battle regalia, this is not the approach of Kripalu Yoga. In Kripalu Yoga, the limitations of ego are treated seriously but handled indirectly. Swami Kripalu taught that only one thing was assured in starting a fight with yourself: you would lose. By attuning again and again to the present

It's Enough to Just Be Present

BY SENIOR TEACHER ARUNI NAN FUTURONSKY

I had been sober for three years when I came to Kripalu Center in 1989. A deep pattern of always striving to be worthy of love spurred me on to success in my professional life as a high school teacher. But it also led me into dark places and addictive behaviors. A twelve-step program helped me to get my life back on track, but I was going forward with the belief that being spiritual meant not having feelings, especially bad feelings. I was living in my head, confused and cut off from my body, looking for God by trying to have the right thoughts.

My experience of Kripalu Yoga as a body-centered spirituality was life changing. It freed up my energy and gave me access to a spontaneity and joy I had not known since childhood. More important, it showed me that my feelings, whatever they are, are not evidence that there is something wrong with me. They are a doorway into the present moment and the healing presence of Spirit. For me, walking through that doorway is what calmed and cleared my mind.

Since becoming a Kripalu teacher, I have been with thousands of people as they go through their own version of this healing journey. They find inner peace by learning how to be fully present in their bodies, not in figuring it all out. They discover that life is not a quest for a perfect outcome. It is an unfolding process of learning and growing, an evolutionary journey that is never perfect. In giving up their need to do it right, they find self-acceptance, compassion, and a great inner strength that allows them to be in reality as it shows up moment by moment and act from a place of connection.

As for me, I continue to mess up, lose myself in anger or self-judgment, and show up less than ideal. But it's different now. I know it's enough for me to be present, to do my best, and that it's safe to let go of the results. In the coming and going, I discover Spirit again and again, and that seems to be my path.

moment and accepting the truth of what is, the flow of life force is diverted away from the false self, which slowly withers. This is not to imply that self-discipline and struggle aren't involved in this process, for they most certainly are, but the ego likes nothing better than a good fight. Refusing to do battle is the better part of valor and requires the capacity to rest in choiceless awareness that Kripalu Yoga calls *Witness Consciousness*, the topic of the following chapter.

C H A P T E R   T W E N T Y

WITNESS CONSCIOUSNESS

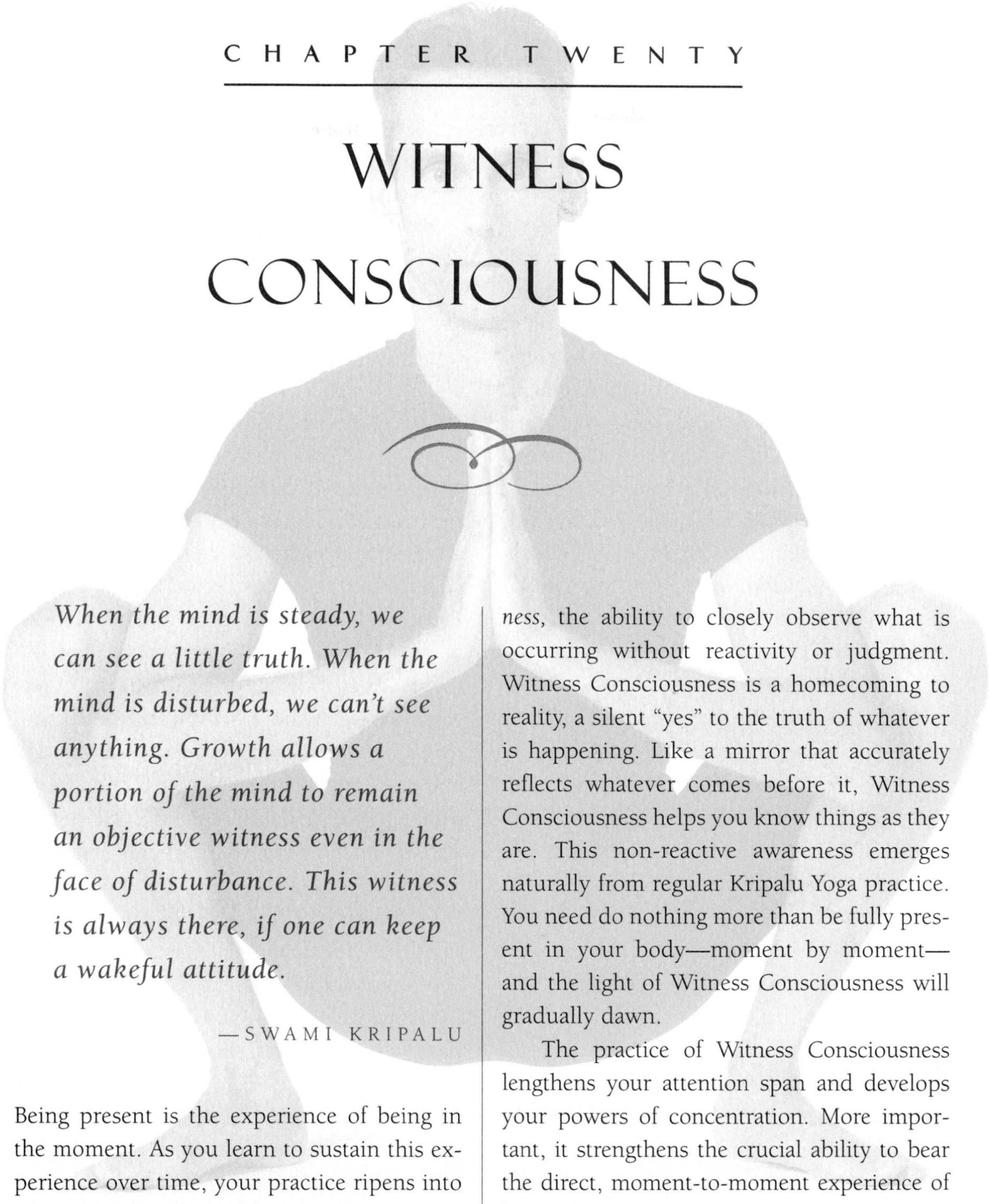

When the mind is steady, we can see a little truth. When the mind is disturbed, we can't see anything. Growth allows a portion of the mind to remain an objective witness even in the face of disturbance. This witness is always there, if one can keep a wakeful attitude.

—SWAMI KRIPALU

Being present is the experience of being in the moment. As you learn to sustain this experience over time, your practice ripens into what Kripalu Yoga calls *Witness Consciousness*, the ability to closely observe what is occurring without reactivity or judgment. Witness Consciousness is a homecoming to reality, a silent "yes" to the truth of whatever is happening. Like a mirror that accurately reflects whatever comes before it, Witness Consciousness helps you know things as they are. This non-reactive awareness emerges naturally from regular Kripalu Yoga practice. You need do nothing more than be fully present in your body—moment by moment—and the light of Witness Consciousness will gradually dawn.

The practice of Witness Consciousness lengthens your attention span and develops your powers of concentration. More important, it strengthens the crucial ability to bear the direct, moment-to-moment experience of being alive. Engaging Witness Consciousness, you can closely feel and watch the inner flow of sensation, emotion, and thought without losing yourself in reaction. As your ability to observe the spectrum of human experience broadens, you can slowly let go of the defenses that protect you from uncomfortable thoughts and feelings, but also drain vitality and wall you off from reality. Witness Consciousness allows you to persist in the face of the so-called distractions that inevitably arise in spiritual practice—obsessive thinking, self-judgment, blame, comparison, and boredom—and learn that they are actually grist for the mill of awakening. At first Witness Consciousness is something you practice, a technique employed to develop your latent capacity for higher awareness. As the witness awakes, you begin to see it as an innate quality of the mind and integral aspect of your being.

> *I found my compassionate witness through Kripalu Yoga. I was thirty and my life was in terrible turmoil. Being in a Kripalu Yoga class helped me endure the emotional roller coaster I was riding. Finding calm and peace even temporarily kept me from totally falling apart.*
>
> *I didn't have any sudden "aha" moments, but rather the slow dawning of being more and more conscious of my thoughts, emotions, inner dialogue, and overall attitude. I saw that I had created the turmoil in my life. Now I had a tool to examine and evaluate it with compassion.*
>
> *Despite years of therapy, self-help study, and group work, I had somehow missed the vital ingredient of a compassionate witness. The ability to look at myself and others with equanimity, yet with a tender heart, opened a whole world for me. I feel like I have a secret to life that makes the world make sense.*
>
> —Carol E. Klammer

Attraction and Aversion

Yoga philosophy teaches that the oneness at the heart of creation expresses in the world as pairs of opposites, or *dvanda*. This spectrum of opposites starts out on a universal scale—spirit and matter, energy and awareness, wave and particle, time and space, day and night. It descends all the way into your personal life—self and other, pleasure and pain, love and hate, happiness and sadness, joy and grief. The dualistic nature of life is not a problem that you can solve; it is simply the way the phenomenal world of time and space manifests.

Confronted by a world of opposites, the mind has a natural desire to want to experience one side of the polarity and not the other. Everyone wants pleasure without pain, happiness without sadness, success without failure. Yoga refers to this tendency as *raga and dvesha*, meaning *attraction and aversion*. Attraction leads the mind to seek out what it likes. Aversion leads it to avoid what it doesn't like.

The instinctive forces of attraction and aversion are natural and healthy. They guide you to make appropriate choices to meet the basic needs of the body. But difficulty arises when you attempt to govern your internal world of thought and feeling through attraction and aversion. Adopting a strategy of seeking pleasure and pushing away pain and discomfort, you find yourself at war with life. No matter how you strive, your internal experience always includes a mix of pleasure, pain, and both sides of life's many polarities.

Contemporary science has proven that space and time, the very building blocks of the universe, are not separate entities but rather smoothly linked parts of a larger whole called the space-time continuum. Yoga has always taught that all pairs of opposites are interrelated parts of an indivisible whole, two ends of the same stick. Witness Consciousness is a practical way to integrate these opposites and harness the energy of wholeness. By neutralizing the dualistic forces of attraction and aversion, it allows you to rest in a non-reactive awareness able to sense the unity underlying diversity. Intimate with whatever is arising, free of any compulsive need to change it, you are able to see reality clearly and embrace both sides of life.

Engaging Witness Consciousness activates the intuitive mind. Over time, it helps you shift into the Authentic Self and realize the True Self.

The internal freedom of Witness Consciousness does not equate to external passivity. In fact, it leads to a greater freedom of action. When a decision is required, you are able to explore your desires, and the thoughts that surround them, with great clarity. Rather than being blindly driven by your likes and dislikes, you are free to make conscious choices and follow through with appropriate action. Giving up the losing battle to have pleasure without pain, you can feel more at ease with the mixed bag of experiences that is life.

A Whole Body Experience

Witness Consciousness is not an intellectual strategy to distance yourself from life. Nor is it a skillful technique to prevent disturbing thoughts and feelings from entering your awareness, or a way to avoid pain and discomfort by dissociating from your body. Witness Consciousness transforms the yoga mat into a laboratory for exploring your internal

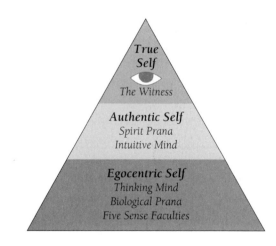

THE WITNESS GOES EVERYWHERE

In *Yoga and the Quest for the True Self*, Stephen Cope identifies six primary characteristics of Witness Consciousness:

1. **The witness does not choose for or against any aspect of reality.** The witness does not split life into good and bad, right and wrong, high and low, or spiritual and not-spiritual.
2. **The witness does not censor life.** The witness allows all thoughts, feelings, and sensations to receive the light of awareness, without discriminating.
3. **Witnessing is a whole body experience.** Instead of an intellectual exercise, the witness receives experience by feeling the reverberations of sensation with the whole physical-emotional organism.
4. **Witness Consciousness is always present at least in its potential form in every human being at every moment.** We don't have to create the witness. This enlightened quality of consciousness needs only to be recognized, evoked, claimed, and cultivated.
5. **The witness is capable of standing completely still, even in the center of the whirlwind of sensations, thoughts, feelings, fantasies—even in serious mental and physical illness.** The witness can objectively observe dramatic or intense experiences even as we're having that experience.
6. **The witness goes everywhere.** The witness is connected to the quantum field of mind and matter, standing outside time and space, living in the eternal now.

world of feeling and thought. Engaging Witness Consciousness, you stand right in the middle of your experience. Encountering the pull of attraction and aversion, you do not follow its lead, choosing instead to remain present in your body and awake to whatever is arising. By learning how to face challenges on the yoga mat, you gain the ability to remain present when the inner storms of life are raging off the mat too.

The Self dwells in me as pure witness consciousness, in equilibrium, without form, and without the divisions of time and space.

—Yoga Vasistha

The Witness Can See It All

As practice deepens, Witness Consciousness helps you recover parts of yourself that have been split off and locked away to protect you from powerful emotions like anger, fear, shame, and guilt. Over time, you discover a remarkable truth: there is nothing the witness cannot see, feel, acknowledge, and embrace. Good and bad, light and shadow, things you are proud of and things you would not do again, there is no limit to what the witness can hold in the light of consciousness. As this awareness dawns, you are freed from the deep fear that there is something inherently inadequate, unlovable or unacceptable about you. Witness Consciousness makes room for all parts of you to be present at the banquet table of life.

Meditation is integral to yoga. Because people are different, various approaches to meditation have evolved to suit their needs. Seekers should experiment with a variety of techniques until they find one to their liking. But if there is no meditation in the practice, it cannot be called yoga.

—Swami Kripalu

When I can be the witness,
all manner of miracles occur—
old wounds heal, the past
reveals itself to be released,
present dramas play themselves
out without sinking emotional
talons into my soft skin. The
witness welcomes truth and
dares to meet reality on its
own terms. It is the ground
in which the seeds of
transformation take root
and finally flower. When
the witness is awake, the
lake of mind is still, and
in that mirrored surface
I see my own true face as
Spirit smiling back at me.

Sitting Meditation

In the early days of the Kripalu Yoga community, the practice of sitting meditation was largely neglected. Yoga postures were seen as sufficient to access deeper states of consciousness. In the late 1980s, the community was exposed to the Buddhist practice of Vipassana meditation and gained a host of benefits from calming and focusing the mind through regular meditation practice. A decade later, Kripalu Center pioneered a series of Yoga and Buddhism conferences that explored the interface of these two traditions. While continuing to recognize that absorption and insight can occur in either movement or stillness, Kripalu Yoga has evolved to emphasize the value of sitting meditation.

> *I had always been afraid of meditating. That may sound ridiculous, but when I first began practicing yoga, even brief periods of sitting still were torture to me. I had this inexplicable feeling that I would simply cease to be if I really got still. In addition to that, I was terrified of what I would see if I really looked into the contents of my mind, and afraid that God would condemn me for what I really was. Then I was invited to join a group of friends who were meditating every morning for an hour. An hour? I couldn't imagine getting through it. But I "borrowed" strength I didn't actually have from the group, and started meditating.*
>
> *I found it confrontive and not easy. I squirmed. My body screamed. My mind was all over the map. Others described the tranquility of their meditations. That wasn't my experience. It took every bit of willpower I possessed to keep from running out of the room. But my friends just sat there, so I sat there too. It turns out I didn't disappear. I didn't die. I didn't become enlightened, but I did learn to witness the outrageous array of thoughts and feelings that could display themselves behind closed eyes in the course of an hour. Where yoga helped me get more familiar with my body, meditation taught me to become comfortable with the contents of my mind.*
>
> —Danna Faulds

All meditation techniques use some focal point to aid concentration. It can be a word repeated over and over as a mantra, the movement of breath in and out of the body, a physical object like a candle flame, a geometric design known as a *yantra,* a bodily location such as the point between the eyebrows, a visualized image such as a deity, or even awareness itself. In Kripalu Yoga sitting meditation, it is typically the breath.

Beginning meditators are often frustrated at their inability to stay with the breath. Within moments, they find themselves lost in thought. Initially the process of returning to the breath again and again is the core of the practice. Bringing the mind back to the breath is like lifting a barbell. It is the act that trains the mind and strengthens the faculty of concentration. Instead of cause to berate yourself, each moment of awakening from the hypnotism of the thought stream should be celebrated.

Regular meditators may encounter various yoga experiences, including shifts in body awareness, vivid emotions, visual images, and a wide range of mind states. The practice is to simply be with each experience, whether pleasant or uncomfortable, allowing it to arise and pass through your spacious awareness like clouds in the sky. If you become lost in the

EXPERIENCE: SEATED MEDITATION

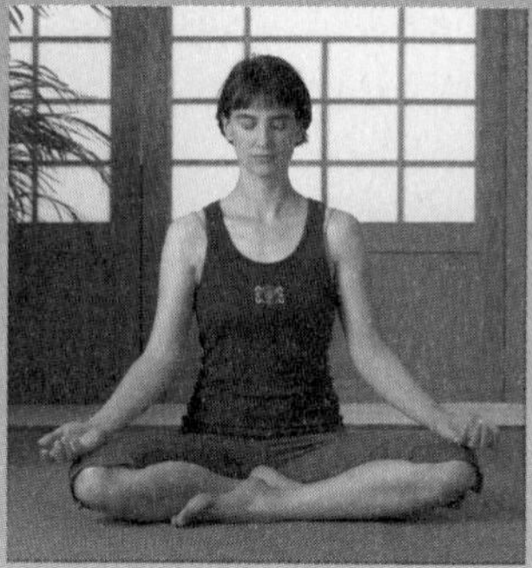

SETTLE IN

Sit comfortably on the floor or a straight-backed chair. Press the sitz bones down, level the chin, and extend through the crown of your head to elongate the spine. If you are sitting in a chair, resist the tendency to lean against the chair back, which compresses the abdomen and restricts breathing.

BRING YOURSELF FULLY PRESENT

To bring yourself fully present in your body, use the five steps of breathe, relax, feel, watch, and allow.

DEEPEN THE BREATH

Gradually deepen the breath until you are taking slow Three-Part Breaths. Do this slowly so as to avoid any sense of strain. Take ten or more Three-Part Breaths to deeply relax the body, oxygenate the blood, and free up the breathing process.

WATCH THE BREATH

Let go of any effort to control the breath. To begin meditation practice, rest your attention on the natural flow of breath. This can be done by attending to the tip of the nostrils, where the movement of air in and out of the body is easy to discern. Resting the awareness on the lower belly and noting its rise and fall is another effective technique. No effort is applied to control the breath. At times it may be rhythmic and deep. At other times it may be irregular and shallow. This is simply a process of watching the breath flow naturally and spontaneously.

BROADEN YOUR AWARENESS

As concentration deepens, broaden your focus to include all the sensations associated with the process of breathing. As the breath shifts and changes, let your attention rest on the area of strongest sensation, be that belly, chest, nose, or elsewhere. Gradually broaden the scope of your awareness still further to include the full spectrum of sensations, feelings, and thoughts passing through you. Remain intimate with the flow of your moment-to-moment inner experience.

Remember that seated meditation is not a disembodied practice. Remain present, awareness anchored in the breath. Ride the Wave and use the compassionate witness to resist the tendency to censor uncomfortable thoughts and feelings. See up close and personal the tendency to cling to what is pleasant, and push away what is painful; let go of any need to change your experience in any way. If you become lost in thought or story, simply come back to the breath to regain focus. Anchor yourself, and gradually allow awareness once again to broaden outward. You are likely to repeat this many times in a single sitting.

LET GO OF ALL TECHNIQUE

At the end of every sitting, reserve some time to drop all technique and release any effort to focus the mind. For a few precious minutes, just be. Rest there, ending your session with a prayer or affirmation of gratitude for your experience, whatever it was, and for the opportunity to practice.

experience, simply come back to breath and body to regain focus. Then gradually allow awareness to broaden outward. Meditation ends with a period in which you drop all technique and simply be. As much as possible, surrender any attempt to focus the mind or control your experience in subtle ways. Learn to savor the joy of effortless being.

Conscious Living

By learning to rest in choiceless awareness, you gain the willpower needed to fully exercise the power of choice. Out from under the unconscious sway of attraction and aversion, you can live consciously. In touch with your inner authority, dogmatic belief systems and moralistic thinking play less of a role in guiding your behavior. The need for conformity is replaced by a heightened sensitivity to values and preferences that are uniquely yours. No one can guide you down the pathless path of a life that is consciously chosen. Rather than a belief system or even a practice, yoga becomes the consciousness in which you live, a way to express your authentic self through action.

Help for an Aching Heart

BY SENIOR TEACHER KONDA MASON

Raised by a wonderful family in a real neighborhood, I was a kid with a wide open heart. I was friends with everyone and even knew heaven in the choir of our Baptist church. Then at twelve we moved to the suburbs, the second black family on the block. As I encountered racism, my heart closed down. I entered Cal Berkeley in 1974 and learned about sexism, classism, environmental degradations, corporate greed, and social activism. College was great, but it didn't help my heart much. I found myself asking: How do you live with an open heart in a world that is so messed up?

That's what brought me to yoga, and I came with the unspoken request "Please, please, fix me." Some people come to fix their butts. I came to fix my heart. It's the same thing, really. Kripalu Yoga taught me to not avoid the ugly stuff that comes up, to delve into it with full awareness, to watch the patterns in the mind and see layers of tension fall away one by one. Experiencing the profound results of deeply letting go through Witness Consciousness, all I could say was "Wow." And then another layer would come up and I would say "Uh-oh," and if I could hang in there I'd get another "Wow." I was hooked.

Eventually my yoga left the mat and entered my life. As I worked to integrate yoga with activism, Vipassana meditation became important to me. Buddhism taught me that the equanimity sought through Witness Consciousness should not be confused with its not-so-distant cousins: denial, resignation, complacency, emotional deadness, and privileged distance.

When I encountered the teaching "Equanimity gives to love an even, unchanging firmness and loyalty, and love imparts to equanimity its selflessness and fervor," it really hit home for me. This was the answer to my question asked so long ago. Now I know that real equanimity includes an open heart and requires dynamic action to make the world a better place. That remains the path I am on.

CHAPTER TWENTY-ONE

MEDITATION-IN-MOTION

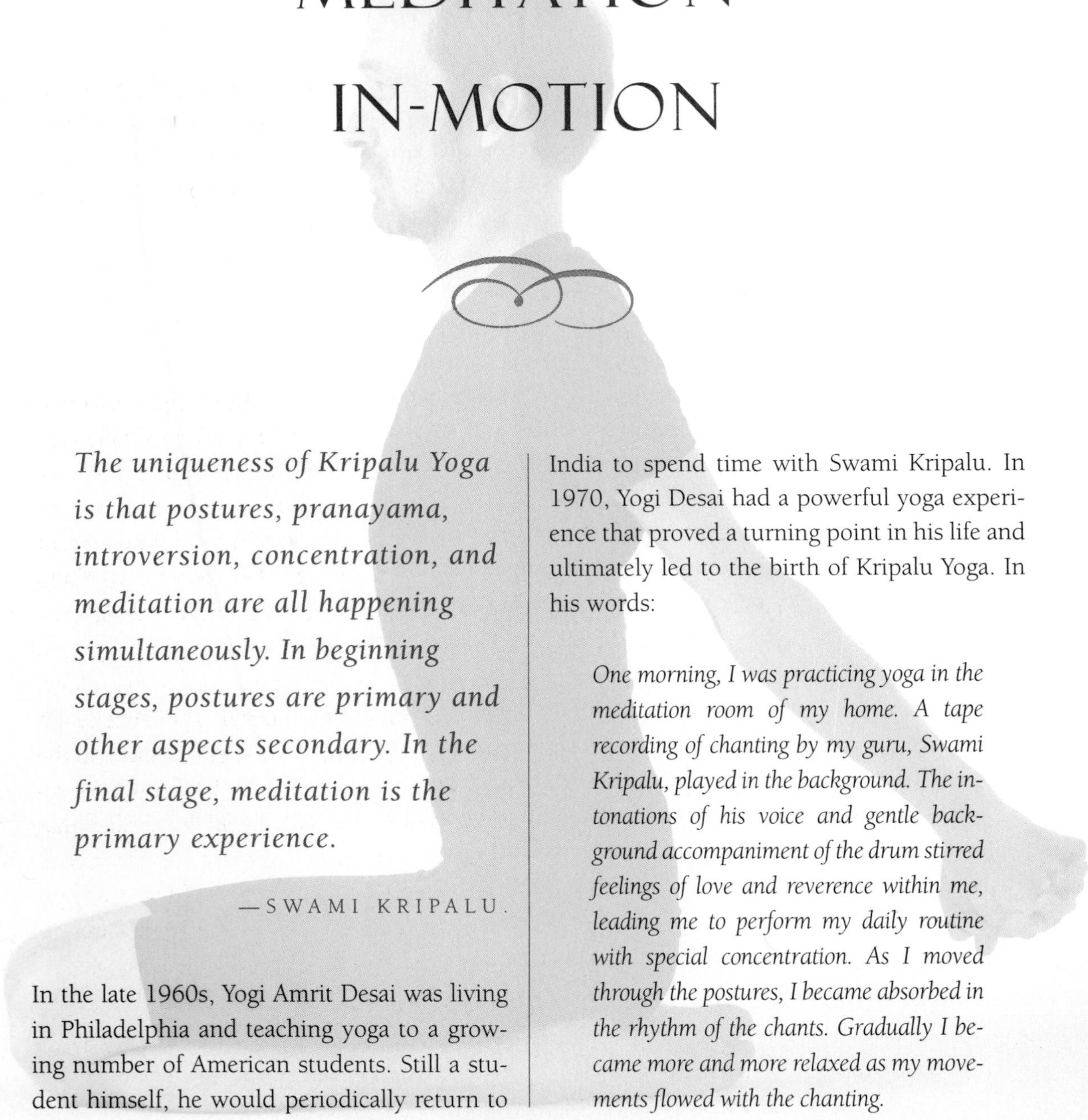

The uniqueness of Kripalu Yoga is that postures, pranayama, introversion, concentration, and meditation are all happening simultaneously. In beginning stages, postures are primary and other aspects secondary. In the final stage, meditation is the primary experience.

—SWAMI KRIPALU.

In the late 1960s, Yogi Amrit Desai was living in Philadelphia and teaching yoga to a growing number of American students. Still a student himself, he would periodically return to India to spend time with Swami Kripalu. In 1970, Yogi Desai had a powerful yoga experience that proved a turning point in his life and ultimately led to the birth of Kripalu Yoga. In his words:

> *One morning, I was practicing yoga in the meditation room of my home. A tape recording of chanting by my guru, Swami Kripalu, played in the background. The intonations of his voice and gentle background accompaniment of the drum stirred feelings of love and reverence within me, leading me to perform my daily routine with special concentration. As I moved through the postures, I became absorbed in the rhythm of the chants. Gradually I became more and more relaxed as my movements flowed with the chanting.*

Suddenly, like an unexpected spring downpour, bliss flooded throughout my entire being, and I felt myself being irresistibly drawn to another level of consciousness. My mind was drawn inward, and the external surroundings dissolved far into the background. I began to feel that I was no longer the performer of the exercises—they were being performed through me. A new flow of energy coursed throughout my system, and with no conscious effort on my part, my body spontaneously began to twist and turn on its own, flowing smoothly from one posture to the next.

The movements were effortless and free, a command and a gift from a newly opened, higher dimension of my being. I was not aware of giving any direction to the movements and felt like I was moving in perfect rhythm with the whole universe. One after another the postures flowed. Some of them were traditional yoga exercises; others were movements I had never seen before. At the end of this flow of postures, my body naturally entered the Lotus Position. A deep stillness penetrated every level of my being. A second explosion of ecstasy spread through me, and I became engulfed, overwhelmed, by a state of complete inner bliss.

After a time, my consciousness began to slowly return to normal. With considerable effort, I was able to open my eyes, discovering to my amazement that it was about thirty minutes later, and I was still in my own home. In twenty-two years of yoga practice, I had never entered such a deep and blissful state, even in meditation. My great desire was to formalize an approach that would give others an opportunity to have this experience.

Yogi Desai spent the next twenty years working with a skilled cadre of teachers and a large community of practitioners to develop Kripalu Yoga into an effective approach to enter *Meditation-in-Motion*.

Awakening Prana

Learning how to relax and invite prana to step into the driver's seat is the key to Meditation-in-Motion. Swami Kripalu described this phenomenon as *spontaneous, effortless, and automatic. Spontaneous* means the impetus for movement comes from a source other than the thinking mind's control over the voluntary skeletal muscles. Once they get in the groove, many people experience this when they dance or make love. *Effortless* refers to the mental experience of not striving or "efforting." Muscles contract and the body exerts, but the overall felt sense is of relaxing and letting go. *Automatic* implies that the movement from one posture to the next is not planned or premeditated. If you are lying in bed and need to go to the bathroom, the mind thinks "bathroom" and the body gets itself up. The way you roll over and come to standing is automatic. Gain entry through any one of these doorways, and you will soon become familiar with all three.

EXPERIENCE: SPONTANEOUS MOVEMENT PRACTICE

Traditional Chinese medicine includes a simple and highly effective technique of prana awakening called *Spontaneous Movement Practice*. This is a version for self-healing that anyone can do, taught by Roger Jahnke, Doctor of Oriental Medicine:

1. Stand with your feet hip-width apart and knees slightly flexed.

2. Relax the body and take a few deep breaths.

3. Allow yourself to wiggle, shake, bounce, flow, massage, stand, sit, or jump. Let out sighs or other sounds. Shake your hands, snap your fingers, and move in ways that release tension.

4. Follow your inner guidance. This may seem awkward at first, but you will soon discover that this is the easiest practice because it is completely spontaneous. There is nothing to learn. Respond to inner urges and an intuitive sense of what is needed.

5. Move gently or vigorously, focusing on remaining relaxed and allowing the breath to be slow and deep. Imagine that energy is flowing to places that have been blocked or stuck.

6. After a while, stop and turn your attention inward. Feel the energy circulating within you.

Adapted from *The Healer Within* by Roger Jahnke (Harper San Francisco, 1999).

> *Substituting technique for conscious awareness has a dumbing effect on our delicate inner guidance mechanism. Devoting yourself to a formulaic and impersonalized practice of yoga can easily displace trust in your ability to know and act upon what is right for you.*
>
> —Don Stapleton

It is common to assume that imperfect health, limited flexibility, insufficient self-discipline, or some other deficit in self-worth prevents the awakening of prana. This is simply not true. Self-doubt is the biggest hurdle. If you are alive and breathing, prana is active in your body, and you can find a way to allow it to express more fully. The ability to connect with prana and allow it to direct the movement of your body is a great boon. You grow intuitively aware of what postures to practice, how to enter them in ways tailored to your body's needs, the best way to breathe in them, how long to hold, at what level of intensity, and how to rebalance after releasing. This raises the therapeutic and transformative power of your practice to a new order of magnitude.

> *When a person is in deep slumber, he is not conscious of turning over. Singers, musicians, sculptors, orators, and other artists become so engrossed in their work that they do not notice when they change postures. In the same natural way, the yogi shifts from posture to posture. Prana takes care to see that the body remains comfortable, and performs various activities to nurture and develop it. It does not need instructions from the mind. A person watching would believe that one is purposefully doing these activities, but one's experience is different.*
>
> —Swami Kripalu

BE THE ENERGY

Trust the energy that courses
through you. Trust—then take
surrender even deeper.
Be the energy.

Don't push anything away.
Follow each sensation back to
its source and focus your awareness
there. Be the ecstasy.

Be unafraid of consummate wonder.
Emerge so new, so vulnerable,
that you don't know
who you are.

Be the energy, and paradoxically,
be at peace. Dare to be your own
illumination, and blaze a trail across
the clear night sky like lightning.

How to Practice

There are several ways to enter Meditation-in-Motion, and you can explore them all. The first is a stage one approach, entering the basic form of a posture as a springboard to explore the body's range of motion. Be creative, using micromovements to flow into variations that just feel good. Exploring beyond the bounds of the known and habitual compels you to deeply attune to the body. Allow it to guide you into a movement meditation of its own making.

You can also use a stage two approach, choosing a posture for prolonged holding that is not too physically taxing. Enter it slowly, and don't go to your maximum stretch right away. Work into a full stretch gradually, progressively relaxing and letting go of surface tensions, then deeper tensions. As you hold, sustain a flowing breath, engage Witness Consciousness, and Ride the Wave. When you have held to your limit, come out of the posture slowly, paying close attention to all the feelings associated with release. Notice if your body is prompting

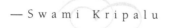

A Return to the Roots of Yoga

BY SENIOR TEACHER DON STAPLETON

The final years of the ashram were profoundly painful for me. I had taken yoga on as a lifelong practice, but for the first time I allowed my responsibilities and the many conflicts arising in the community to interfere with my practice. An injury to my spine compounded matters, and I found myself living in chronic pain. While the breakup of the ashram community was devastating, it freed me to come back to prana and the very exploration that had drawn me to Kripalu in the first place.

I resumed my daily practice, compelled to get out of bed in the night or the wee hours of morning by the force of energy moving through my body. Cradling muscles and joints, I drew more deeply than ever before from the counsel of prana. This required venturing into new territory to allow inner wisdom to truly guide me. Witnessing my experiences and letting go of any attempt to control them, insights unfolded as gifts from the teacher within. Any remnant of doubt about the evolutionary intelligence of the body was subsumed in the miracle of physical, mental, and emotional transformations occurring within the cocoon of my practice.

More than just healing, that post-ashram time laid the foundation for a whole new creative, connected, and conscious life. Ultimately it freed me from the illusion that "truth" exists outside of me, or resides in the authority of any expert or teacher. Just knowing that this life is my own unique and personal journey, and that there is no "right" way to practice yoga, provides its own comforting peace.

you into a compensatory stretch. At first the urge to move may be so mild or subtle that it is easily overlooked, but when you feel it don't hesitate to follow. On the other hand, if you release the posture and find yourself moving quickly or vigorously, let that happen too. You may be surprised to find yourself entering Meditation-in-Motion quite easily. When it naturally ends, choose another posture and repeat the process.

You can also enter Meditation-in-Motion directly in what Kripalu Yoga calls a *posture flow*. This is a yoga ritual, a devotional practice of surrendering to the indwelling spirit, often experienced as a prayer spoken with your whole being. A Kripalu Yoga posture flow is a doorway to the high states of consciousness achieved by yogis, in which all of life is experienced as happening spontaneously, free of any sense of being the

EXPERIENCE: POSTURE FLOW

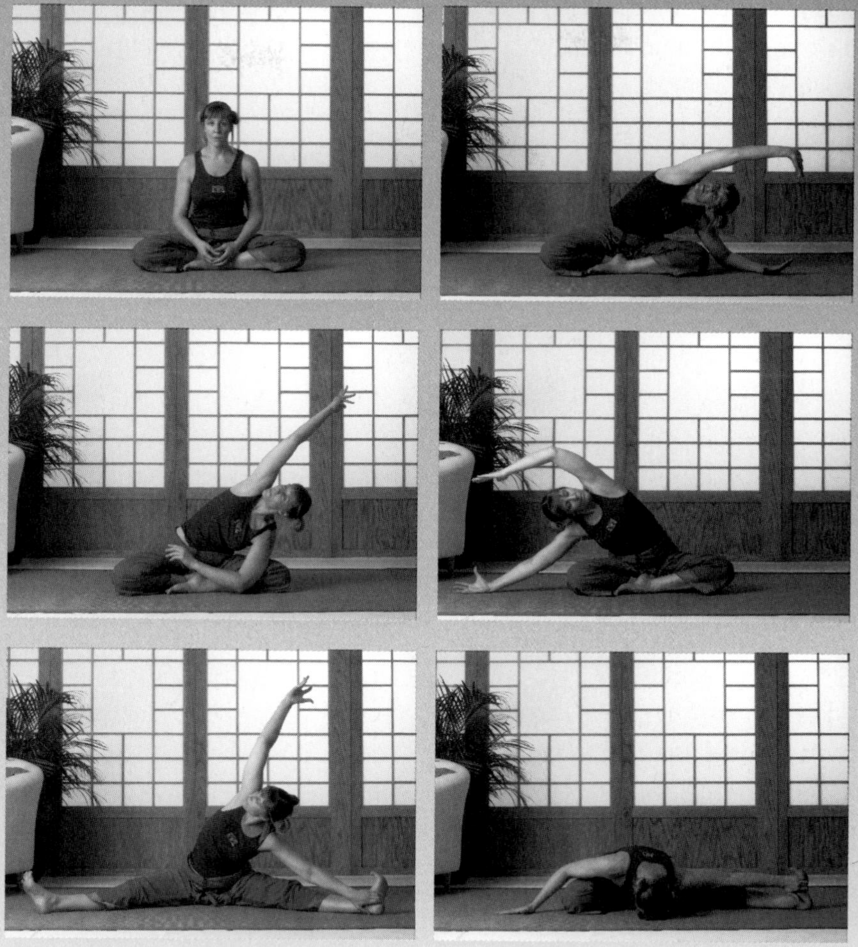

1. Choose a time when you will not be interrupted. You may want to turn off the phone, close the door, and dim the lights. If you enjoy music, select something soft and flowing, conducive to relaxing and slowing down. You may want to light a candle. Taking external steps like these puts you in a receptive frame of mind to focus inward and dive deep into experience.

2. Begin by doing a sequence of warm-ups to prepare the body for movement. You may want to include one or more breathing exercises to charge the body with prana. Then sit in stillness, saying a prayer or affirming your connection to spirit. If prayer does not come naturally, set an intention to enter Witness Consciousness and observe the inner flow of prana and the external movements it prompts. Take

several long flowing breaths, consciously softening the muscles of the belly, chest, shoulders, and face. Let yourself become receptive to the stirring of energy in your body. Then consciously lift your mind's control over prana, freeing the energy of your body to do its work.

3. Sit quietly until you feel an urge to move. If the urge comes, follow it into whatever stretch or movement the body is calling for. This may be a traditional yoga posture, a position you have never seen before, or some form of flowing movement. Neither suppress nor exaggerate the movements. Try not to make anything happen, but also don't prevent anything from happening. Stay relaxed, letting your mind be the witness. If no urge comes, start a simple movement and let it flow to its natural completion. Repeat this again and again as needed, using flowing movement as a tool to sensitize you to the ability of prana to direct the body's movements.

4. As energy awakens, your sensitivity to the body's instinctive urges becomes pronounced and the body may begin to flow, move, turn, and twist. Gentle movements guided by prana are unhurried and have a timeless quality. Vigorous movements can be intense while also effortless.

5. At some point, your flow of postures will naturally draw to completion. Allow your body to come into stillness, sitting or relaxing for a few moments. Notice if an inner flow of energy continues. Be grateful for whatever experience came your way.

doer of the actions. Instructions are set out above.

In a mature practice, the boundaries between the three stages of Kripalu Yoga are fluid, and you can move through all three in each session. Start with willful practice as you warm up and become present in the body. Deepen your inward focus by holding one or more postures to release tensions and attune to prana. Let micromovements and natural sounds emerge from the body. Then allow prana to lead you into intermittent periods of Meditation-in-Motion. If your mind starts to wander, return to stage one, and start over. Trust yourself to create a practice that has just the right mix of will and surrender for you.

CHAPTER TWENTY-TWO

A LIVING RELATIONSHIP WITH SPIRIT

In my first Kripalu Yoga class, I touched the tender, peaceful center of myself and through the postures discovered my connection to the Divine in a very direct and physical way. This deep connection to the best part of myself has sustained my practice ever since. Twenty years later, I can truly say that yoga has transformed my life.

—LESLIE OSTER

Spiritual life is often depicted as an arduous journey to an enlightenment that ends all suffering. Others say there is nowhere to go and nothing to do; it's a moment-to-moment openness to what's here and now. Still others praise a gradual growth process that bestows wisdom, compassion, and spiritual maturity. There is truth in each of these perspectives.

Strictly speaking, there is no yoga or meditation technique capable of enlightening you. As long as there is a *doer,* a practitioner applying a technique to achieve a result, there is something less than the effortless being and oneness of non-duality. Practices can do many things. They can free you of obstacles that dull sensitivity and awareness. They can amplify energy and teach you how to rest in a state of equipoise between attraction and aversion. They can even focus the mind on the infinite, but spiritual awakening only arises from *non-doing*, the release of struggle and striving.

Expressed in the affirmative, this is *surrender*, an attitude of your entire being that embraces the mystery of life unfolding without making anything happen, or stopping anything occurring naturally from flowing to completion. Although it may sound restful and comforting, true surrender is a journey into the unknown that tears your story to shreds and compels you to face insecurity and the shadow aspects of your psyche. Surrender is a precursor of spiritual awakening, not the experience itself. To pass from two-ness into oneness, a shift in identity is required that is not easily pinned down or captured in words.

During Kripalu Yoga Teacher Training, a group of us were led in the experience of holding the posture. After a few minutes of holding the Side Warrior with conscious breathing, we were invited to either release the posture and flow into other stretches or continue to hold the posture and Ride the Wave of energy and awareness.

I decided to continue holding the posture. Staying with the breath, I was able to relax and feel at ease. The energy of the breath seemed to hold me. My feet and lower legs were engaged, but from the knees up I felt light as a feather. I kept breathing and the solid sense of my body dissolved and I became pure breath. And then I was gone. There was no sense of "I." I did not feel a sense of peace. I was peace. When my sense of self returned, there were enormous tears rolling down my face.

For as long as I can remember, I have been a worrier. Having known few if any moments of peace during my life, it was quite something to feel this ultimate peace and to realize that peace is what I really am. Afterward, I spontaneously knelt down and thanked the universe. Since then, how I have opened. How I have learned. How I have been freed.

—Yvette Bulger

Two Paths

Yoga recognizes two paths to the radical shift that underlies a range of non-dual states most often described as *oneness*. The first is the way of negation, described by the Sanskrit credo *neti-neti* which means *not this, not this*. Negation disentangles spirit from a false identification with matter by enumerating what we are not:

I am not this body, or its sensations and feelings
I am not this mind, or its thoughts and desires
I am not intuition or insight
I am not this sense of self
I am Spirit, the Absolute

Seeking spirit through negation casts desire and the alluring world of the senses as profane, a distraction from the holy life. It often leads seekers to label the human dimension of existence as illusory and unreal. Anyone employing the practices of yoga to walk the path of negation tends to adopt an attitude, consciously or unconsciously, of withdrawal from the tasks and challenges of everyday life.

The second path is the way of affirmation, described by the credo *asmi-asmi,* which means *this too, this too.* This path embraces everything as a manifestation of the Divine, dispelling the myth of separateness that divides reality into artificial distinctions like matter and spirit. Its approach is expressed in this chant from the Kripalu Yoga tradition:

All is spirit
These thoughts are spirit
These memories are spirit
These feelings are spirit
This body is spirit
The world is spirit
These others are spirit
All is spirit

The stark contrast of these paths reflects the paradox of depth spiritual experience. Spirit is transcendent, an all-pervading consciousness that exists beyond the confines of time, space, matter, and mind. Spirit is also immanent, closer to you than breath or heartbeat, the primordial source of all creation. Although seemingly contradictory, both paths share a common root. They are thought-trails of contemplative practitioners who passed beyond the limits of mind by inquiring deeply into the true nature of self and psyche. As the Zen poet Basho advises, we should not so much seek to follow in the footsteps of past masters as to seek what they sought.

THE SEEDS OF MY AWARENESS

You mean to say that I am
plugged into the same socket
as that electric blue sky, so
vibrant that I want to lose
myself in its azure height?

You mean that the same juice
that runs the universe flows
through me like a love song
or a bolt of lightning?

You mean life isn't about
being good or perfect or
virtuous, but daring to
freely follow energy?

Are you trying to say in your
slow and patient way that the
presence of God is everywhere,
and that the seeds of my
awareness are sprouting,
even now?

However accessed, any deep non-dual experience makes it clear that no one has to earn a connection to spirit. You were born divine, the energy, awareness, and love of spirit made manifest. Seen in this light, spiritual awakening is not a rarified mind state. It's the direct

There When I Needed It

BY SENIOR TEACHER SHANTIPRIYA MARCIA GOLDBERG

Being with my dad for six days before he died, and at the moment he left his body, was one of the peak experiences of my life. It transformed my whole experience of what death is, and who I am too. As I sat at his side, I tuned in to my breath, feeling its rhythm in my belly anchoring me into the present moment. My awareness heightened and my thoughts became still. My awareness expanded to include my father's breath, his hand holding mine, and our deep heart connection. Time stopped and I was present with myself and my father in a way I had never experienced before. As I felt him slip out of his body, I was aware of peace around me and within me. I knew he was not his body, but spirit—and so was I. I am so grateful for my Kripalu Yoga practice of many years, which was automatically there for me when I needed it.

experience of who and what you really are. While stress, illness, self-judgment, and a host of other factors can leave you feeling distant from spirit, none of these can alter the truth of your identity. You are spirit.

Focus, Flow, Let It Go

Yoga's description of the inner process that leads to spiritual awakening is remarkably straightforward. The mind is led into three states of absorption called *dharana* (one-pointedness), *dhyana* (one-flowingness), and *samadhi* (oneness). This trio is often translated as concentration, meditation, and realization.

Initial practice relaxes the body and calms the thinking mind. As awareness grows steady, it becomes possible to maintain a one-pointed focus on an object of concentration, such as the breath, a mantra, or a visualized deity. Concentration activates the intuitive mind, and dharana gives way to the highly lucid flow states of meditation. Thoughts continue, but your once-scattered awareness increasingly streams in a single direction. This is the state mystics call *communion,* often accompanied by sublime feelings of peace, bliss, exaltation, or love. As dhyana deepens, these feelings completely absorb the mind.

While enlightenment is often equated with powerful feelings or crystal clear insights, spirit can never be known by the mind. It can only be *realized* by a radical shift in identification. Like an acrobat who must let go of one trapeze bar to grasp another, realization requires you to release all concepts and fixed identities. The call to spiritual awakening is a radical assertion that it is possible to live from a direct and real-time connection to reality, free of the static produced by the machinations of mind. Although unusually vivid and compelling, yoga experiences are magnified versions of normal perception in which the awareness of self and other remains. Realization is a union, a profound connectedness in which the rigid distinction between subject and object falls away. Some traditions describe this direct perception of reality as the *Divine* or *Self,* others as *emptiness* or *no-self,* and arguments over what is the highest state rage on for centuries. Regardless of the label attached, it is clear that *samadhi* (joining together) is a quantum leap beyond the intuitive, authentic self and mind states associated with meditation.

Personal accounts vary, with some practitioners describing a dramatic falling away of barriers that separate self and world to reveal a vast unbroken wholeness. Others dissolve into a blissful ocean of being. A dramatic energy experience propels one into an entirely new state of consciousness; a gentle homecoming restores another to the remembrance of what has always been true. While characterized differently, all report an experience that goes completely beyond the body, mind, and processes of thinking, feeling, intuition, and insight. As the doorway of immanence swings open, it reveals an interior depth that is truly transpersonal. An experience of the true self, no matter how short-lived, reacquaints us with the sacred presence that underlies not only our bodily existence, but all of creation. It is the direct experience that spirit dwells within you, *as you.*

> *I was led into Locust and remember going into the posture with a lot of focus. While holding, I felt my body start to shake and vibrate. It got so pronounced that I thought people might be noticing me, shaking all about. I opened my eyes slightly to see what was really happening, but the parts of my body I could see looked normal. At the end of the class, I went really deep in meditation. Opening my eyes, I felt profoundly connected to the others in the room, to the point where I could not discern a difference between me and the next person. I looked outside and felt no separation between me and the sky. I was stunned.*
>
> —Pamela K. Myers

Embodying Spirit

Yoga experiences of all kinds are catalysts for change. They speed up the rate of a transformative process that requires years to run its course. Non-dual experiences are especially potent. In some cases, they usher in ecstatic periods of rapid growth. Along with positive effects, powerful breakthroughs also pose a real danger. They can leave practitioners inflated and complacent, willing to cash in their chips and declare themselves done when blind spots, insecurity, and grandiosity remain.

The goal of Kripalu Yoga is more nuanced and practical than a one-time enlightenment experience. Kripalu Yoga helps you develop a strong and healthy body, an open caring heart, and a clear and creative mind. All along the way, it recognizes that you were born divine and connected to spirit. Bringing you back again and again to the experience of being mentally present and spiritually awake in a relaxed body, Kripalu Yoga helps you weave spiritual awareness into the fabric of your everyday life and being. This process of embodying spirit is not only reflected in what happens on the yoga mat or meditation cushion. In many ways, a better measure is the presence of positive qualities like peace, joy, love, creativity, wisdom, humility, generosity, fearlessness, compassion, and courage in your life.

If there's a Kripalu Yoga definition of enlightenment, it is the ability to live in deep connection with self, life, and others. Each moment arises fresh and we are free to respond. Do we react with fear and defensiveness? Or respond with openness, curiosity, and gratitude? More than a search to encounter the absolute or transpersonal, the Kripalu Yoga path is about marrying the absolute and the relative in a deeply integrated life.

After three decades of practice, you might find it surprising that no one in the Kripalu community claims a full and final enlightenment. What are the results? The community as a whole demonstrates a genuine realness, warmth, and sincerity. Some individuals have blossomed into brilliant teachers and capable leaders. Many have developed their skills and talents to high levels. A critic could say that the majority remains normally neurotic, but a deeper look reveals that most are well-adjusted and engaged in an active growth process. Almost to a person, mature Kripalu Yoga practitioners have come to view spiritual life as a process of continual awakening to deeper levels of wholeness and connection, versus a search for the holy grail of enlightenment.

> *I used to think an enlightened being wouldn't suffer at all. Now I believe the only difference between us mortals and a realized soul is their lack of reaction and judgment to the inevitable suffering of life. Jesus and Buddha suffered, as did Swami Kripalu. Yes, life is suffering but I know from my yoga practice that it's only a ripple on the surface. In sacred moments, I can peek through the gaps and see that love is the real me, and that my life is just God playing.*
>
> —Dharmadas Anthony Conard

Traditional yoga advises a practitioner to stick with one approach, pursuing it diligently to the desired end of enlightenment. There is real wisdom in this advice, as all of us are apt to move on to other things whenever we come up against the daunting hurdles that present themselves in the process of self-transformation. Once steeped in Kripalu Yoga, many mature practitioners have found it valuable to "cross train" in other contemporary approaches like

Yoga Is for Everyone

BY SENIOR TEACHER MAYA BREUER

My grandmother used to tell me "Stay close to God and stay out of trouble." This was good advice. Born into an African American and orthodox Jewish family, I always felt different from those around me: none of my black friends prayed morning and evening, or spent every Sabbath in the temple. But under the watchful eye of my grandparents, I took refuge in spirit and grew up in a loving yet structured religious environment.

My challenges came later in life, as my career as a jazz singer, the nightlife, and the demands of raising three children by myself pulled me away from spirit. A desire to reconnect to my self and spirit is what drew me to Kripalu Center. There, once again, I found I was different, often the only black face in the room, but I didn't care because I was entranced with yoga and it was bringing my spirit alive again. Feeling alone in the ashram didn't stop me from becoming a disciple, a devoted practitioner, and eventually a full-time teacher.

At first my focus was teaching Kripalu Yoga with its resplendent yet simple emphasis on breath and easy movement in and out of postures. Then I was invited to go to India and study in the village where Swami Kripalu had built a temple and spent years in seclusion and intensive practice. Something happened to me there, life energy awakening and dancing through my being and deepening my understanding of compassion, yoga, and life.

When I returned to the States, I was on fire with Swami Kripalu's message that the whole world was one family. This had become my mission, and I refocused my teaching to serve others like me—people of color—who needed the holistic and healing benefits of yoga as much as, if not more than, the white majority. Free yoga at the public library, Saturday morning yoga and breakfast, fostering diversity in the world of yoga became my practice.

It took energy, some friends, and lots of patience, but eventually the Kripalu community awoke to the need for greater diversity at Kripalu Center and in the American yoga movement. I took a deep breath and submitted a proposal to lead a healing retreat for women of color at Kripalu Center. It was accepted, and I was as amazed as anyone to see the program fill to capacity and spill over into a lengthy waiting list. Today I know that Swami Kripalu was right. No matter what our color, culture, socioeconomic status, or position in life, we all need to breathe and to learn how to take care of our bodies, ease our minds, and connect to the divinity that lives within us. This yoga is for everyone.

Ashtanga, Anusara, Bikram, and Iyengar Yoga. Those drawn to pursue a depth awakening often immerse themselves in the liberation teachings of Kundalini Yoga, Patanjali's classical yoga, Advaita Vedanta, the various schools of Buddhism, and mystical Christianity and Judaism. Others grow fascinated with quantum physics, transpersonal psychology, or gardening. Each person embodies spirit in their own way. While sharing a commitment to focused spiritual practice, eclecticism has become part of the Kripalu Yoga approach.

> *It is worth remembering that there is only one yoga. True, aspirants are of different natures and resort to various doctrines and practices to progress along the path. But one who completes the process understands its different paths and sees that the practice of various disciplines leads to the same place. In the end, all yogas lead to one great yoga.*
>
> — Swami Kripalu

A Living Relationship with Spirit

Spirit has a unique quality. It is transpersonal, absolutely the same in you and others, and entirely free of egocentric concerns. Cut off from a vital spiritual connection, it seems we are separate, independent, and disconnected. Sages from all traditions have taught that this sense of separateness is the root of human suffering. As you begin to recognize spirit in yourself, you increasingly see it shining in others, and reflected in the world around you. As separation falls away, so does suffering.

Swami Kripalu taught that the highest spiritual attainment is reflected in the maxim *Vasudeva Khatumbhakam,* which means *The Whole World Is One Family*. A proverbial saying in his youth, it became a revealed truth that inspired a profound life of love, service, ardent practice, artistic expression, and joyous celebration. To realize this truth for ourselves, Swami Kripalu gave some simple advice: *Practice spiritual disciplines, love your family with a pure heart, and selflessly serve your community, nation, and the world.*

At Kripalu Center, we believe practices like yoga have a part to play in addressing our current dilemma as people and as a planet. With 25,000 guests passing through our doors each year, we have seen firsthand their power to tear down the walls that separate us from ourselves and others. The healing and growth that results empowers us to play our parts in establishing the extraordinary culture and conditions needed to heal our world. If yoga can actually lead us to love ourselves and see the world as one family, perhaps other shifts in heart and mind may be possible, and humankind can realize the astounding potentials of life on earth.

5. EVOLVING YOUR PRACTICE

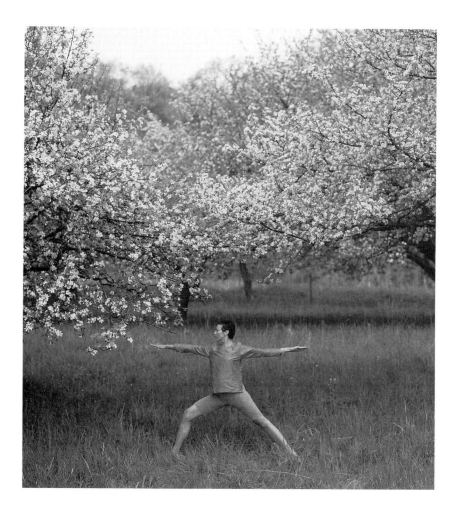

CHAPTER TWENTY-THREE

CREATING POSTURE SEQUENCES

Only through the faithful practice of elementary yoga is the advanced yoga generated.

—SWAMI KRIPALU

The litmus test for an evolving practice is whether your time on the mat produces a palpable sense of forward movement and inspiration. Many people experience this in the early stages of yoga practice. Sustaining this type of positive momentum over time is a fine art, and learning how to create your own yoga sequences is an essential aspect of yoga mastery.

You can feel the "body logic" underlying a good yoga sequence. Easier stretches flow seamlessly into moderate and then more challenging postures. Vigorous effort is balanced by moments of rest, gentle movements that relieve strain, and complementary stretches that restore balance. Over the course of a session, the whole body is warmed up, powerfully stimulated, and cooled back down. As the flow of postures draws to an end, relaxation comes naturally. The overall result is a profound sense of rejuvenation and balance. Proper sequencing is critical to fostering this balance—and avoiding injuries.

Sun and Moon Series are intended to provide an in-your-body experience of postures done with proper sequencing. After becoming familiar with them, begin to personalize the routines by paying close attention to what works—and what doesn't work—for you. Give yourself permission to freely adapt the postures based on the felt sense of your body. If a certain posture causes you to strain, modify it or substitute an easier form of the same stretch. If another is too easy, replace it with one that's a little more challenging. If the sequence is too long, shorten it.

An evolving practice has a growing edge. Gains in strength, flexibility, and focus naturally draw you to explore and ultimately master postures previously beyond your reach. Beyond regular practice, a willingness to experiment is all that is needed to learn the finer points of yoga sequencing. Who could know your body and discern its needs better than you?

Traditional Sequencing

The posture sequences preserved and taught in most traditional yoga schools are suited to physically adept practitioners. After minimal warm-ups, often repetitions of the Sun Salutation done at a brisk pace, the practitioner moves through a series of classic yoga postures. Multiple postures that stretch the spine intensively in one direction are followed by another set of postures that provide the opposite stretch. This method of sequencing pos-

EXERCISE PLATEAU

No matter how good the exercise routine, you can't repeat it day after day and continue to get the same results. Your body adapts to the demands made upon it. A well-worn routine ceases to be a healthy challenge and loses its ability to stimulate you to higher levels of fitness. Progress levels off in a phenomenon called *exercise plateau*. As a once-cherished routine goes stale, it becomes hard to keep your mind focused and engaged. When boredom sets in, your love affair with yoga can start to feel like a rut. This is why experts recommend that you alter an exercise regimen every six weeks, the approximate time it takes the body to adapt to a new routine. The key to skillfully working with exercise plateau is simple: mix it up! Learn new postures that work different parts of the body. Hold the postures you already know a little longer to ramp up your intensity. Vary the order and manner in which you do things to open doorways into greater spontaneity and self-expression.

tures is known as *pose* and *counterpose*. Postures that are relatively challenging for an average practitioner—like Cobra and Locust—are used to warm the body up for advanced poses like Bow and Camel. Little time is allotted between posture groupings for rest or compensatory movements that relieve strain.

Beginning students are often guided to start practicing the traditional sequence by simply doing their best and omitting any postures that prove too challenging. Through disciplined repetition, it is expected they will develop the fitness required to perform the full routine properly. Preparatory exercises that build the core strength required to safely perform many classic yoga postures may be neglected. Easier versions of the postures may not be taught in a process of progressive strengthening.

Kripalu Yoga Sequencing

Kripalu Yoga refers to a good sequence as a *yoga flow.* This implies that there is an underlying logic to the arrangement and unfolding of exercises that makes sense to the body. On the most basic level, it's a layered movement from simpler stretches to challenging postures to closing movements that soothe and integrate. Focused time is spent on strengthening the core muscles of the torso that support the proper alignment of the spine. Every Kripalu Yoga sequence includes *the six movements of the spine:* backward bends, forward bends, lateral stretches of both sides, and twists that rotate the vertebrae right and left. A balanced mix of these movements is yoga's prescription to maintain the natural curvature of the spine.

In a short sequence of fifteen minutes, the six movements of the spine may be repeated a single time. In a thirty minute practice session, the six movements may be done twice, with simpler warm-up movements followed by slightly more challenging ones. In a spacious session, the six movements may be repeated three or four times in layers of warm-ups, easier poses, and challenging postures. In addition to articulating the spine, a sequence should aim to stimulate the body's musculature by including postures that work the abdomen and chest, the back, legs and hips, arms and shoulders, and neck. Even in a short sequence, inversions can be used as "cooldowns" to trigger the relaxation response.

From Easy to Challenging

Nothing could be simpler than the idea behind posture progression: gentle postures prepare the body for moderate postures, which prepare the body for vigorous postures. Yet the practical importance of this simple concept cannot be overstated.

Each yoga posture exists on a spectrum of difficulty. Grasping this fact, you can layer your practice to move from easy to challenging. Start out with simple warm-ups that take you through the six movements of the spine. Then add a second layer, choosing postures from a few of the categories set out in the chart on pages 320–321 that are easily within your capacity. Staying within these categories, end with a third layer of postures that are healthy challenges. Come to completion with a few minutes of integrating and compensatory movements to help you flow smoothly into relaxation.

Posture progress often occurs in the following manner. At first, the classic posture may need to be modified in ways that make it easier to enter, hold, and release. With practice, the classic form of the posture comes into reach and can eventually be done without a great deal of effort. Then variations of the posture emerge, each enhancing the basic stretch in some way, which keeps the learning process alive. Eventually, the next posture on the progression list beckons and the process repeats. The first posture remains part of your repertoire, and can now be done earlier in the session as preparation.

At some point, everyone reaches their healthy limit, which reflects in part a genetic potential. Very few practitioners develop the ability to do the "pretzel postures" traditionally considered to constitute an advanced posture practice. Yet almost everyone can progress to a moderate practice sufficient to maintain a high degree of health and well-being, and one that offers the variety of exercises needed to be fulfilling over time. Moreover, a moderate posture practice is all that's needed to facilitate psychological growth and spiritual awakening—the deeper benefits yoga was designed to pursue.

POSTURE PROGRESSIONS

(Easier to Vigorous Within Each Category)

Core Strengtheners
Single Leg Lifts
Side Leg Lifts
Half Curl Up
Balancing Cat
Waterwheel
Scissors
Toe Touches
Plank and Side Plank
Upward Boat

Hip Openers
Inverted Frog
Lunge
Happy Baby
Figure Four Stretch
Gate
Squat
Frog
Pigeon

Side Stretches
Quarter Moon
Half Circle
Gate
Half Moon
Triangle
Bent Knee Side Stretch
Lateral Angle
Rotated Triangle

Supported Backbends or Belly Downs
Serpent
Half Locust
Sphinx
Boat
Cobra
Diagonal Stretch
Half Bow
Bow
Full Locust

Backbends
Parabola
Bridge
Inverted Table
Bridge Variations
Dancer
Standing Bow Pulling
Half Camel
Camel
Wheel

Forward Bends
Downward Dog
Standing Angle
Lying Hamstring Stretch
Hands to Feet
Great Seal
Posterior Stretch
Seated Angle

Spinal Twists
Supine Twist
Knee Down Twist
Straight Legged Spinal Twist
Seated Spinal Twist
Folded Leg Twist
Half Lotus Twist

Inversions
Dead Bug
Half Shoulderstand
Three-Quarters Shoulderstand

Practice Templates

Like any artistic endeavor, learning posture sequencing begins with mastering a form. All of the above sequencing principles can be distilled into two templates for a full practice session. By varying the exercises selected from the posture progression list, the intensity of the session can be adjusted to produce a gentle, moderate, or vigorous practice. The first begins with standing warm-ups. The second begins with warm-ups done on the floor. You are likely to recognize these templates, as they form the basic skeleton of the Sun and Moon Series. Although sharing much in common, each has a noticeably different feel. Alternating from one to the other helps provide some of the variety needed to spice up your practice and prevent boredom.

Standing Warm-Ups	Floor Warm-Ups
Standing Postures	Core Strengthening
Core Strengthening	Standing Postures
Belly Downs and Backbends	Inversion Option
Forward Bends	Belly Downs and Backbends
Twists	Forward Bends
Inversion Option	Twists
Relaxation	Relaxation

ANOTHER ALTERNATIVE

Another effective way to structure a yoga sequence is to work yourself slowly in and out of a challenging posture. Let's assume you are deepening your backbends and exploring Wheel posture. A supportive sequence might look like the following:

1. A set of warm-ups that engages the breath and includes all six movements of the spine. Begin gently, gradually increase the intensity of effort, and end with one or more core strengthening exercises.
2. A set of easier belly down backbends, done slowly and consciously, such as Serpent and Half Locust, which work the upper then lower spine.
3. One moderate backbend, such as the Boat, which works the whole spine. Follow the Boat with a complementary posture such as Child Pose. Further compensate by coming onto your back and bringing the knees into the chest. Reach your arms out to the sides into a wide T. Allow the knees to rock to the right and come into a gentle twist, breathing deeply. Repeat on the opposite side. Rest for a minute in Corpse Pose.
4. Come into Bridge Pose, holding the posture for ten or more deep breaths. Release and bring the knees into the chest. Reach up around the knees and interlace the fingers, rocking gently side to side to massage and soothe the low back. Come into Corpse Pose and rest until the breath returns to normal.
5. Come back into Bridge and move directly into Wheel Posture. Hold at your relaxed edge with a flowing breath, teasing out the effort from the let go. When the time is right, release and once again bring the knees into the chest. Reach up around the knees and interlace the fingers, rocking gently side to side to massage and soothe the low back. Come into Corpse Pose and rest until the breath returns to normal. Continue to compensate and restore balance with other gentle forward bends and twists that feel good to your body.
6. Close the session by coming into Half Shoulderstand, then Knee Down Twist.
7. Relax in Corpse Pose.

These same principles can be applied to move in and out of any postures that offer you a healthy challenge.

Experiment with the practice templates on page 321, but don't treat them as rigid rules. Use them to enhance but not limit a personal exploration of what works for you.

A Curious Journey

Your ability to create yoga sessions may unfold so organically that it is easy to overlook. After holding a posture at your edge, its release is often accompanied by an urge to move that naturally leads you into the next stretch your body is calling for. Hold that stretch at your edge, letting micromovements and sounds emerge. Then follow your body into another posture. Practicing in this manner, you are likely to find yourself automatically flowing from posture to posture in accord with the sequencing principles just discussed. Why is this so? It's because you are being guided by the actual needs of your body, and the same anatomical factors that led the early yogis to discover these principles in the first place. After a hectic day, you are likely to find yourself creating a practice that is slow and soothing. In the morning, you might gently ease away morning stiffness and then do a series of vigorous standing postures that send you off into your day feeling energized.

A curious journey begins when a practitioner really catches on to sequencing. At first, it feels as if the secret language of yoga has been decoded. New and different postures can now be assembled into many coherent "sentences" or flows. With continued practice, the conception of a "sequence" begins to break down. It now seems that the language is not composed of sentences at all, but shorter phrases of "posture clusters." These are complementary postures that fit nicely together, consistently feel good to your body, and can be strung together in all sorts of creative ways.

As prana awakes, the body begins to speak its own language. Now even the idea of posture clusters falls away and the root language of yoga is heard as an authentic response to the immediate needs of the body, heart, mind, and spirit. Postures and movements arise naturally from a deep attunement to self, free from conditioning and without regard for abstract principles. This ability to attune to what is true for you in the moment is what transforms yoga into a joyous form of self-expression. Yoga becomes simplicity itself, a free response to the guidance that is always flowing from within.

A GALLERY OF WARM-UPS AND POSES

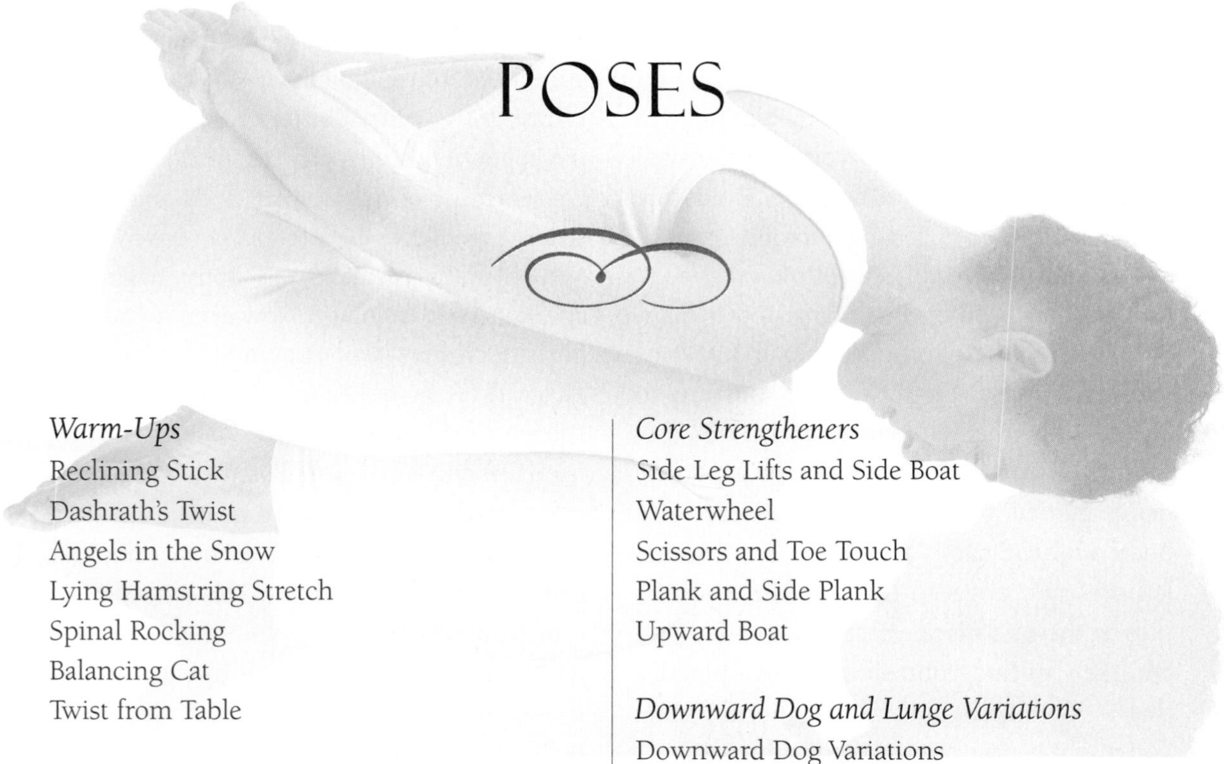

Warm-Ups

Reclining Stick
Dashrath's Twist
Angels in the Snow
Lying Hamstring Stretch
Spinal Rocking
Balancing Cat
Twist from Table

Hip Openers

Gate
Frog
Figure Four Stretch
Happy Baby
Squat
Pigeon
Pigeon Variations

Core Strengtheners

Side Leg Lifts and Side Boat
Waterwheel
Scissors and Toe Touch
Plank and Side Plank
Upward Boat

Downward Dog and Lunge Variations

Downward Dog Variations
Basic Lunge Variations
Deeper Lunge Variations

Standing Postures

Parabola
Standing Hands to Feet
Dancer
Standing Bow Pulling

Eagle
Bent Knee Side Stretch and Lateral Angle
Rotated Triangle

Belly Downs
Cobra
Diagonal Stretch
Locust Series
Half Bow
Bow

Backbends
Inverted Table
Bridge Variations
Half Camel
Camel
Wheel

Forward Bends
Pyramid and Rotated Pyramid
Yoga Mudra
Chin to Knee
Seated Angle

Twists
Half Lotus Twist
Folded Leg Twist
Seated Spinal Twist

Inversions
Three-Quarters Shoulderstand and Fish

Sitting Poses
Thunderbolt
Adept's Pose
Half Lotus
Hero

WARM-UPS

RECLINING STICK

(Yastikasana)

1. Lie on your back with the legs extended, feet hip-width apart, and arms at the sides. Exhale fully.

2. Inhale and slowly sweep the arms out to the sides and overhead. Bring the palms together and stretch the body long by pressing out through the heels and fingertips. Resist the tendency for the spine to arch by pressing the low back and area between the shoulder blades into the floor, while keeping the chin slightly tucked.

3. Exhale and slowly sweep the arms back to the sides. Relax as you take a deep breath in and out.

4. Come into several repetitions of this flowing movement. Coordinate breath and movement, inhaling the arms overhead and exhaling them back to the sides. Rest for a deep breath in and out each time the arms return to the sides.

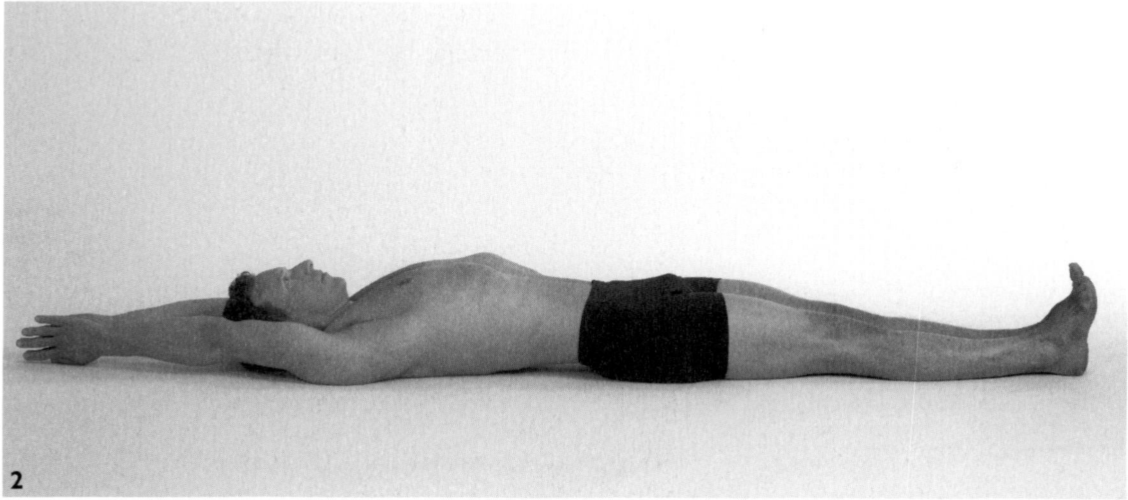

5. On the final repetition, hold the stretch with arms overhead for several long and flowing breaths. Flex the feet and press the heels away. Press the lower and mid-back into the floor. Keep the chin slightly tucked as you extend through the crown of the head. To release, slowly exhale the arms back to the sides.

Be Aware:
The Reclining Stick is part posture and part pranayama. Taking a deep breath in and out between each repetition makes this exercise both energizing and relaxing.

DASHRATH'S TWIST

(Dashrathasana)

1. Lie on your back with the feet close to the buttocks and hip-width apart.

2. Reach up to grasp the elbows with opposite hands. Bring the elbows directly above the shoulders.

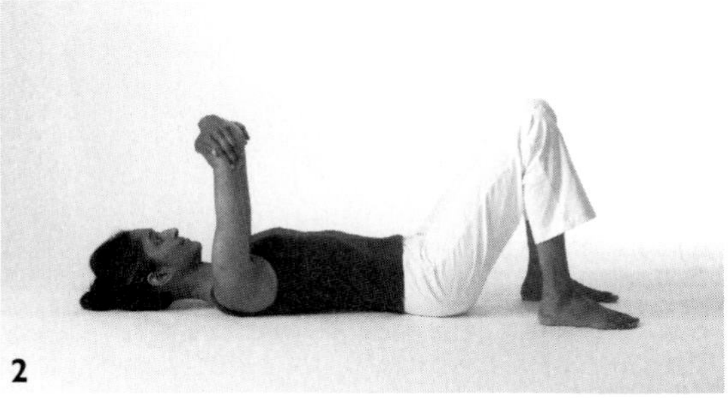

3. Take a deep breath in. As you exhale, let the arms move as a unit to the right, bringing the right elbow toward the ground. Allow the eyes to follow the movement of the elbows and eventually look right. Simultaneously let the knees rock to the left while keeping both feet on the floor.

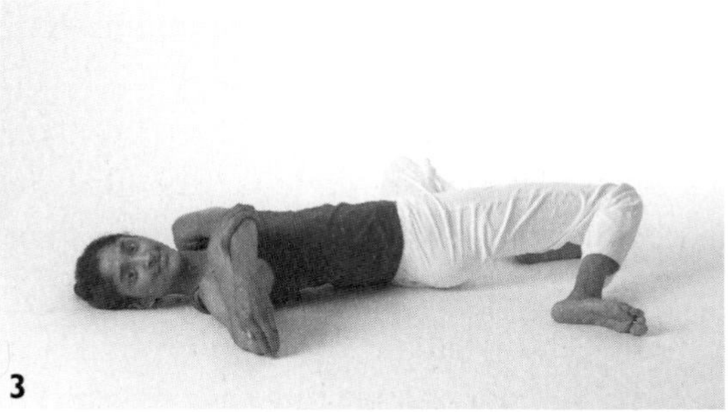

4. Inhale the arms, head, and knees back to center, and exhale to the opposite side.

5. Move smoothly from side to side. As much as possible, keep both shoulder blades resting solidly on the floor.

Be Aware:
This warm-up works the hips, shoulders, and neck in one flowing movement. It is named after a sage in the Kripalu tradition named *Dashrath*.

ANGELS IN THE SNOW

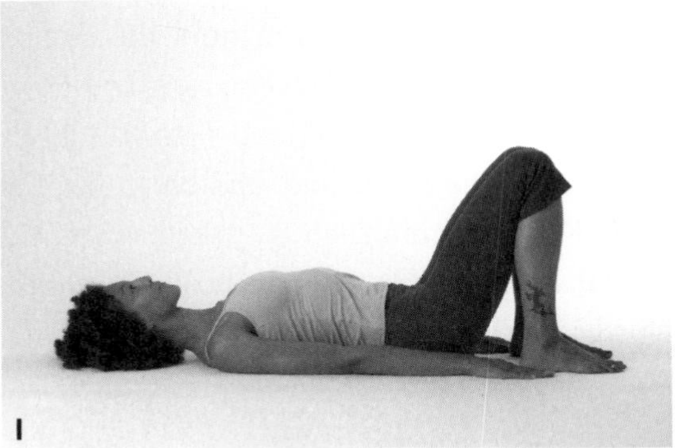
1

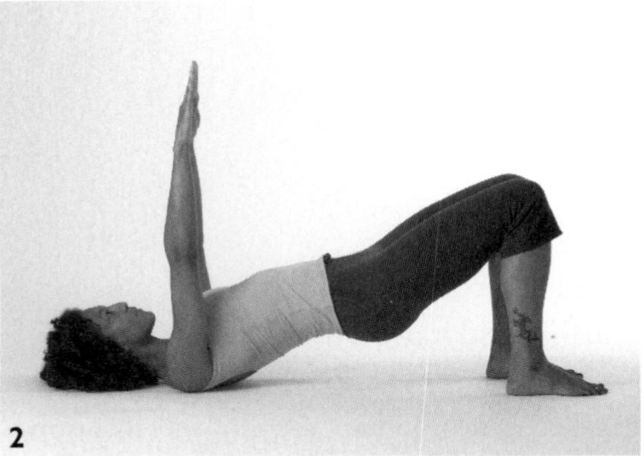
2

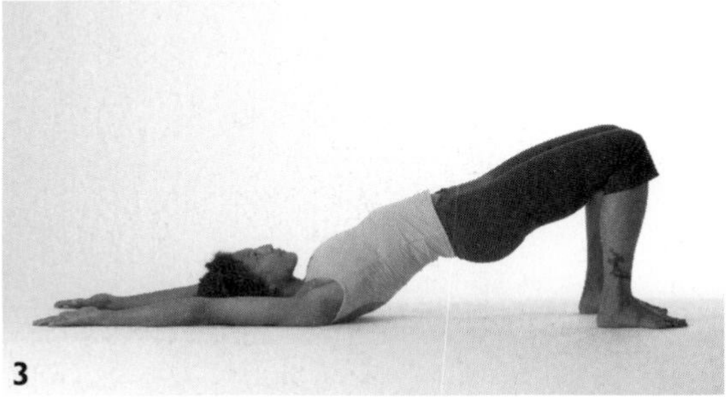
3

1. Lie on your back with the feet close to the buttocks and hip-width apart. Bring the arms to the sides, palms down. Exhale completely.

2. Inhale and press into the feet to lift the hips and buttocks off the floor, simultaneously lifting your arms toward the ceiling.

3. As the hips lift to their maximum, bring the arms all the way overhead.

4. Exhale as you slowly lower the hips and sweep the arms out to the sides along the floor, as if you were making an angel in the snow.

5. When the hips and arms have returned to the starting position, inhale and repeat, coordinating breath and movement.

6. Come into the movement a final time, pausing with the hips lifted high and the arms overhead, weight resting on the feet and shoulders. Take several deep breaths in this position. Slowly release on an exhale, returning to the starting position.

Be Aware:

This series of flowing movements warms up the legs, hips, abdomen, spine, and shoulders. It is an especially good sequence to prepare for Bridge pose. As you lift the hips high, make sure your body weight rests on the feet and shoulders, and not the back of the neck. Resist the tendency of the knees to splay out to the sides by keeping them hip-width apart and directly over the ankles. If your low back is sensitive, bring the knees into the chest and rock gently side to side as a compensatory stretch.

LYING HAMSTRING STRETCH

(Supta Padangushtasana)

1. Lie on your back with the feet close to the buttocks and hip-width apart.

2. Lift the right foot toward the ceiling. Reach the hands up to hold the back of the right thigh. As much as possible, keep the sacrum, hip bones, and low back resting solidly on the floor. Flex the right foot and press the heel away to lengthen the leg.

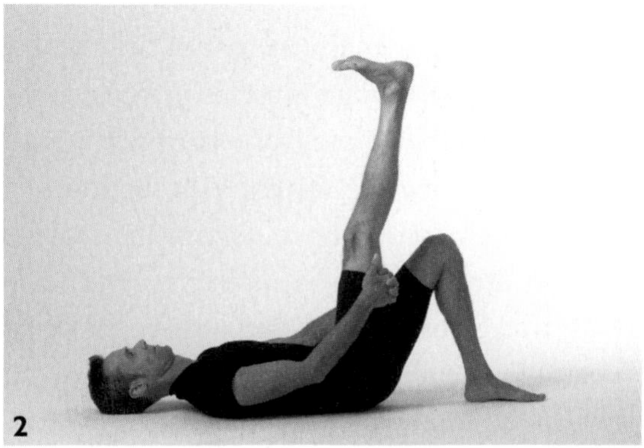
2

3. Take a deep breath in. As you exhale, slide the hands up until you feel a stretch to the back of the right leg. Let the breath flow freely as you hold. You may want to come into micro-movements by letting the right leg sway just a few inches side to side to explore the stretch. Come back to center.

4. If you want to go a little deeper, take another deep breath in and as you exhale slide the hands a little farther up the leg. Flex the right foot and press the heel away.

5. If you want to go even deeper, straighten the left leg out onto the floor. Maintain a steady stretch to the back of the right leg.

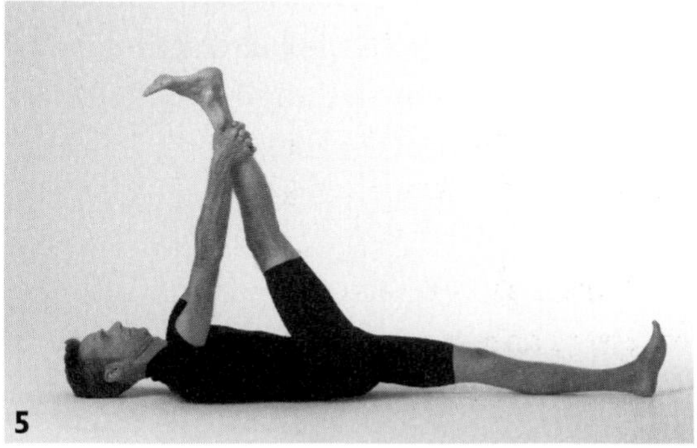
5

6. To release, bring the left foot back onto the floor near the buttocks. Lower the right leg, returning to the starting position.

7. Repeat on the opposite side.

Be Aware:
A measure of hamstring flexibility is required to practice forward bending postures. To compensate for hamstring inflexibility, there is a tendency to force your body into the posture by overstretching the low back. This stretch helps you safely isolate the stretch in the hamstrings by using the support of the floor to stabilize the low back.

SPINAL ROCKING

1. Sit with your knees bent, feet hip-width on the floor in front of you. Reach the hands between the knees to clasp the feet. Tuck the chin slightly and extend through the crown to lengthen the neck.

2. Begin to gently roll backward, shifting the weight smoothly from the buttocks across the low back and onto the mid-back. Roll back until the majority of the back is on the floor.

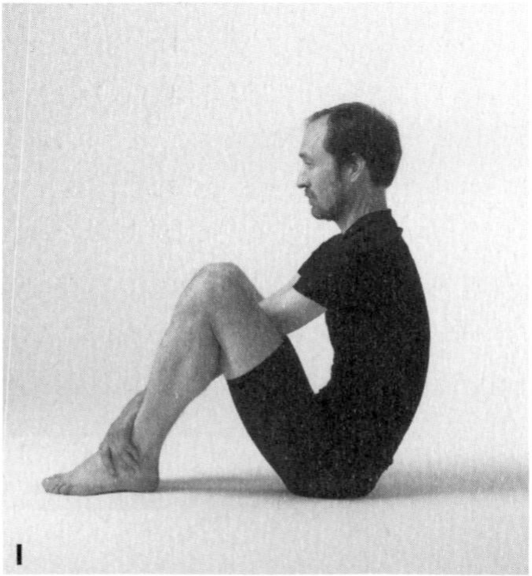

1

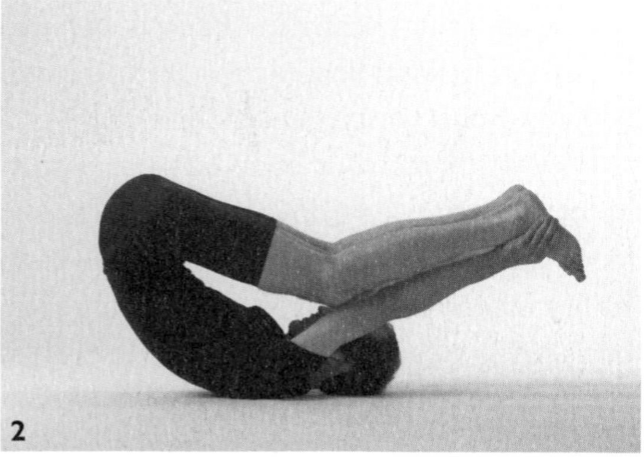

2

3. Then rock forward, reversing the motion and returning to the starting position.

4. Keep some portion of the spine in constant contact with the floor, moving like the curved base of a rocking chair. Avoid any "bumps" by rocking smoothly, especially across the low back.

5. Rock smoothly back and forth, building modest momentum and massaging the entire spine. When you get a feel for the movement, coordinate breath and motion. Exhale as you rock backward, and inhale as you rock forward.

Be Aware:

Spinal Rocking uses the weight of the body to massage the paraspinal muscles that run along both sides of the spine. Done correctly, it uses the floor to bring the vertebrae of the low and middle back into proper alignment. Do not rock so strongly that you bring significant body weight to bear on the upper spine and especially the back of the neck. Focus your rocking on the area of spine between the tailbone and shoulder blades.

If you have difficulty clasping the feet, you can reach the hands behind the knees, grasping one wrist with the opposite hand, or simply hold the knees. Once you are familiar with this movement, you can move directly into Spinal Rocking from a position on the floor by initiating a rocking with the feet and lower legs. You will quickly build enough momentum to come into the full movement, but always be sure to rock smoothly through the low spine.

BALANCING CAT

1. Come into Table Pose, hands directly under the shoulders, fingers spread wide, and knees directly under the hips.

2. Slide your right hand forward and the left foot back, keeping the palm and top of the foot touching the floor. Focus your gaze at a point on the floor in front of you to help establish your balance. Exhale.

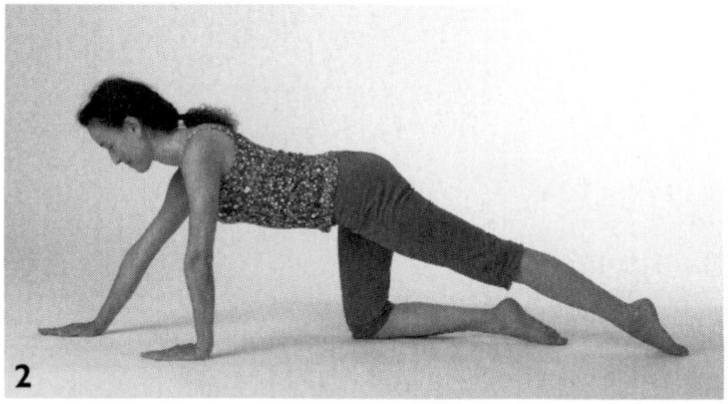
2

3. Inhale and lift the right arm and left leg parallel to the floor. Press the fingers forward and the toes back, stretching diagonally across the spine. Breathe deeply as you hold.

4. Release slowly on an exhale, returning to Table Pose.

5. Repeat on the opposite side.

Be Aware:
Balancing Cat strengthens a range of back muscles, offering a diagonal stretch across the back that helps maintain the balanced muscle tone needed to hold the spine in alignment. If you have difficulty balancing, come partway into the posture by keeping the hand and foot on the floor. Eventually you will find your balance point and be able to smoothly lift up. Balancing Cat is a great warm-up for sessions that include balancing postures done from standing.

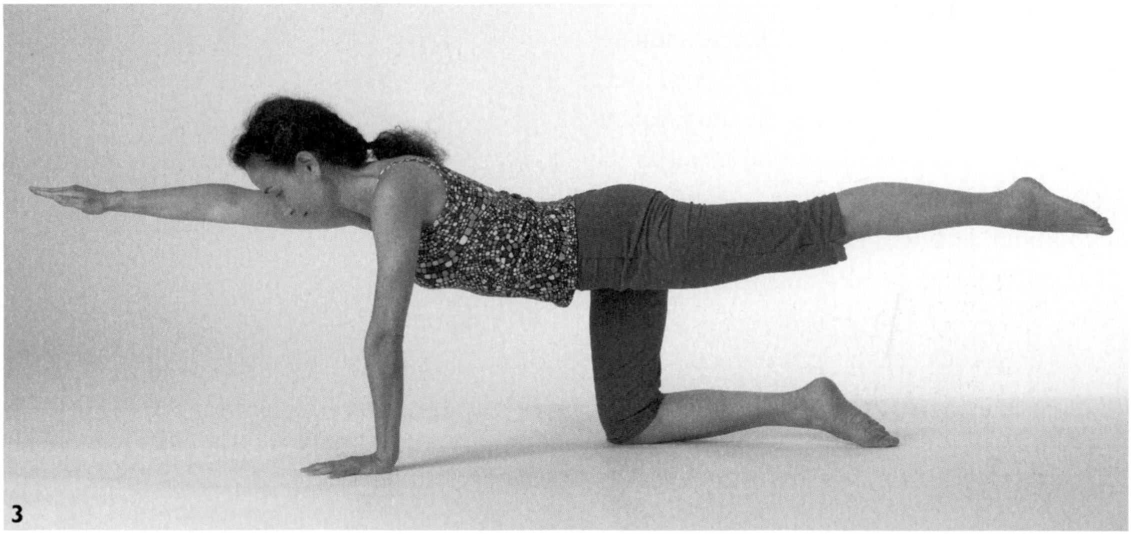
3

TWIST FROM TABLE

1. Come into Table Pose, hands directly under the shoulders, fingers spread wide, and knees directly under the hips.

2. Place the back of the right hand on the floor.

3. Take a deep breath in. Exhale and slide the back of the right hand along the floor, threading the needle between the left hand and left knee. Allow the right shoulder to come down to the floor as the spine twists.

4. Inhale up into the Table Pose. Place the back of your left hand on the floor and exhale to the other side.

5. Flow smoothly from side to side, twisting the spine one way, then the other.

6. If you want to go deeper, thread the needle to the left and carefully place the right shoulder and then right ear on the floor. Press both knees and right shoulder into the floor to create a stable base that allows you to reach the left hand up toward the ceiling. Breathe deeply as you hold, feeling the twist to the spine and the opening to the left shoulder joint.

7. To release, exhale the left hand back to the floor. Inhale and press the hand into the floor to come up into Table Pose. Exhale and repeat on the opposite side.

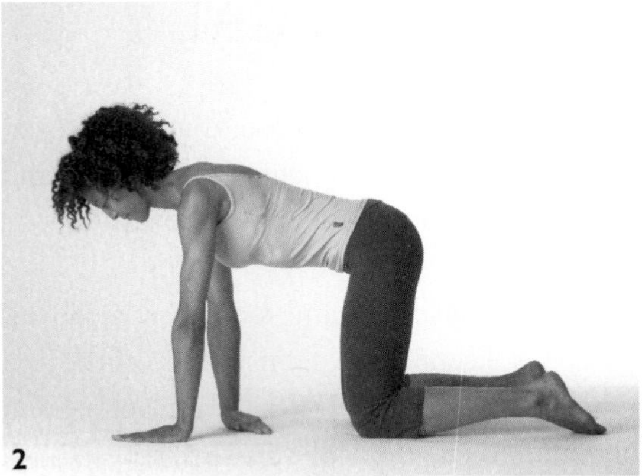
2

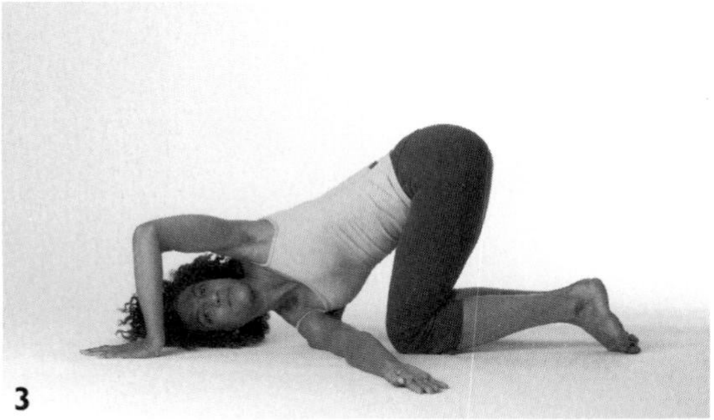
3

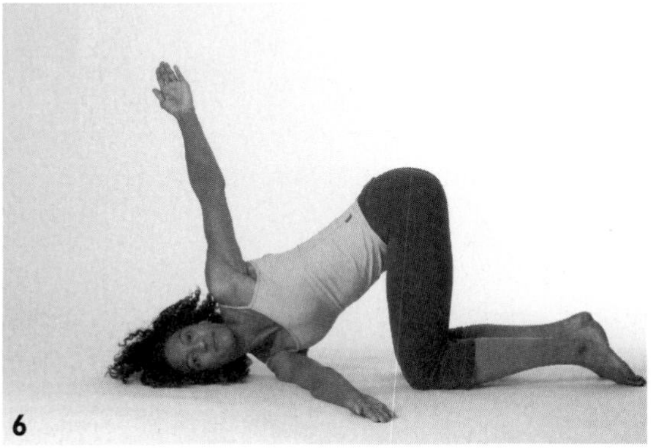
6

Be Aware:

Steps 1–5 of this warm-up gently twist the spine right then left. Coordinate breath and movement, exhaling as you twist and inhaling back up to Table Pose. Steps 6 and 7 provide a deeper twist and shoulder stretch. It is important to carefully place the shoulder then the ear on the ground, making sure that the shoulder, and not the neck, bears the weight of the upper body as you lift the opposite hand. Once the hand is lifted, you can explore micromovements by circling the upraised hand.

HIP OPENERS

GATE

(Parighasana)

1. Come into a kneeling position with the knees hip-width apart. The tops of the feet rest on the floor directly behind the legs.

2. Step the right foot out to the side, keeping the left knee directly under the left hip. Position the right heel so it is in line with the left knee, and flex the foot so the toes point toward the ceiling. Take care not to hyperextend the right knee, keeping the knee bent slightly if needed to avoid strain.

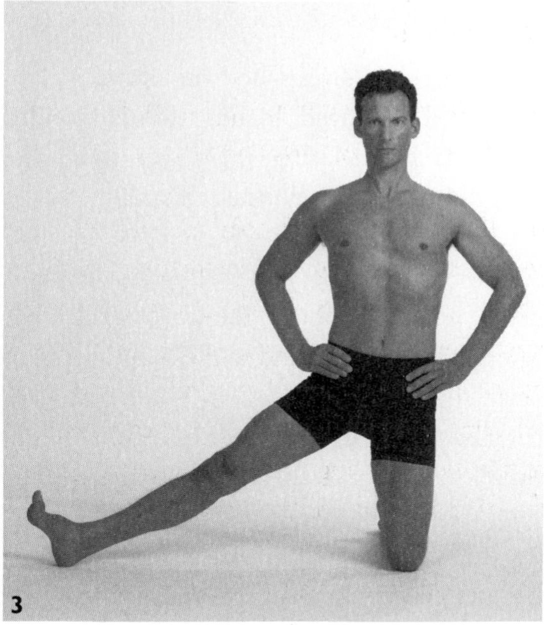
3

3. Bring the hands to the hips. Square the hips and chest to the front. Stabilize the core by pressing the tailbone down, leveling the pelvis and gently contracting the muscles of the pelvic floor. Elongate the spine by lifting out of the waist and extending through the crown.

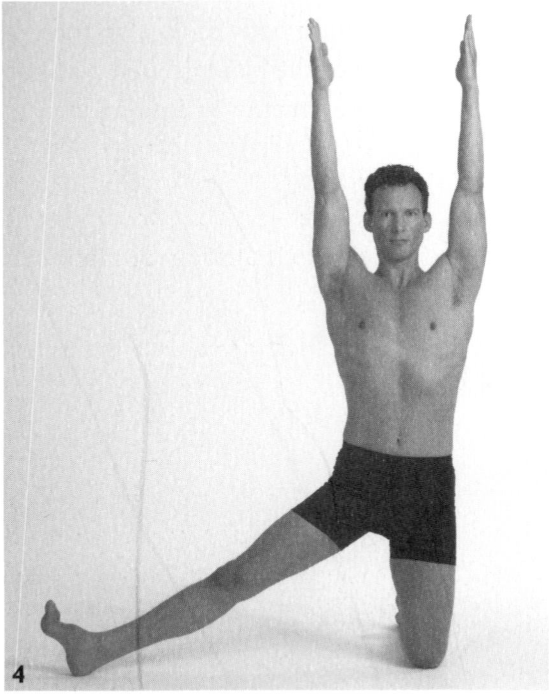

4

4. Inhale and sweep both arms out to the sides and overhead, hands shoulder-width apart and palms facing. Press up through the fingertips to further elongate the spine.

5. Keeping the hips and chest facing forward, exhale and press out on the left hip point, allowing the torso to bend to the right.

6. Lower the right hand to rest lightly on the right leg. Breathe deeply as you hold.

7. To release, inhale and bring the torso back to center and arms overhead. Lower the arms to the sides and return to kneeling.

8. Step the left foot out and repeat on the opposite side.

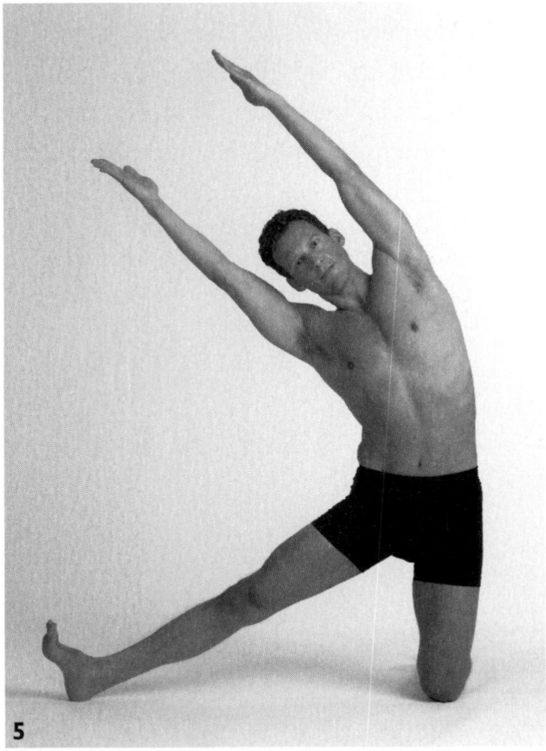

5

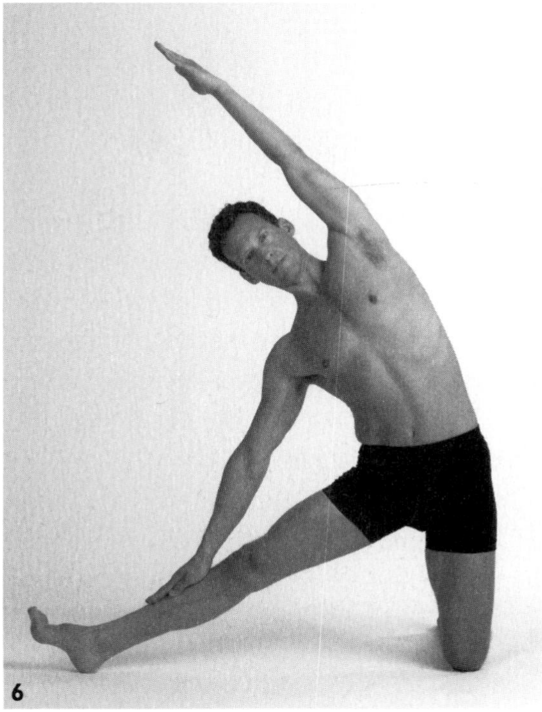

6

Be Aware:

The stable position of the lower body in Gate makes it easy to flex the spine laterally and deeply stretch the hips and sides. This makes it good preparation for standing side stretches like the Half Moon and Triangle. Gate is also a good side stretch to mix in with floor postures, which tend to be forward bends, backward bends, and twists. If bearing weight in a kneeling position causes pain, discontinue practice and substitute other hip openers and side stretches. If you feel pain in the knee of the extended leg, try pointing the toes and bringing the sole of the foot onto the floor. Some people find this foot position easier on the knee.

FROG

(Mandukasana)

1. Come into Table Pose.

2. Bring the forearms to the floor, elbows directly under the shoulders, and interlace the fingers. Press into the forearms to establish a stable base to support the weight of the upper body.

3. Take a deep breath in. As you exhale, gently slide the knees apart. Turn the feet out to the sides, and slide the lower legs out until they are in line with the knees. The hips, knees, and ankles form three ninety-degree angles.

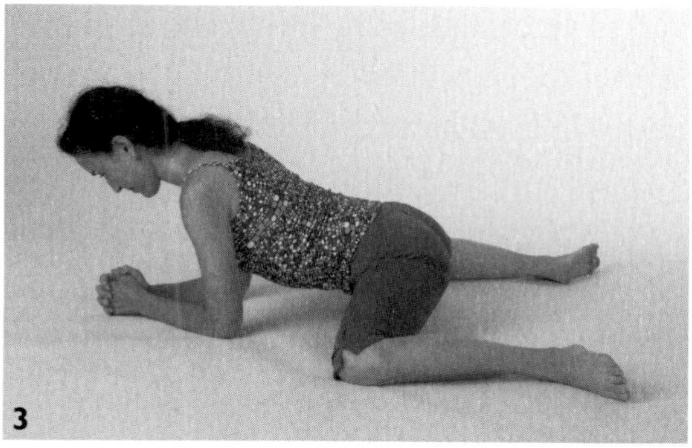

3

4. Press the buttocks toward the heels to deeply stretch the hip joints. If your hips are flexible, you may need to walk the elbows back a little so they remain directly under the shoulders. Keep the spine elongated by rolling the tailbone under and extending through the crown. Breathe deeply as you hold.

5. To release, press firmly into the forearms and draw your body weight a little forward, making it possible to walk the knees back under the hips. Release the interlaced fingers and press up into Table Pose.

Be Aware:

The Frog provides a deep stretch to the hips, pelvis, groin, legs, and feet. Move into the posture slowly, breathing deeply and allowing muscles and connective tissues to gradually open. Resist the tendency to drop the belly toward the floor and sway the low back. Instead work to keep the spine elongated. Some people find that breathing deeply while holding Frog creates a state of introversion that allows them to access deeply held feelings. Stay present in your body and focused on the flow of sensation.

FIGURE FOUR STRETCH

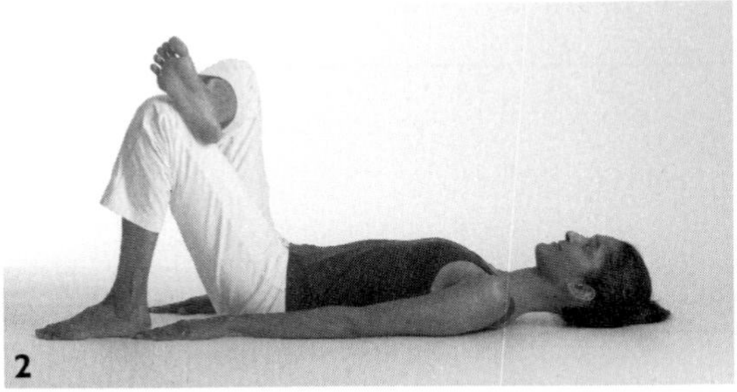

2

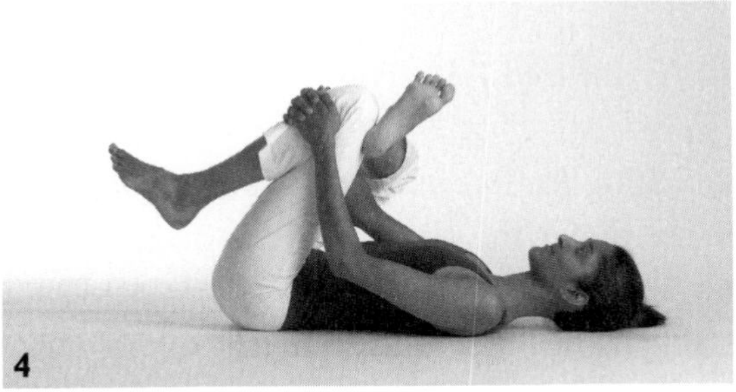

4

1. Lie on your back with the feet close to the buttocks, feet hip-width apart. Bring the arms to the sides, palms down. Tuck the chin slightly and extend through the crown.

2. Lift the right leg and place the outside of the ankle just below the left knee. Your legs will roughly form the figure four.

3. Take a deep breath in. As you exhale, lift the left foot off the floor and bring the knee up toward the chest.

4. Reach the hands up and interlace the fingers around the left knee. The right hand reaches under the right calf. You can also hold the back of the left thigh just above the knee. Pause for a moment to breathe and let your body adjust to this position.

5. Take a deep breath in. As you exhale, gently draw the left knee toward the chest, feeling the stretch in the upper right leg, hip, and buttocks. Come into tiny micromovements, rocking the left knee an inch or two from side to side, allowing any tight muscles to relax.

6. Come back to center. Take a deep breath in and as you exhale come into your full expression of the stretch by gently drawing the left knee a little closer to the chest.

7. Exhale and release the posture, returning the left foot to the floor and lowering the right leg and foot back to the starting position.

8. Repeat on the opposite side.

Be Aware:
This is a great stretch for those wanting to learn to sit in a cross-legged position. For most people, the main obstacle to sitting comfortably on the floor is hip—not knee—flexibility. If the hips are open, you can sit tall with the legs crossed. Before giving up on ever sitting in Easy Pose or Half Lotus, practice this stretch and Happy Baby pose for a month. Proceed slowly and gently to protect the low back; hip flexibility cannot be forced.

HAPPY BABY

(Ananda Balasana)

1. Lie on your back with the feet close to the buttocks, feet hip-width apart. Tuck the chin slightly and extend through the crown.

2. Draw the knees into the chest. Press the sacrum toward the floor to support the low back. Let the knees splay out just to the sides of the torso, and bring the feet directly over the knees so the shins are roughly vertical. If possible, reach up and grasp the outside of the feet with the hands, elbows near the inside of the knees. If you cannot grasp the feet, hold the outside of the shins.

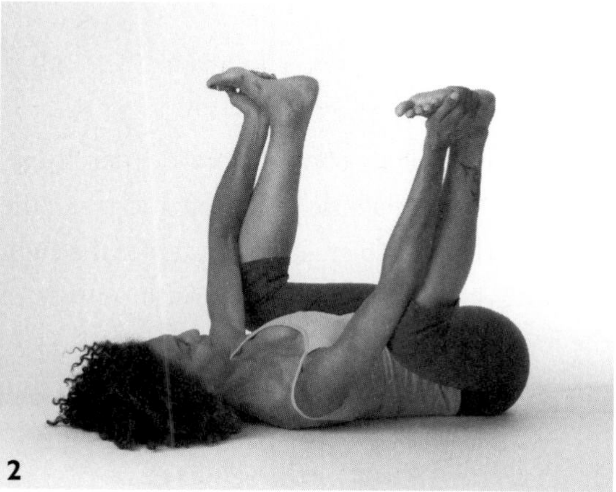

2

3. Take a minute or more to explore micromovements, rocking a few inches from side to side, allowing any tight muscles to relax. Then come back to center.

4. Take a deep breath in. As you exhale, gently pull the knees toward the floor with your hands. As much as possible, keep the sacrum pressed down and let the low back rest solidly on the floor. Breathe deeply as you hold.

5. To release, take a deep breath in. As you exhale, gently release the hands and return the feet to the floor by the buttocks. Bring the hands to rest on the belly and notice any sensations in the pelvis, hips, and groin.

Be Aware:
This is another valuable posture for those wanting to learn to sit cross-legged. Keeping the sacrum pressed down as you pull the knees toward the floor stretches and strengthens the muscles of the low back.

SQUAT

(Malasana and Baddha Trikonasana)

1. From Table Pose, curl the toes under and press back into a supported squat. The heels are lifted, and the palms or fingertips rest on the floor. Take a few deep breaths as the body adjusts to this position.

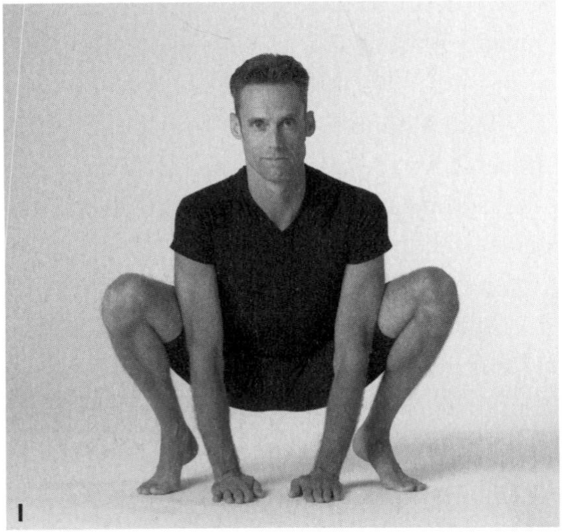

2. Walk the feet a little wider than hip-width apart and slightly splayed out to the sides. Shift your weight back and bring the heels to the floor if possible. Raise the hands into Prayer Position. Use the elbows to work the knees apart, bringing the forearms into a straight line. Press the knees into the elbows and the palms of the hands together. Extend through the crown to elongate the spine. This is Prayer Squat, a variation of Garland Pose. Breathe deeply as you hold.

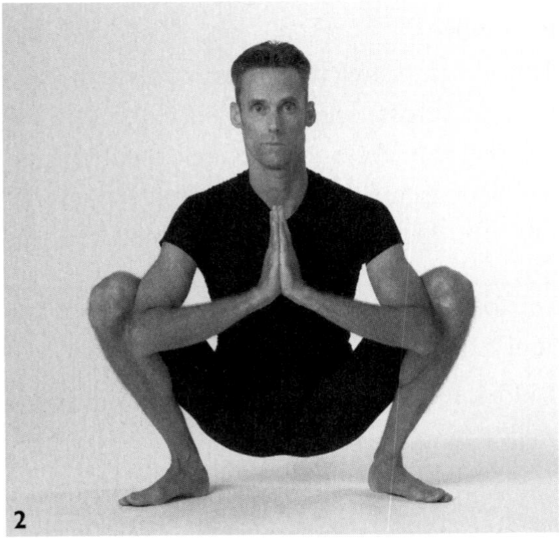

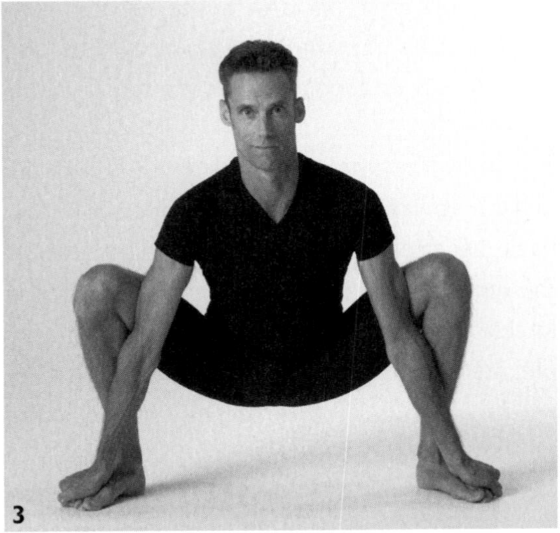

3. If you want to come into a deeper squat, rock your weight a little to the left and reach the right hand down to grasp the instep of the right foot. Work the fingertips under the outside of the foot to give you a firm grip. Maintaining the grip with your right hand, rock your weight a little to the right and reach the left hand down to grasp the left foot in the same way.

4. Press the sitz bones down and pull on the feet to deeply stretch the hips and groin. Press the sternum forward and extend through the crown to elongate the spine. Bend your arms slightly if needed to avoid any elbow strain. This is Bound Triangle. Breathe deeply as you hold.

5. To release, bring the hands onto the floor in front of you. Rock your weight forward and bring the knees onto the floor to return to Table Pose.

Be Aware:

In many traditional cultures, chairs were unknown and squatting was the primary manner of sitting. Use Squat to stretch the hips, groin, and back. If these areas are tight, begin practice by holding the supported squat in step 1. When you are able to bring the heels to the ground, move on to Prayer Squat and then Bound Triangle. Spend a few minutes squatting every day, and you may be surprised to find your body becomes able to move through this entire series.

PIGEON

(Kapotasana)

1. Come into Table Pose, hands directly under the shoulders and knees directly under the hips.

2. Slide the right knee forward between the hands, letting the outside of the right knee and foot come onto the floor. Bring the right heel in line with the left hip bone. Take a deep breath in. As you exhale, slide the left foot and leg back, allowing the hips to sink toward the floor.

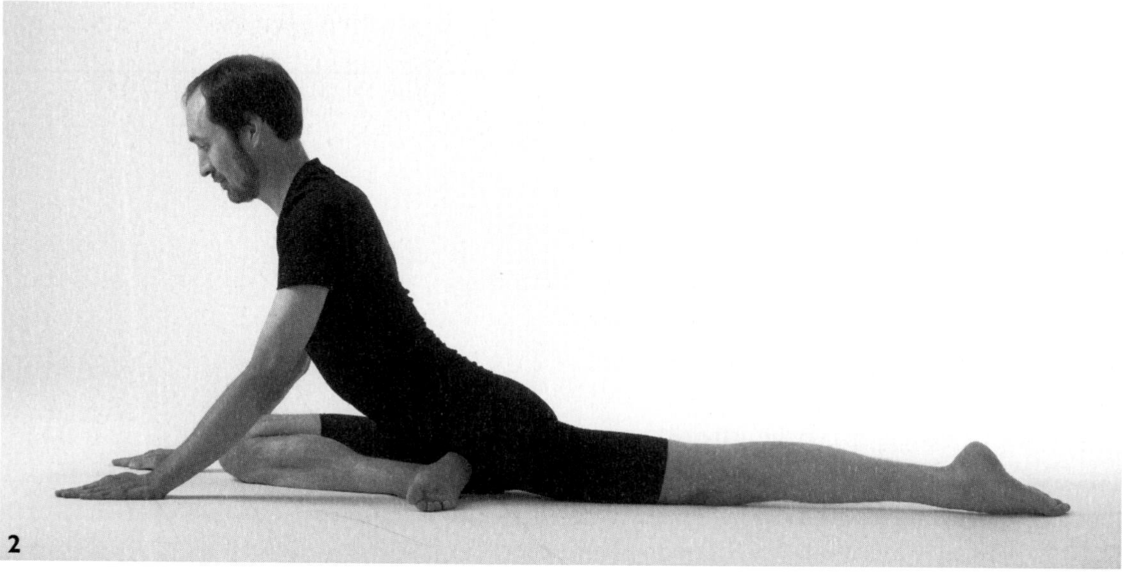

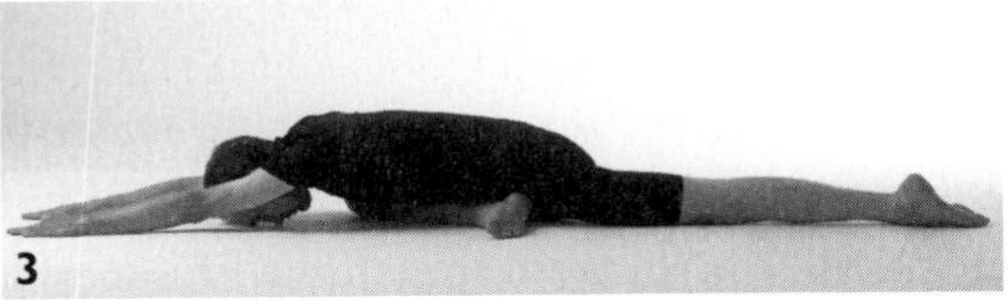
3

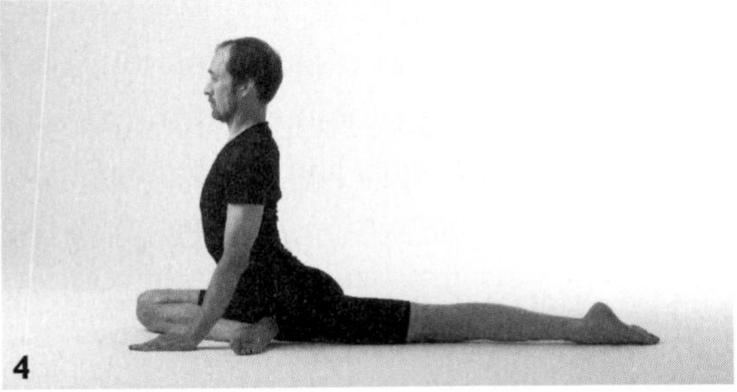
4

3. Take another deep breath in. As you exhale, slide both hands forward, extending the torso over the bent right knee and extending through the crown to keep the spine long. If comfortable, allow the forehead to rest on the floor and relax the thighs, hips, buttocks, and low back. This is Resting Pigeon.

4. Slide the palms back under the shoulders, elbows close to the sides and fingers spread wide. As you inhale, press gently into the palms and use your back muscles to lift the torso. Square the hips by pressing both hip bones down and the left hip forward. Elongate the spine by lifting out of the waist and extending through the crown. Press the sternum forward to open the chest and allow the spine to arch back. Breathe deeply as you hold.

5. To release, press into the hands and slide the right knee back and the left knee forward, returning to Table Pose.

6. Repeat on the opposite side.

Be Aware:
This posture takes its name from the puffed-out chest characteristic of pigeons. But before you can enjoy the deep chest stretch that advanced variations of this posture offer, you must first work to expand hip flexibility. The position of the legs in Pigeon deeply stretches the hips on alternate sides. If you have knee sensitivity, proceed carefully. If coming into this posture causes knee pain, substitute the Frog and other hip openers.

PIGEON VARIATIONS

(Kapotasana)

1. Come into Pigeon Pose.

2. Lift the hands and sweep the arms out to the sides. Let the hips sink down, press the sternum forward, and extend through the fingertips.

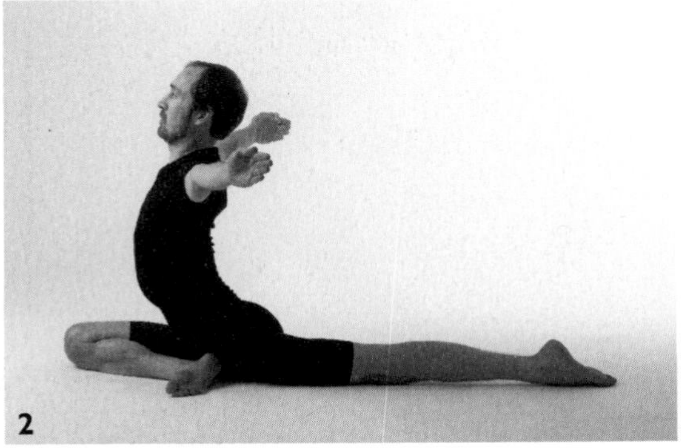
2

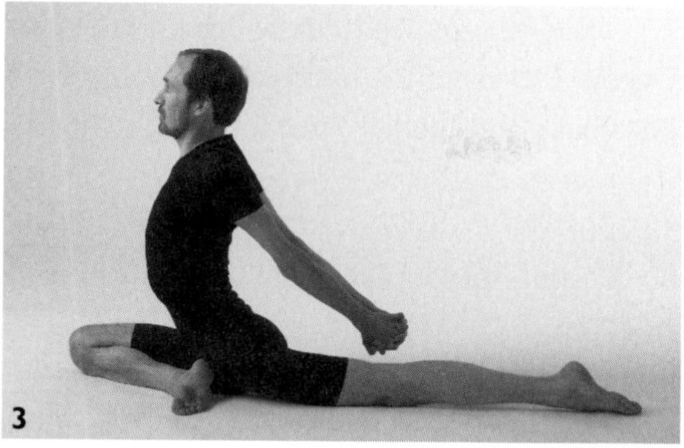

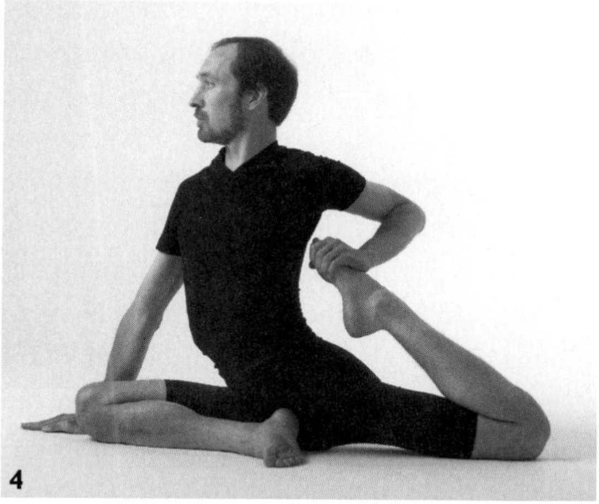

3. Reach the arms behind you, interlacing the fingers. Press the knuckles back and the sternum forward to open the chest. Then press the pinky side of the hands up toward the ceiling to stretch the shoulders.

4. Release the hands, bringing the right hand to rest on the floor just outside the front right knee. Press into the right palm to help keep the spine elongated, as you bend the back leg and reach the left hand back to clasp the top of the foot. Use the handhold to press the heel toward the buttocks, deeply stretching the quadriceps.

5. Begin to straighten the back left leg, eventually resisting the movement with a straight left arm. Square the chest to the front as much as possible. Lift the right arm up parallel to the floor and extend forward through the fingertips. Keep pressing the left leg back and right fingertips forward to stretch the chest.

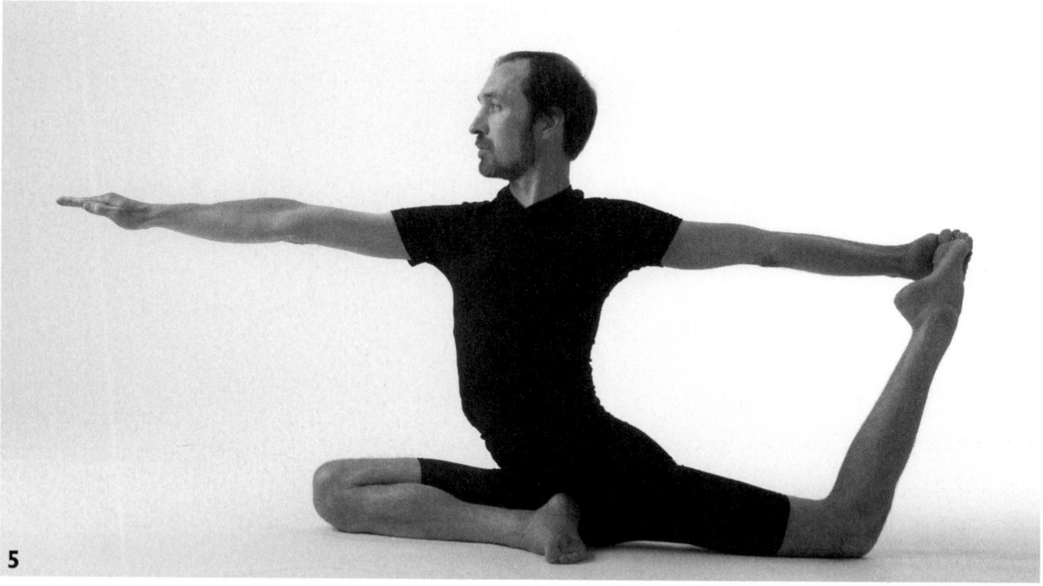

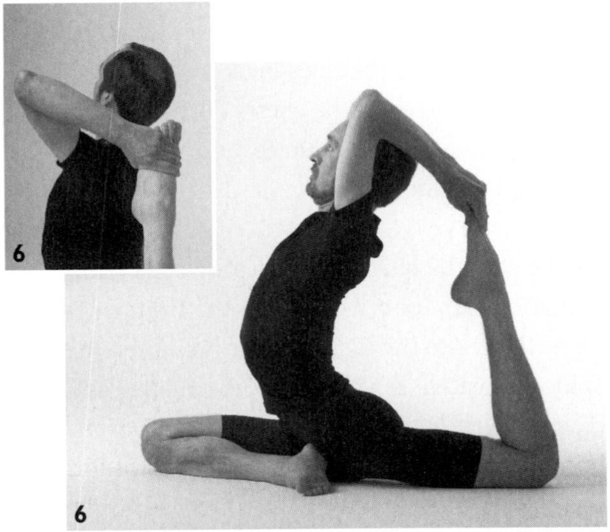

6

6

6. Turn to the left and grasp the outside of the left foot with the left hand. Slowly roll the left shoulder forward, lifting the elbow, hand and foot. Reach the right arm overhead and back to grasp the left foot. Lift the crown of the head toward the ceiling and pull the sole of the foot toward the back of the head, resisting any tendency to collapse the neck back. Breathe deeply as you hold.

7. To release, return to basic Pigeon or resting Pigeon. Press into the hands and slide the right knee back and the left knee forward, returning to Table Pose.

8. Repeat these variations on the opposite side.

Be Aware:

The Pigeon is an extremely versatile posture, offering a wide range of variations that stretch different areas of the body. As you become comfortable in the basic posture, explore these variations. With practice, you can move through a number of variations in just a few minutes. Resist the tendency to overemphasize the position of the hands or arms by compromising the alignment of the lower body. Keep both hips pressed down and the hip bone of the back leg pressed forward to stabilize the body. Emphasize the inhalation to expand and stretch the chest.

CORE STRENGTHENERS

SIDE LEG LIFTS AND SIDE BOAT

(Parsva Navasana)

1. Lie on your right side. Reach the right arm overhead along the floor, pressing through the fingers to lengthen the entire right side of the body. Bend the right arm at the elbow, cradling the head with the hand. Place the left hand on the floor in front of the belly. Bend the right knee ninety degrees to create a stable base for the posture. Lift the left leg up to hip height.

2. Inhale and lift the left leg toward the ceiling. As the leg lifts, the hip joint rotates and the toes eventually point toward the head. Exhale and lower the leg back to hip height, side of foot parallel to the floor. Coordinate breath and movement, lifting and lowering the leg, pressing the right hip into the floor to keep the lower body as stable as possible.

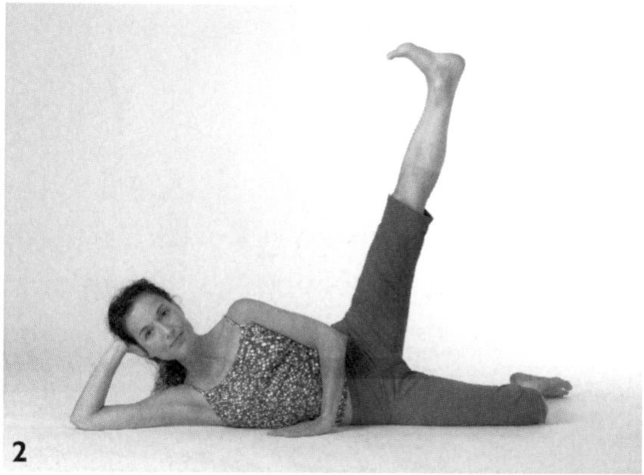
2

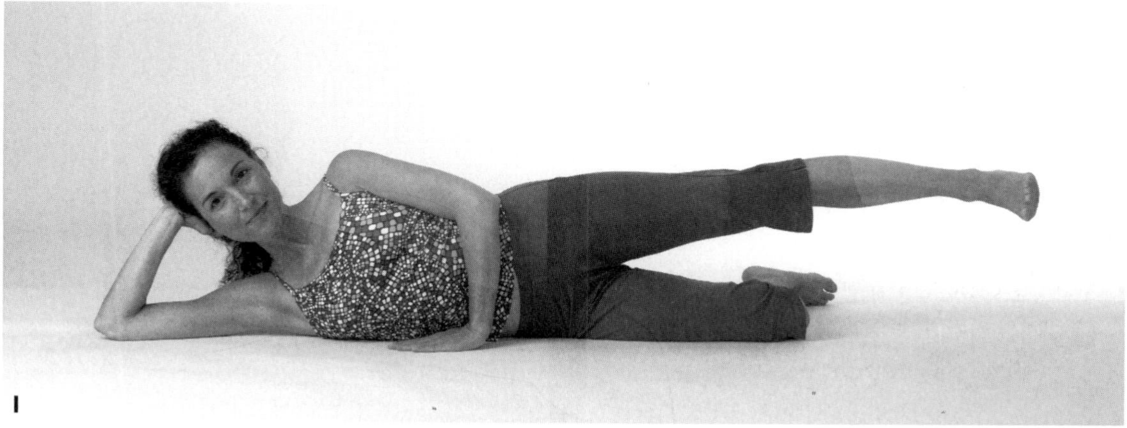
1

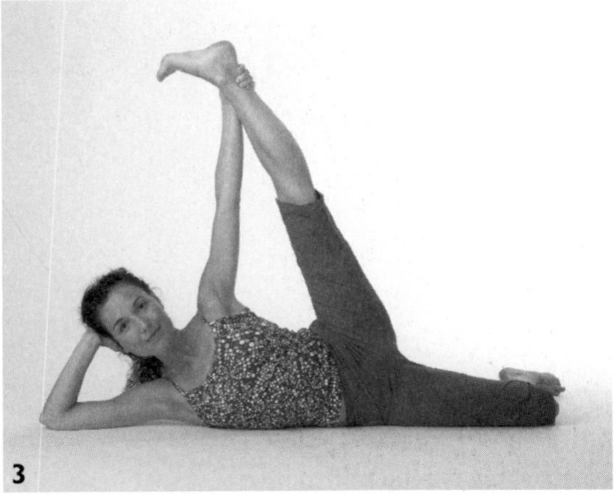
3

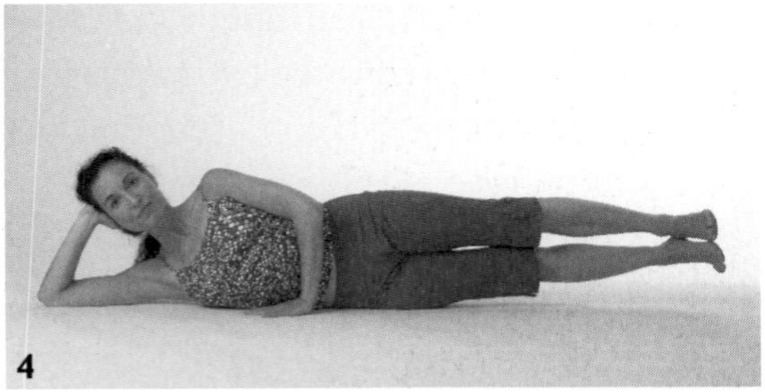
4

3. Pause with leg lifted, flexing the foot to accentuate the stretch to the back of the leg. Reach the left hand up to hold behind the left knee. Take a deep breath in, and as you exhale slide the hand up the leg until you feel a good stretch to the back of the leg. Hold the stretch for several deep breaths.

4. To come into Side Boat, lower the left leg and then straighten both legs. Align your body so that the heels, knees, hip joints, shoulders, and right elbow form a straight line. Take a deep breath in. Exhale and press the right hip point into the floor and lift both legs. Breathe deeply as you hold.

5. To release, slowly lower the legs to the ground.

6. Roll over to the left side and repeat.

Be Aware:

Side Leg Lifts strengthen a set of abdominal muscles on the sides of the body called the obliques. Side Boat works the abductor and adductor muscles of the hips and legs. Finding your balance in Side Boat may be challenging. Align the body in a straight line, positioning the upper hip directly over the lower hip. Then press the lower hip point into the floor, which makes it possible to lift the legs. Side Leg Lifts and Side Boat combine nicely with Single Leg Lifts for a simple yet effective core strengthening routine.

WATERWHEEL

1. Lie on your back with the hands palms down at the sides. Bring both knees into the chest, feet hip-width apart. Walk the hands under the sides of the buttocks until the thumbs touch just below the tailbone.

2. Inhale and begin to circle the feet by extending the legs, then lifting the feet until the soles point toward the ceiling, then exhaling as the knees bend and come back into the chest. Start with small circles. As your body becomes accustomed to the movement, let the circles gradually grow larger. Move slowly and smoothly, lower body circling like the waterwheel of an old-fashioned mill.

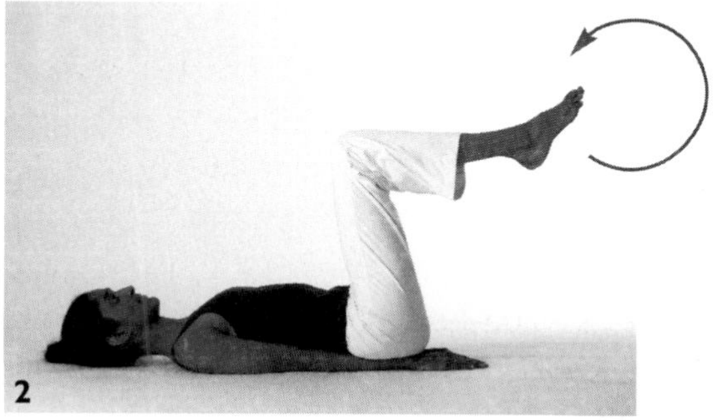
2

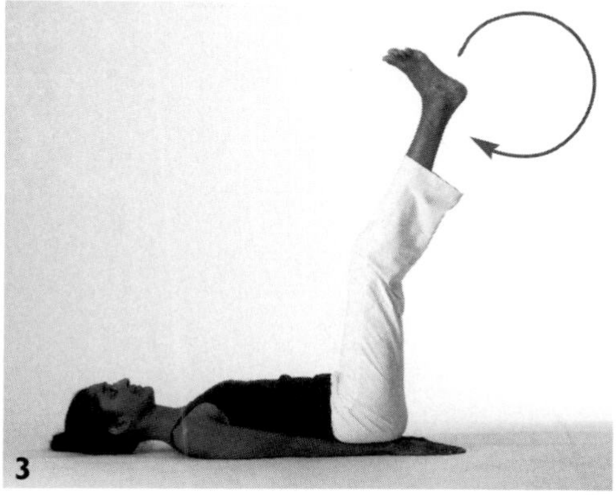
3

3. Pause with your feet pointing toward the ceiling. Take a deep breath in, and as you exhale reverse the direction of the circles. Lower the legs and bend the knees, bringing the knees back into the chest, and then lifting the feet up to the ceiling. Start small and gradually let the circles grow larger.

4. End by returning knees to chest. Reach the arms up around the knees, interlacing the fingers. Rock gently from side to side, massaging the low back.

Be Aware:

The position of the hands and thumbs in Waterwheel supports the low back, allowing the sacrum to rest solidly on the floor throughout the exercise. If you feel your low back starting to tip, buckle, or arch off the floor, reduce the size of the circles. This is one of the primary benefits of Waterwheel, in that it gives you the ability to adjust the intensity and safely work at the healthy edge of your abdominal strength and low back stability. Move slowly and smoothly, gradually expanding the size of your circles. Practiced regularly, Waterwheel helps prepare your body for a host of challenging postures that require a mix of abdominal strength and low back stability to practice safely.

SCISSORS AND TOE TOUCH

1. Lie on your back and bring both knees into the chest. Reach the arms out to the sides in a T, hands palms down. Extend the legs until the soles of the feet point toward the ceiling. Let the sacrum rest solidly on the floor. Flex the feet to straighten the legs.

2. Take a deep breath in. As you exhale, let the legs smoothly spread to the sides in a split.

3. Inhale the legs back together and cross the right leg over the left. Exhale the legs back out to the sides and into a split. Bring the legs back together and cross the left leg over the right. This movement is the Scissors. Repeat several times, coordinating breath and movement.

4. End the Scissors by pausing for several breaths with the legs in a split, letting the muscles of the legs and groin relax and lengthen.

5. To come into Toe Touch, bring the legs back to center, sacrum resting solidly on the floor. Lift the arms directly above the shoulders and extend through the fingertips.

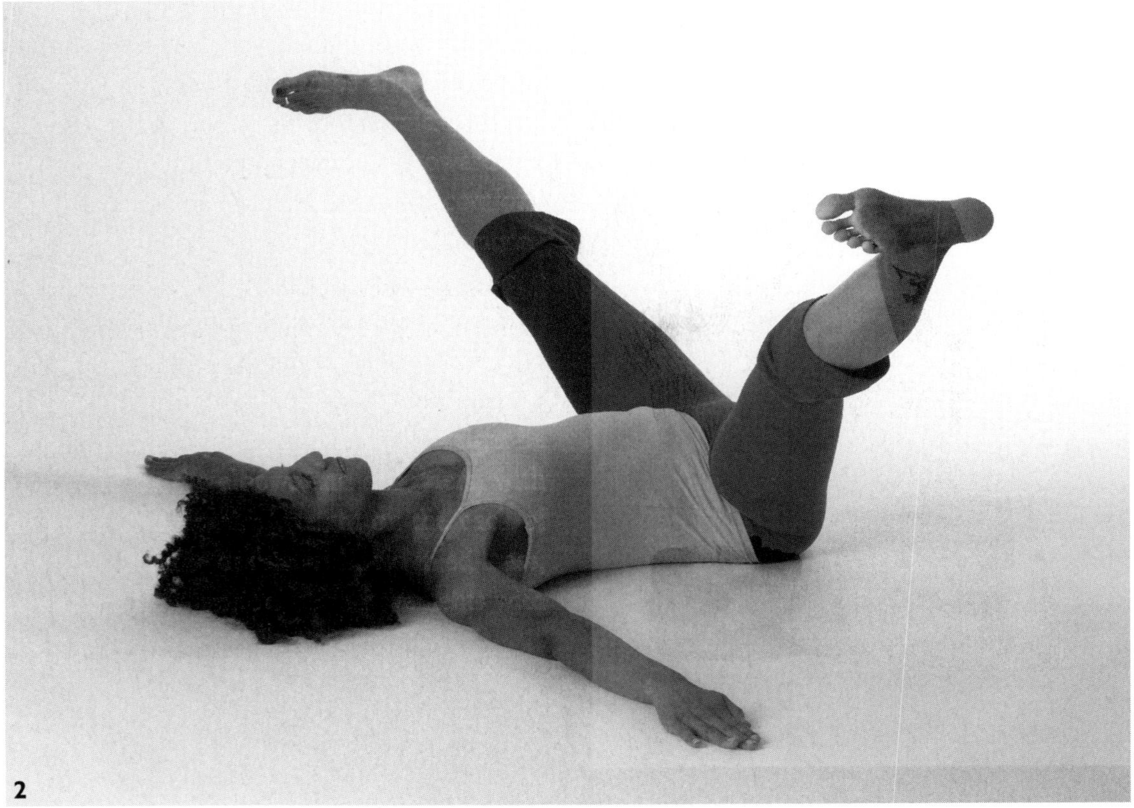

2

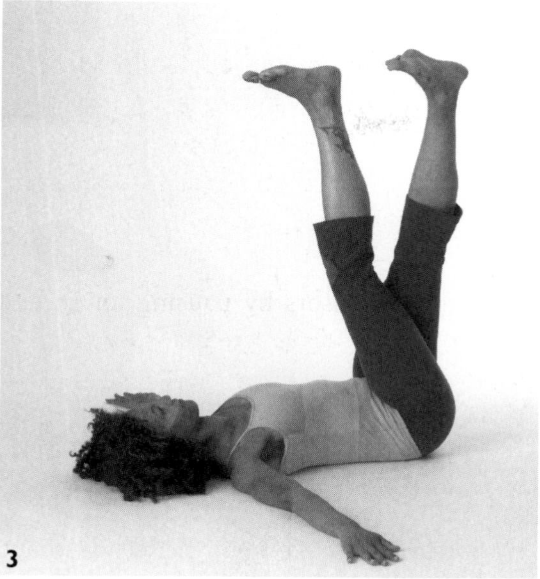
3

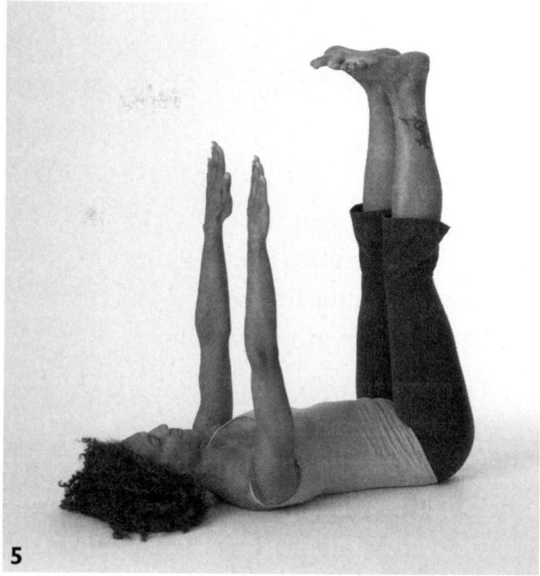
5

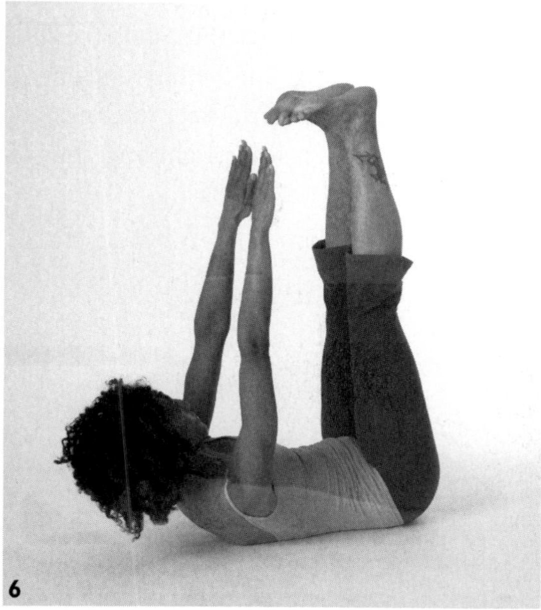
6

6. Take a deep breath in. As you exhale, contract the muscles of the abdomen, press the low back into the floor, and reach the fingertips up as if to touch the toes, lifting head and shoulders off the ground. Keep the neck elongated, which focuses the work on the abdominal muscles. Hold for several breaths.

7. End by returning knees to chest. Reach the arms up around the knees, interlacing the fingers, and rock gently from side to side.

Be Aware:

If Scissors poses a challenge to your low back, practice with the hands under the buttocks, thumbs touching, as in Waterwheel. It is important to move the legs slowly and smoothly, which stretches and strengthens core muscles. Resist any tendency to let the legs drop or fall out to the sides with momentum, as the weight of the legs can generate sufficient force to strain tendons and ligaments. In Toe Touch, make sure to press the low back into the floor as you lift the upper body. Combining Waterwheel, Scissors, and Toe Touches makes for a complete abdominal workout.

PLANK AND SIDE PLANK

(Vashistasana)

1. Come into Table Pose. Make sure the hands are directly under the shoulders and the fingers spread wide.

2. Take a deep breath in. As you exhale, step one foot and then the other back into a push-up position. The hands remain directly under the shoulders. The feet are hip-width apart. Press down into the palms, back through the heels, and extend through the crown of the head. Engage the abdominal muscles. The legs, torso, neck, and head form a straight line. This is Plank Pose. Breathe deeply as you hold.

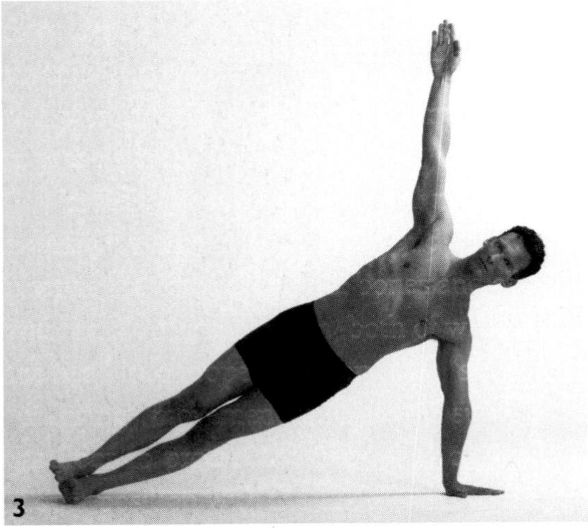

3

3. Shift your weight onto the left hand and sweep the right arm out to the side. Roll onto the outside of your left foot, keeping the sides of both feet touching. Lift the hips and engage the abdominal muscles to keep the legs and spine in one line. Press the right fingertips to-

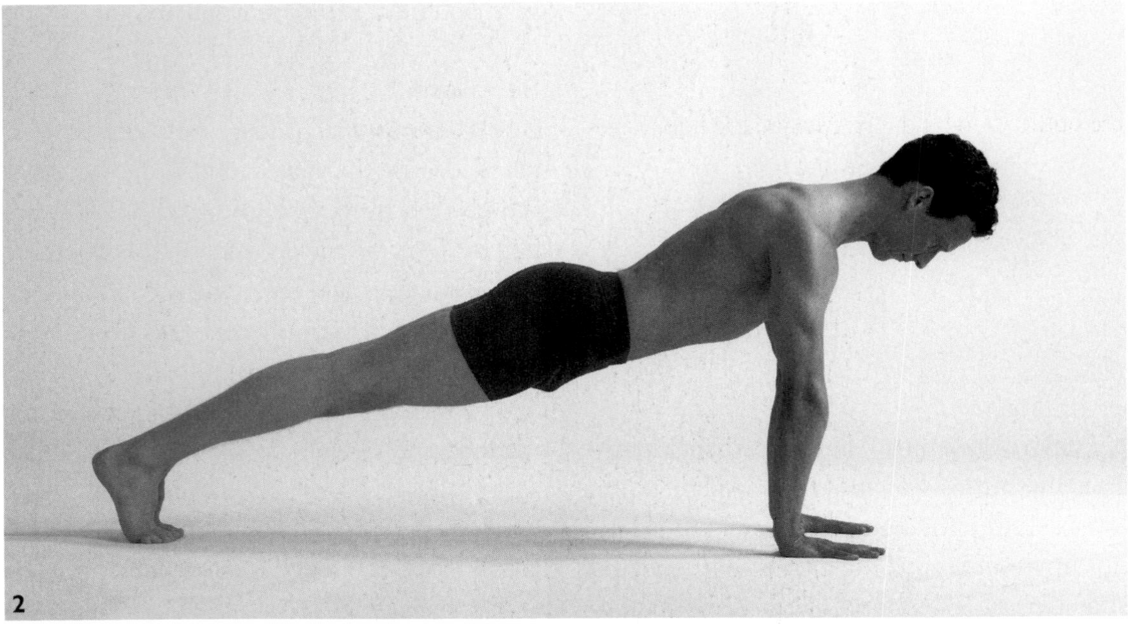

2

ward the ceiling and the left palm into the floor, pulling the shoulder blades down the back. This is Side Plank. Breathe deeply as you hold.

4. To release, lower the right hand and return to Plank. Then lower the knees into Table Pose. Rest until the breath has returned to normal.

5. Repeat this series on the opposite side.

Be Aware:

Plank and Side Plank build core and upper body strength. The transition from Plank into Side Plank is a smooth rotation best done in a single flowing movement. Make sure to keep the hips lifted, which allows the legs, trunk, and neck to form a straight line. If you are unable to keep the hips from collapsing, try coming into a modified push-up position with the legs bent and knees on the floor. Then move into a modified Side Plank as above, but keeping the knees bent. This will help you build the strength required to do the full posture.

UPWARD BOAT

1. Come into a sitting position with the knees bent and feet on the floor, sides of the legs and feet touching. Lightly hold the back of the thighs, just above the knees. Rock the weight back on the buttocks to lift the feet just off the floor. Press down on the sitz bones, lift the sternum, tuck the chin, and extend through the crown.

2. Inhale and slowly extend the legs, keeping the spine elongated and front of the torso long. Flex the feet to lengthen the backs of the legs as much as possible.

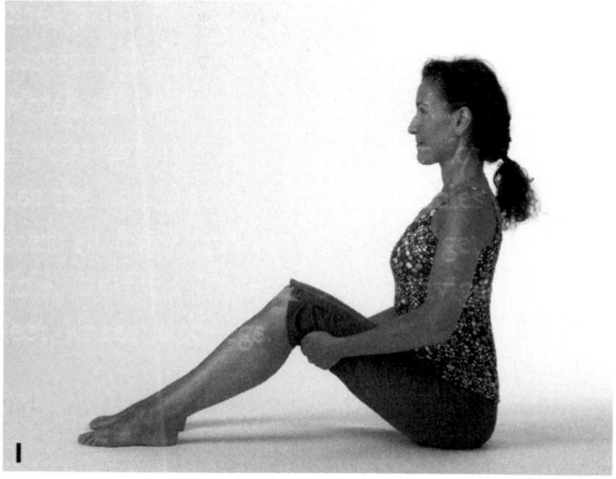

1

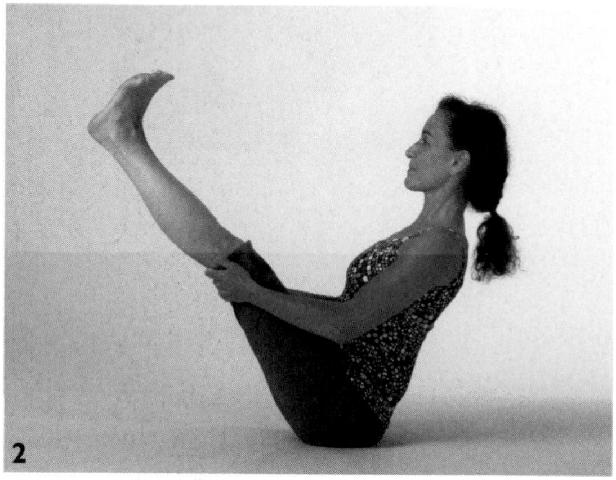

2

3. Slowly release the hold on the legs and extend the arms in front of you, parallel to the floor. Bring the palms facing and press through the fingertips. Breathe deeply as you hold.

4. To release, bring the torso forward and bend the knees. As the knees come in toward the chest, lower the feet to the floor.

Be Aware:
Upward Boat is a vigorous core strengthener. Before attempting its full expression, prepare your body with less vigorous exercises. At first, do not come into the full posture. Keep the hands on the thighs to aid balance, progressively loosening the grip and supporting more of your weight with the muscles of the abdomen, back, and legs. It is important to press the sitz bones down, lift the sternum, and extend through the crown to keep the spine elongated and the front of the torso long. This preserves the natural curve of the low back and prevents excessive arching or rounding. Begin with one repetition and work up to three, holding to your capacity with a flowing breath.

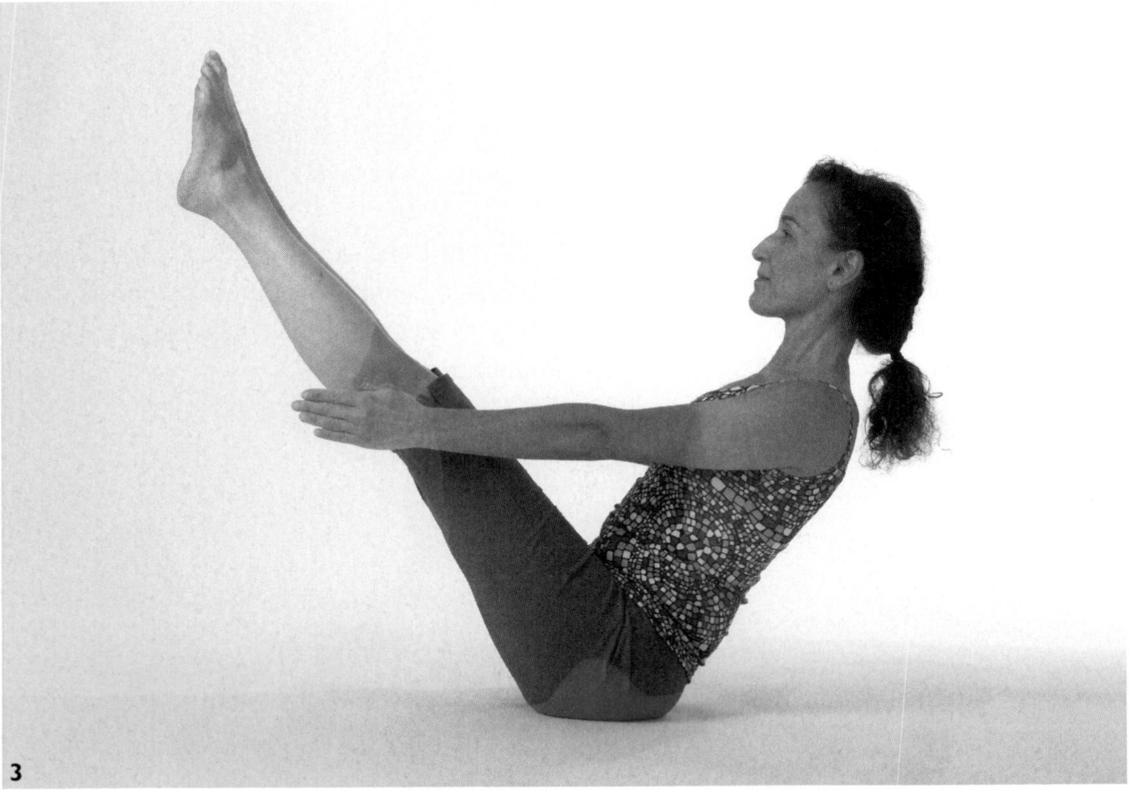

3

DOWNWARD DOG AND LUNGE VARIATIONS

DOWNWARD DOG VARIATIONS

(Adho Mukha Svanasana)

1. Come into Table Pose, hands directly under the shoulders, fingers spread wide, and knees directly under the hips. Curl your toes under and press up into an easy Downward Dog. Let your breath flow as the body adjusts to the basic posture.

2. Shift the weight onto the left foot. Lift the right foot off the floor and extend the leg back

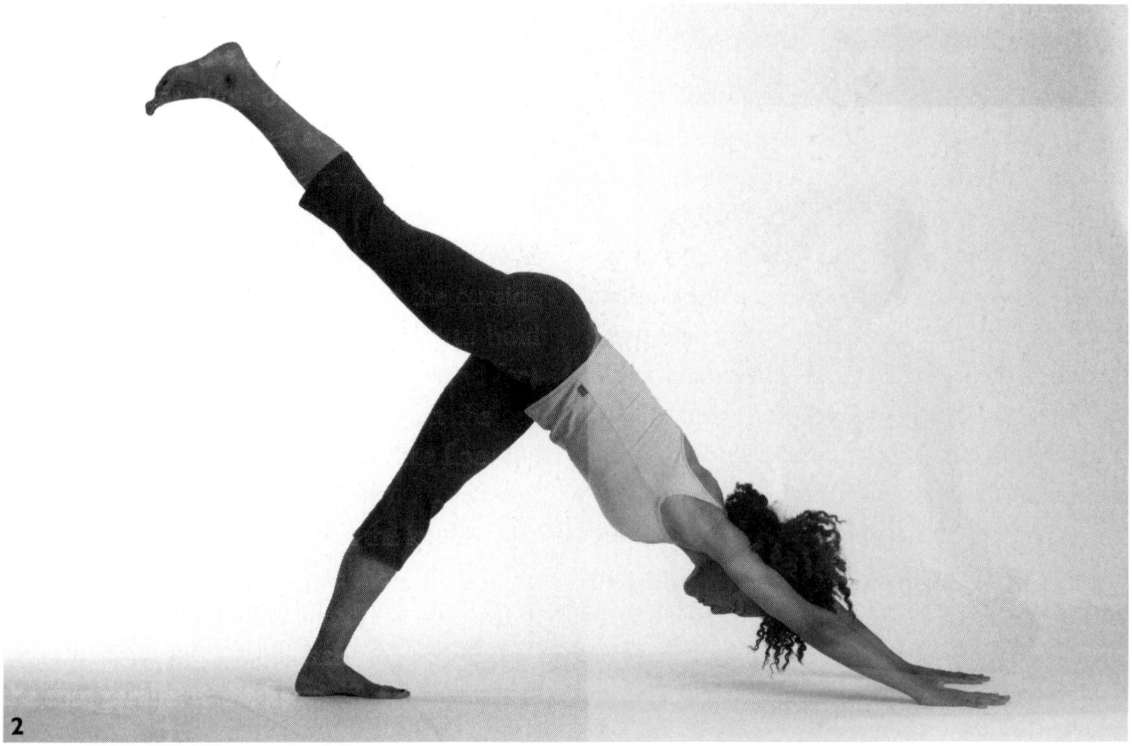

and up, keeping the hips square and level. Press both hands and the left heel into the floor. Extend through the right toes to lengthen the leg, and press up on the right heel to lift the leg until the torso and right leg form a straight line. Breathe deeply as you hold.

3. Slowly let the right hip roll open and the right leg bend at the knee. Press the outside of the right knee toward the ceiling and the right heel toward the opposite buttocks. Breathe deeply as you hold.

4. To release, take a deep breath in. As you exhale, slowly roll down and straighten the right leg. Then lower the right foot back into Downward Dog. Bend both knees to come into Table Pose and rest until the breath has returned to normal.

5. From Table, bring the forearms to the floor, elbows directly under the shoulders. Interlace the fingers so the forearms form an equilateral triangle. Press the hands, forearms, and elbows into the floor to establish a stable base to support the weight of the upper body and curl the toes under. Inhale and press up into Downward Dog. As you exhale, press the hips and buttocks back and heels down, straightening the legs as much as possible. Simultaneously press into the forearms and elbows, feeling the spine being elongated by these two movements. Breathe deeply as you hold.

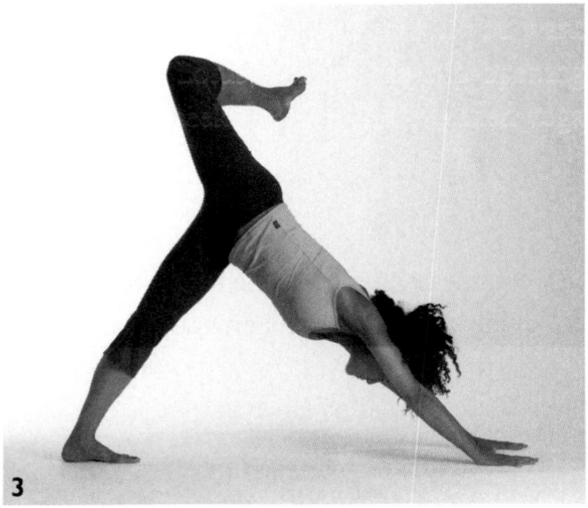
3

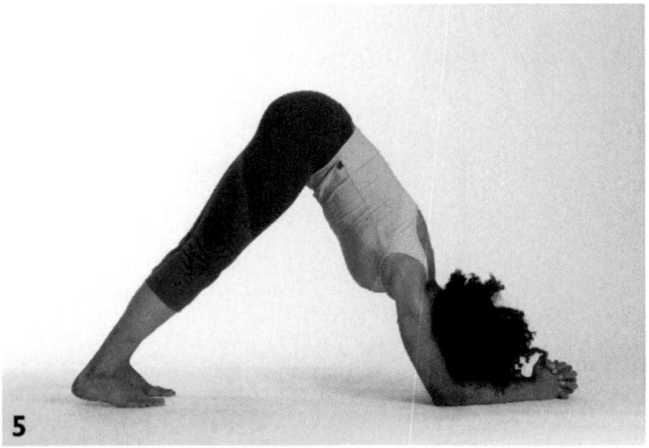
5

6. To release, bend the knees and lower into Child Pose. Rest in Child until the breath has returned to normal, and repeat these stretches on the opposite side.

Be Aware:

These three variations enhance the many benefits of the basic Downward Dog pose. In the first, extend the lifted leg while working to keep the hips square and level. In the second, roll the hip of the lifted leg as high as possible. In the third, keep the hands, forearms, and elbows pressed into the floor to strengthen a different set of upper body muscles.

BASIC LUNGE VARIATIONS

(Anjaneyasana)

1. From Table Pose, step the right foot forward between the hands. Bring the knee directly over the ankle and the shin perpendicular to the floor. Curl the toes of the left foot under and slide the ball of the foot back until the leg is lengthened out behind you. You may want to come up onto your knuckles or fingertips.

2. Inhale and press the left heel back to straighten the leg. Exhale and press both hips toward the floor. Inhale and press the sternum forward to open the chest. Exhale and extend through the crown to elongate the neck. The eyes look down. This is Lunge Pose. Let your breath flow as the body adjusts to the basic posture.

3. Lower the back knee to the floor, and bring the top of the back foot on the floor. Inhale and sweep the arms out to the sides and overhead, arms shoulder-width apart and palms facing. Exhale and let the hips and pelvis sink toward the floor. As you inhale, extend through the crown and fingertips. This is the Supported Warrior Pose. Breathe deeply as you hold.

4. Exhale and bring the left hand back to the floor by the right foot. Place the right hand on the right knee, forearm running along the top of the thigh. Turn to look over the right shoulder, rotating the torso toward the right thigh. If you want more stretch, press the top of the back foot into the floor to lift the knee and straighten the leg. Gently pull with the right hand to rotate the torso into Spinal Twist from Lunge. Breathe deeply as you hold.

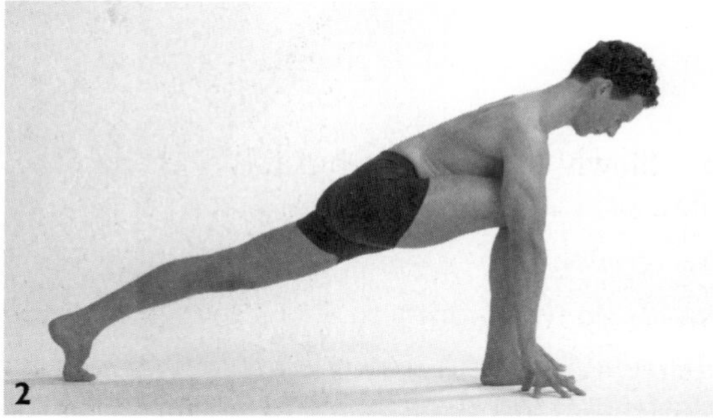

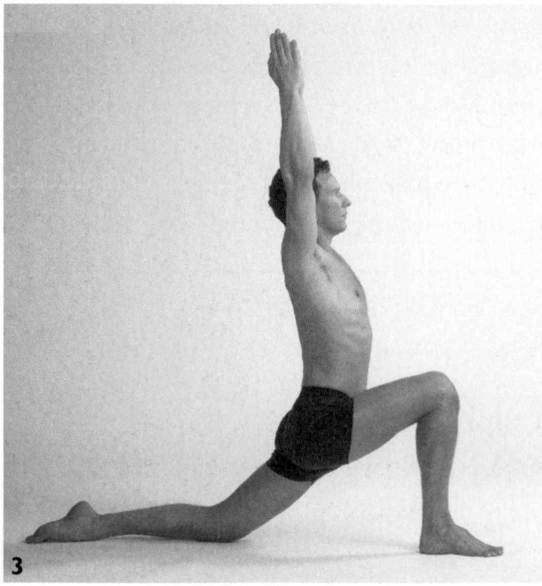

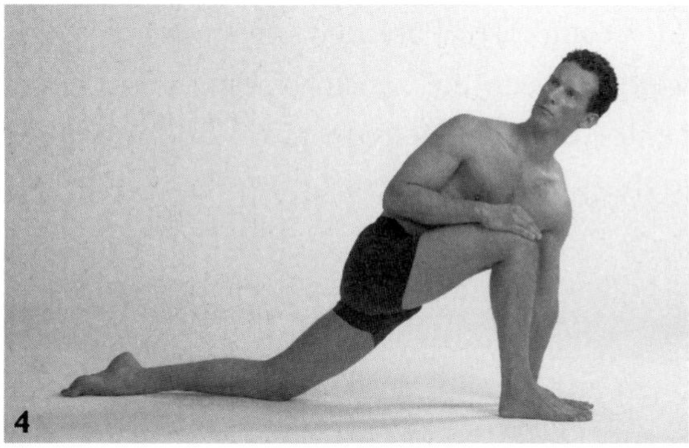

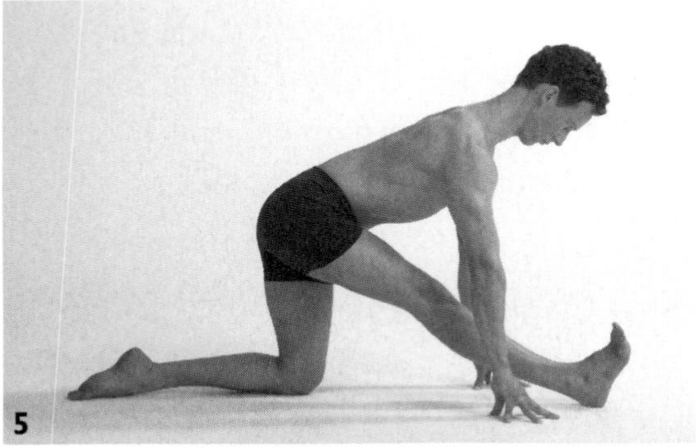

5

5. Lower the right arm and bring both hands on the floor by the right foot. Press into the right foot and slowly straighten the front leg. As the hips slide back, walk the hands so they rest comfortably on either side of the right leg, keeping the torso long. Flex the right foot so the heel rests on the floor and the toes point to the ceiling. Square the hips as much as possible. Gently press the buttocks back toward the wall behind you, and extend through the crown to elongate the spine. Feel the stretch to the back of the right leg. This is Runner's Lunge. Breathe deeply as you hold.

6. To release, slide the front knee forward into Lunge and return to Table Pose.

7. Step the left foot forward, and repeat the series on the opposite side.

Be Aware:
Part of the Sun Salutation, Lunge is a highly versatile posture with many variations. Supported Warrior is a paradoxical posture in which the lower body sinks into the earth while the fingertips reach for the sky, elongating the spine and opening the chest. Spinal Twist from Lunge rotates the torso from hips to neck. Runner's Lunge offers a complementary hamstring stretch.

DEEPER LUNGE VARIATIONS

(Anjaneyasana)

1. From Table Pose, step the right foot forward between the hands to come into Lunge. Let the breath flow freely as your body adjusts to this posture.

2. Press the left hand firmly into the floor. Lift the right hand, twisting the torso toward the thigh and extending the fingertips toward the ceiling. The head turns to gaze at the upturned right thumb. Breathe deeply as you hold this variation of Spinal Twist from Lunge.

3. Lower the right hand to the floor, returning to Lunge. Then lower the left knee to the floor, and bring the top of the back foot on the floor. Rest in this position until the breath returns to normal.

4. Bend the left leg and reach back with the right hand to clasp the foot. Press into the right foot, press into the left hand, and extend

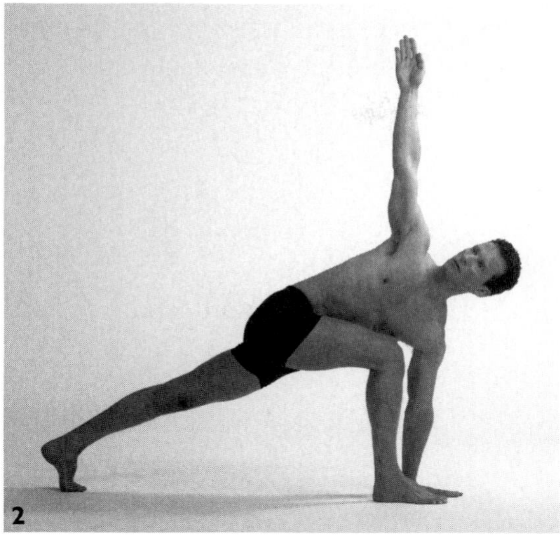

2

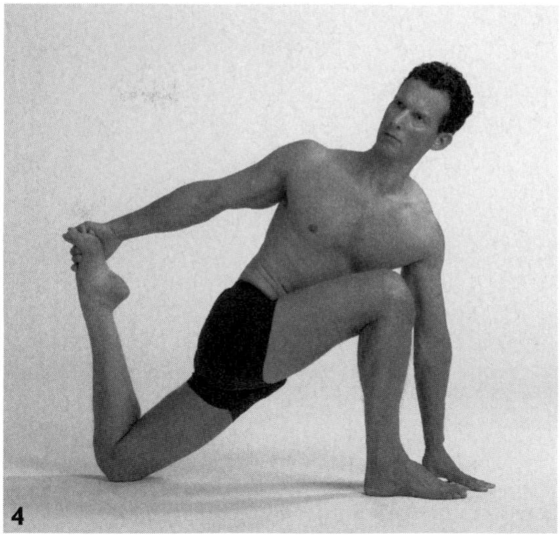

4

through the crown to elongate the spine. Turn the head right to look at the left foot. Press the left leg away to pull on the right arm and stretch the chest. Breathe deeply as you hold this variation of King Pigeon Pose.

5. Lower the left leg to the floor and return to Lunge. Slide the left foot forward about twelve inches, and then press into the right foot and straighten both legs. Turn the left foot out slightly so it rests solidly on the floor. Square the hips to the front. Press into the feet to engage the muscles of the legs. Take a deep breath in. As you exhale, lengthen the torso over the inside of the right leg and extend the crown of the head toward the floor. Breathe deeply as you hold Straight Legged Lunge.

6. Step the right foot back into Downward Dog, holding for several breaths. Then step the left foot forward into Lunge, and repeat this entire series on the opposite side.

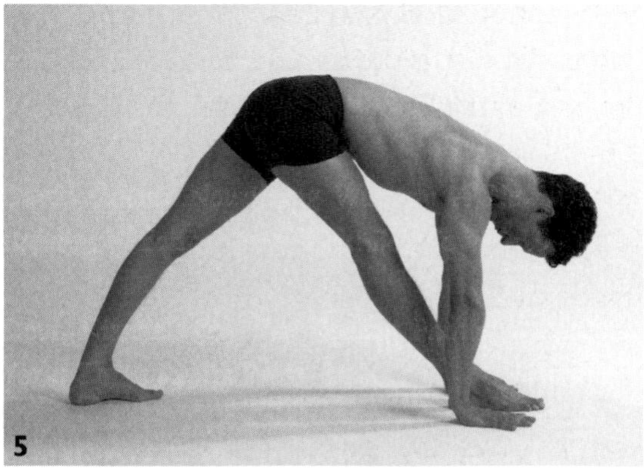

5

Be Aware:

This is a demanding sequence of stretches. You may want to begin by entering each stretch with the right foot forward, and then the left foot forward. Over time you can move through the entire sequence on the right side, then shift to the left side. If you want to take Spinal Twist from Lunge even deeper, reach the left hand over the right knee. Press the palm or knuckles into the floor just outside the right foot, left forearm alongside the right shin. This considerably deepens the twist.

STANDING POSTURES

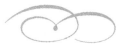

PARABOLA

(Anuvrittasana)

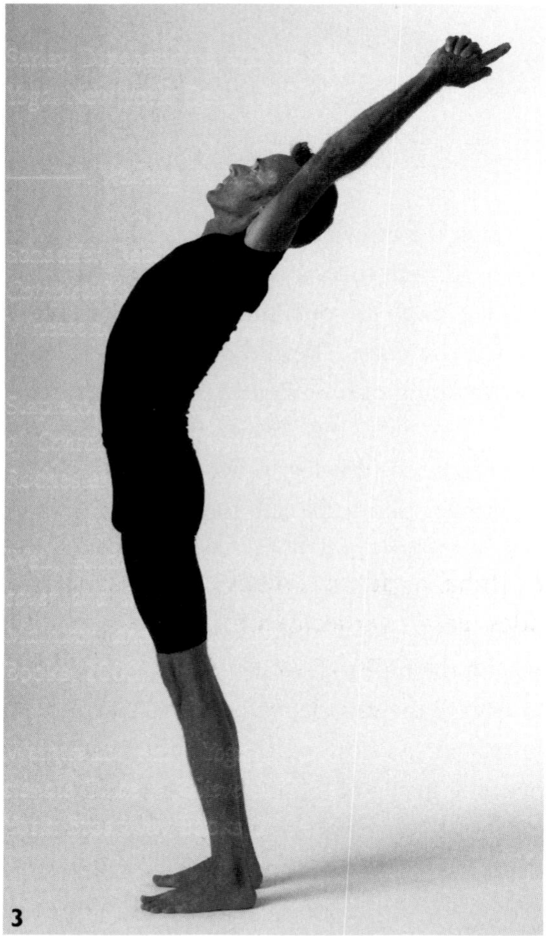

3

1. Stand in Mountain Pose. Press into all four corners of the feet to engage the legs. Stabilize the core of the body and elongate the spine.

2. Inhale and sweep the arms out to the sides and overhead, arms shoulder-width apart, hands in Steeple Position. Press up through the crown and fingertips to further elongate the spine.

3. Press the pubic bone slightly forward to engage the abdominals. Shift the gaze to focus on a point on the ceiling a few feet in front of you and press the sternum forward, allowing the upper spine to arch back. Press the fingertips up and back, so the upper arms come behind the ears. Breathe deeply as you hold.

4. To release, inhale the arms overhead and bring the torso back to vertical. Exhale, and lower the hands to the sides.

Be Aware:

Parabola provides an exhilarating chest stretch and backward bend of the upper spine. Resist the tendency to overstretch the flexible low back and shelter the less flexible chest and upper back. To accomplish this, it is necessary to engage the body's musculature from the soles of the feet to the fingertips. Parabola can also be practiced with the palms together. No matter what hand position you use, don't let the head drop back and neck collapse. Keep the head framed between straight upper arms, which ensures the neck remains aligned with the rest of the spine. Breathe evenly throughout all phases of this posture. If you feel a desire to hold the breath, you are bending back too far. Parabola is a great counterpose to desk and computer work.

STANDING HANDS TO FEET

(Pada Hastasana)

1. Stand in Mountain Pose. Press into all four corners of the feet to engage the legs. Stabilize the core of the body and elongate the spine.

2. Inhale and sweep the arms out to the sides and overhead, arms shoulder-width apart and palms facing. Press up through the crown and fingertips to further elongate the spine.

3. Exhale and lift the tailbone and begin to hinge forward from the hips with a straight spine. Sweep the arms out to the sides like a swan dive, pausing with the back parallel to the floor, arms extended in a T. Bend the knees as needed to avoid strain. Let the eyes look down to the floor, extending through the crown to elongate the neck and spine. Take several breaths in this position.

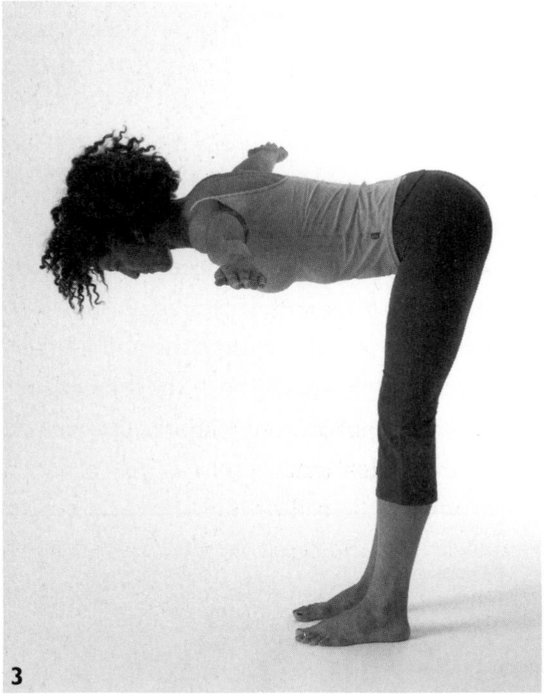

3

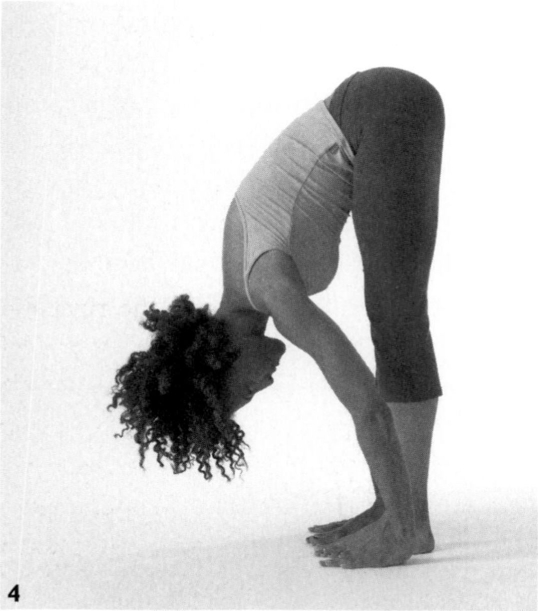
4

4. Continue to hinge at the hips and come forward. Keep the low back straight, while allowing the upper spine and neck to gradually round. Bend the knees as needed to rest the hands on the floor on either side of your feet. Press into the feet and engage the abdominals. If you want more stretch, press the forehead toward the knees or shins. Breathe deeply as you hold.

5. To release, inhale and press into the feet, tucking the tailbone under and hinging at the hips to come up with a straight spine. Let your arms come out to the sides in a T and then overhead in a reverse swan dive. Press the fingertips up to elongate the spine, and exhale the arms down to your sides.

Be Aware:
Forward bending can be challenging if your low back is sensitive. If it is difficult for you to hinge forward while sweeping the arms out to the sides, continue to practice Standing Angle and Forward Fold to build flexibility and strength. If you want more stretch, come into the posture as above. Bend the knees deeply and slide the fingertips under the heels to provide a handhold, and position the elbows behind the knees. On an exhalation, press into the feet and contract the abdominals, gradually straightening the legs. Use your hand and arm strength to enhance the stretch, extending the crown toward the toes and pressing the forehead toward the shins. Keep the breath flowing and take care not to overstretch the low back.

DANCER

(Natarajasana)

1. Stand in Mountain Pose. Press into all four corners of the feet to engage the legs. Stabilize the core of the body and elongate the spine.

2. Focus the gaze on a point eye height on the wall in front of you. Inhale, and lift the left arm overhead, upper arm near the ear, and palm facing forward with the fingers together. Press up through the fingertips to lengthen the arm.

3. Shift your weight to the left foot, pressing the foot into the floor to engage the leg muscles without locking the knee. Bend the right leg at the knee, lifting the foot and clasping it from the outside of the instep with the right hand. The thumb of the right hand will be pointed down. Touch the sides of the knees together, helping you square and level the hips.

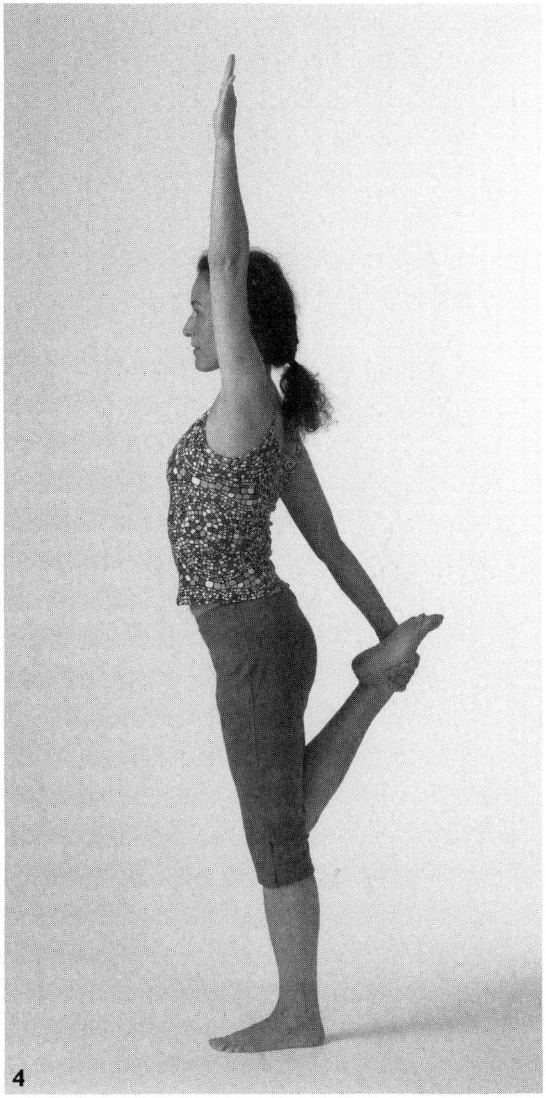

4

4. Inhale and press the right foot back into the right hand. As the press grows stronger, the chest opens and the upper spine begins to arch back. Press the fingertips of the left hand up and the sternum forward to enhance this opening of the chest.

5. As you continue to press the right foot strongly into the right hand, lower the left arm to shoulder height. The chest and shoulders remain square to the front. Keep both hips level and square, resisting the tendency to roll the right hip up. Press the right toes up toward the ceiling. Press the left fingers toward the wall in front of you.

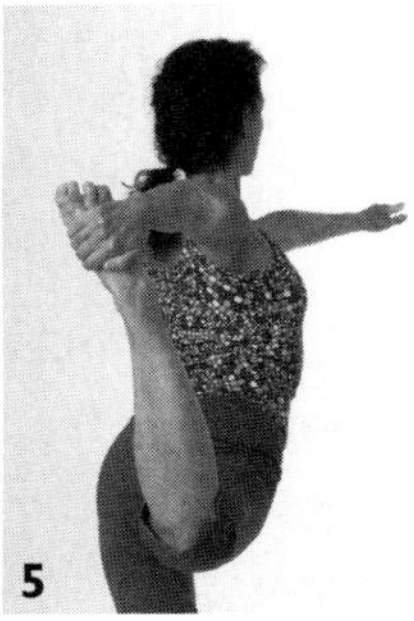

5

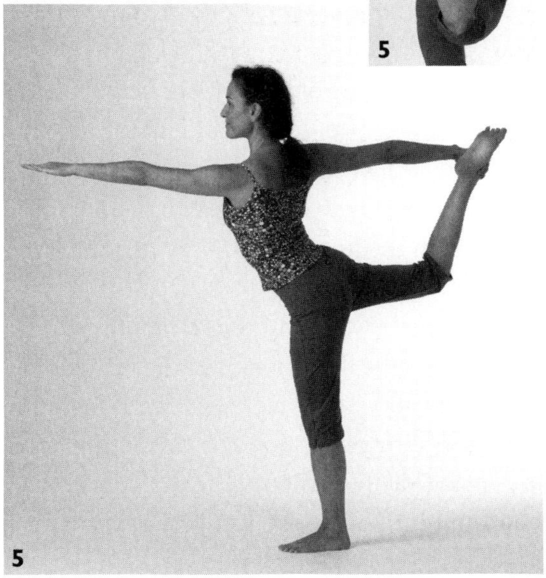

5

6. To release, inhale and bring the torso back to vertical, bringing the knees together. Exhale and release the clasp of the right foot, returning to Mountain Pose.

7. Repeat on the opposite side.

Be Aware:
The Dancer requires that you learn to maintain a dynamic balance, pressing the foot strongly back into the hand while extending through the fingertips. It is a good example of an asymmetrical posture that is practiced on both sides to restore balance between the right and left sides of the body. Start practice with steps 1–3, which is a posture in its own right called Standing Heel to Buttock Pose. As you gain strength and balance, allow the hips to hinge and torso to pivot slightly forward. Provided you keep the shoulders, chest, and hips square to the front, the Dancer provides a deep stretch to the shoulders, chest, and abdomen.

STANDING BOW PULLING

(Dandayamana Dhanurasana)

1. Stand in Mountain Pose. Press into all four corners of the feet to engage the legs. Stabilize the core of the body and elongate the spine.

2. Focus the gaze on a point eye height on the wall in front of you. Inhale, and lift the left arm overhead, upper arm near the ear, and palm facing forward with the fingers together. Press up through the fingertips to lengthen the arm.

3. Shift your weight to the left foot, pressing the foot into the floor to engage the leg muscles without locking the knee. Bend the right leg at the knee, lifting the foot and clasping it from the inside of the instep with the right hand. The thumb of the right hand will be pointed up. Touch the sides of the knees together, helping you square and level the hips.

4. Inhale and press the right foot back into the right hand. As the press of the foot grows

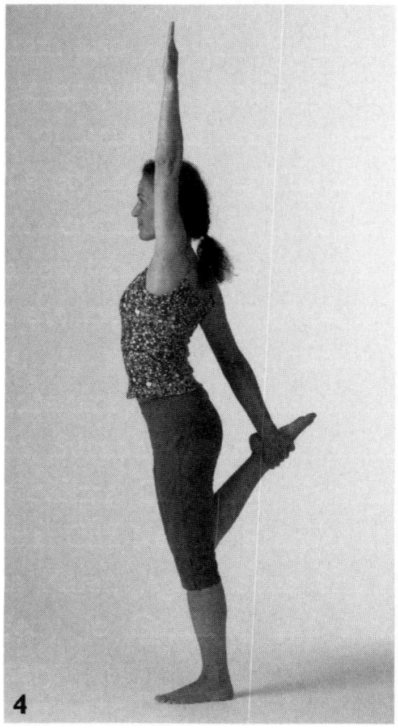

4

stronger, the chest opens and the upper spine begins to arch back. Press the left hand up and the sternum forward to enhance this opening of the chest.

5. As you continue to press the right foot strongly into the right hand, allow the torso to smoothly pivot forward from the hips. The left arm naturally comes down as the torso comes forward. The left shoulder stays forward, fingertips of the left hand pressing toward the wall in front of you. The right shoulder is pulled back by the press of the right leg. Allow the chest to rotate to face the wall to your right. Press the toes of the right foot toward the ceiling, letting the right hip roll up. Extend through the crown, eyes looking straight ahead. Breathe deeply as you hold.

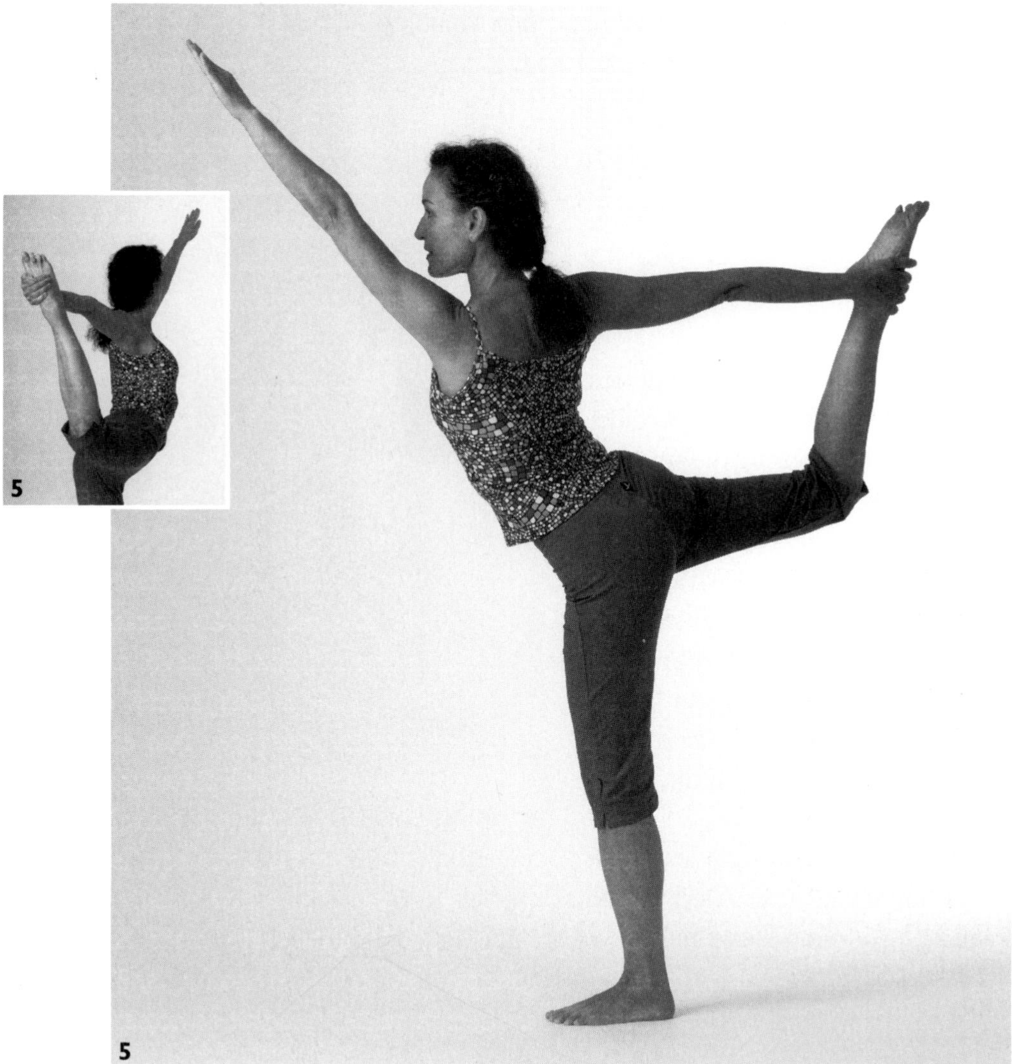

5

5

6. To release, inhale and bring the torso back to vertical, bringing the knees together. Exhale and release the clasp of the right foot, returning to Mountain Pose.

7. Repeat on the opposite side.

Be Aware:
Standing Bow Pulling and the Dancer are similar but different postures. Their starting positions are the same except for the hand positions. In Standing Bow Pulling, the instep is clasped from the inside with the thumb facing up. This hand position aids the rotation of the chest and shoulders, the upward opening of the hip, and the pressing of the toes toward the ceiling. In the Dancer, the clasp of the instep from the outside with the thumb facing down aids in keeping the shoulders, chest, and hips square. Both postures require you to maintain a dynamic balance. Where Dancer offers a torso stretch, Standing Bow Pulling provides a strong hamstring stretch.

EAGLE

(Garudasana)

1. Stand in Mountain Pose. Press into all four corners of the feet to engage the legs. Stabilize the core of the body and elongate the spine.

2. Inhale and sweep the arms out to the sides. Exhale and swing the arms back down, crossing the right elbow under the left elbow and entwining the forearms. As much as possible, bring the palms together. Press the elbows down toward the navel, and bring the hands in close to the face, with the tops of the fingers near the nose.

3. Focus your gaze on a point eight to ten feet on the floor in front of you. Take a deep breath in. As you exhale, bend both knees and lower the buttocks.

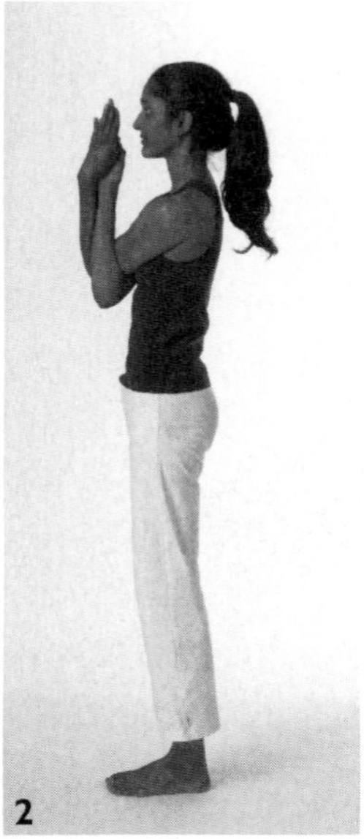
2

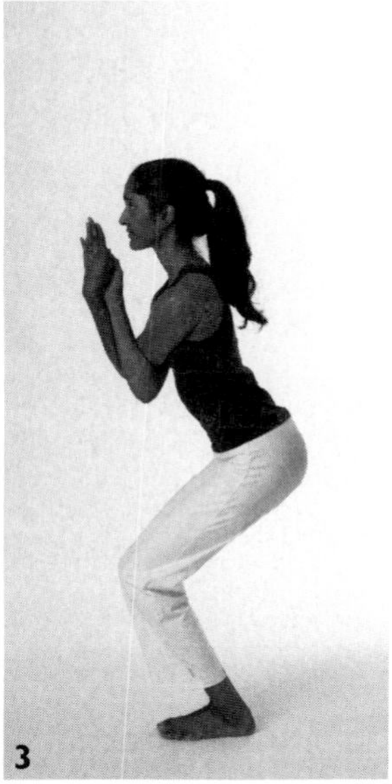
3

4. Shift your weight onto the left foot and smoothly lift the right leg up and cross it over the left leg at the knee. If possible, wrap the right leg around the left leg, bringing the right big toe just above the left ankle. Squeeze the

knees together, and sink a little deeper in the posture by bending the left leg a little farther.

5. Keep the spine elongated and crown lifted. Square both hips to the front by pressing the left hip slightly forward and right hip slightly back. Adjust the knees so they are aligned under the elbows at the centerline of the body. Breathe deeply as you hold.

6. Release on an inhalation by slowly straightening the left leg and unwinding the right leg to come back to standing. Let the arms unwind and come back to the sides. Let the breath flow in and out to integrate the effects of the posture.

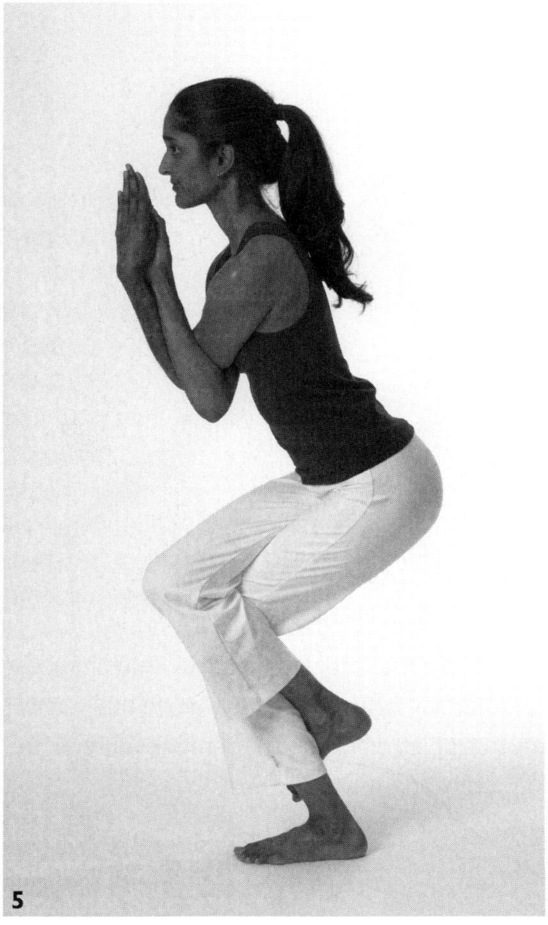

5

7. Come back into Mountain Pose. Inhale and sweep the arms out to the sides. Repeat on the opposite side, swinging the left elbow under the right, and lifting the left leg over the right.

Be Aware:

The Eagle articulates all the major joints of the body. Although challenging, the posture's many benefits justify the discipline required to master it. Start by simply working with the arm position, which braids the forearms like two strands of a rope. If you cannot bring the palms together, grasp the wrist or thumb of the upper hand. Interlacing the fingers and wriggling the hands back and forth is one way to gradually join the palms. Circling the elbows with the arms in Eagle position offers a great arm and shoulder stretch. Work with the legs in similar fashion. At first, simply cross the legs at the knees and don't worry about wrapping the lifted leg around the calf of the standing leg. Explore wrapping the legs together when sitting in a chair at home or work. Gradually work to hook the big toe just above the ankle and just under the calf muscle.

BENT KNEE SIDE STRETCH AND LATERAL ANGLE

(Parshvakonasana)

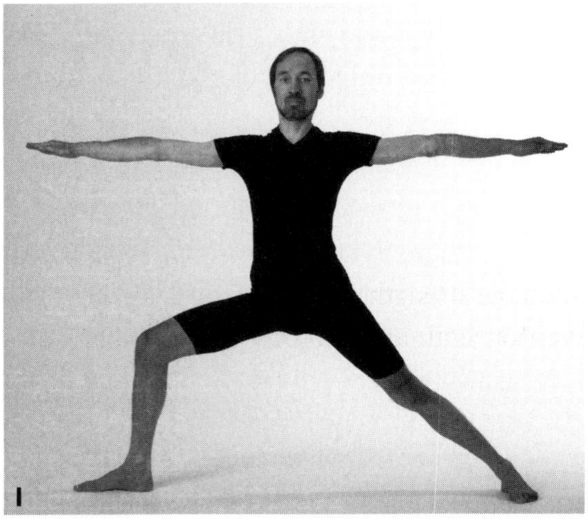

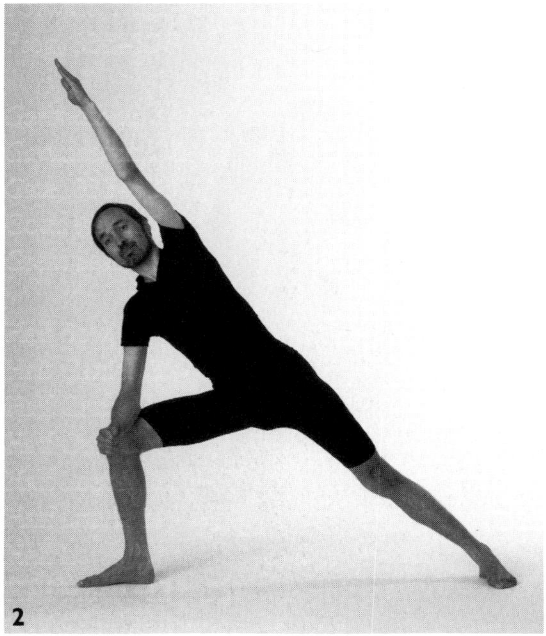

1. Step the feet slightly wider apart than your legs are long. Turn the right foot out a full turn of ninety degrees, and turn the left foot in a quarter turn. Come into Side Warrior Pose. Let the breath flow freely as your body adjusts to this posture.

2. Take a deep breath in. As you exhale, bend the right arm at the elbow and rest the forearm on the thigh just above the knee. Press the forearm into the thigh, and sweep the left arm overhead, bringing the upper arm close to the left ear. Press down on the outside of the left foot and extend through the left fingertips, deeply stretching the left side of the body. This is Bent Knee Side Stretch. Breathe deeply as you hold.

3. To come into Lateral Angle, reach the right arm down to press the palm or knuckles firmly into the floor just inside the right foot. Roll the left hip and shoulder back, opening the pelvis and chest. Press down on the outside of the left foot and extend through the left fingertips, deeply stretching the left side of the body. Breathe deeply as you hold.

4. To release, inhale and press into the right foot, slowly bringing the torso back to vertical and arms parallel to the floor. Straighten the right leg, and lower the arms.

5. Reverse the direction of the feet, turning the left foot out a full turn and the right foot in a quarter turn. Repeat on the opposite side.

Be Aware:

Bent Knee Side Stretch and Lateral Angle build upon the strength and flexibility gained in Side Warrior. Both are vigorous postures that combine a deep side stretch with a rotation of the hips, rib cage, shoulders, and neck. As you begin practice, experiment to discover the proper distance to separate your feet. The right stance allows the front knee to be directly over the ankle when the thigh is parallel to the floor. Don't be afraid to step the feet quite far apart. Most people make the mistake of assuming too narrow a stance, especially for Lateral Angle, which makes a challenging posture even more difficult. Resist any tendency to sag in Bent Knee Side Stretch, by pressing firmly into the bent elbow to keep both sides of the torso elongated.

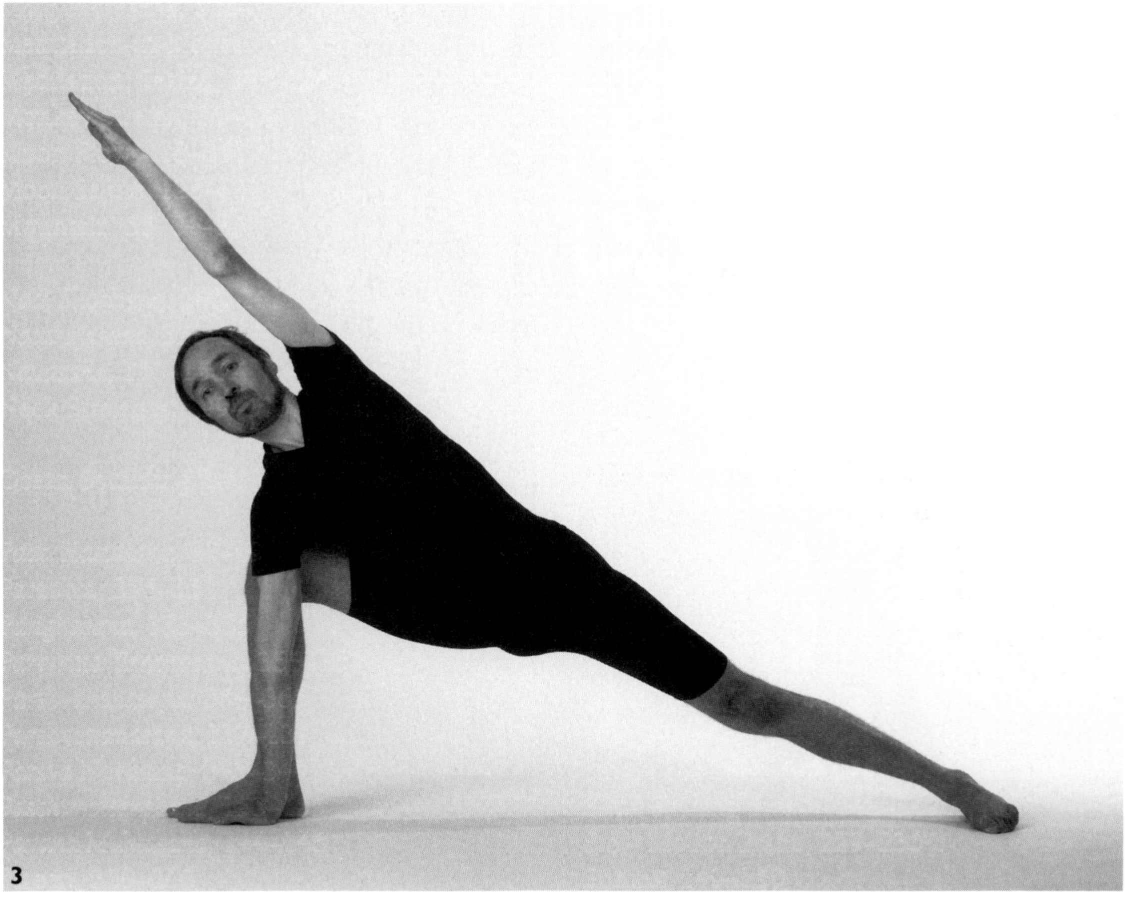
3

ROTATED TRIANGLE

(Parivritta Trikonasana)

1. Step the feet as wide apart as your legs are long. Turn the right foot out a full turn of ninety degrees, and turn the left foot in a quarter turn. Come into the starting position for Triangle Pose.

2. Take a deep breath in. Pressing firmly into the feet, exhale and rotate the hips, torso, and shoulders as far as possible to the right. Then slide the right arm out to the right, pressing the fingertips away to keep the arms straight and horizontal to the ground. Allow the right knee to bend slightly if necessary to avoid strain, but continue to press into the foot to keep the leg muscles engaged. Extend through the crown of the head to keep the spine elongated.

3. When you have rotated and reached as far as possible without strain, pivot from the hips to place the left hand outside the right foot. Inhale and press the fingertips down, coming into a deep standing twist. Gaze straight ahead. If your balance is steady, you can turn the head to gaze at the thumb of the lifted right hand. You can also gaze down to the floor. Pull your shoulder blades together and down your back. Extend through the crown. Breathe deeply as you hold.

4. To release, inhale and press into the feet to lift and unwind the torso back to the upright starting position for Triangle. Return the feet to the starting position. Exhale and lower the arms. Rest until the breath returns to normal.

5. Rotate the left foot out a full turn of ninety degrees, turn the left foot in a quarter turn, and repeat on the other side.

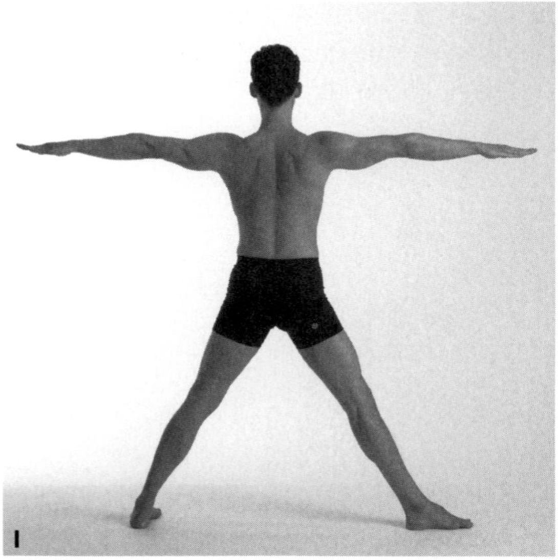
1

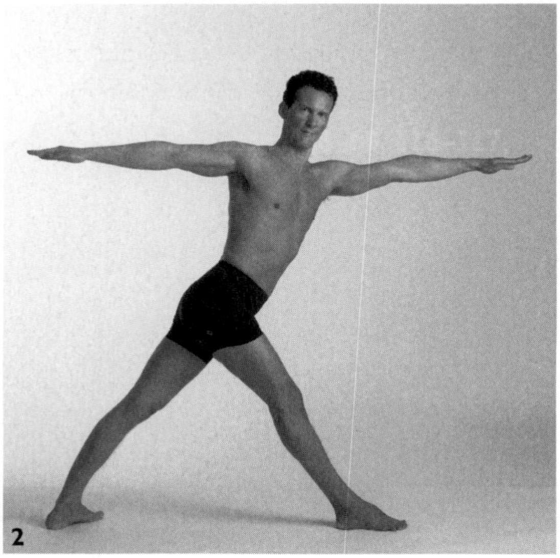
2

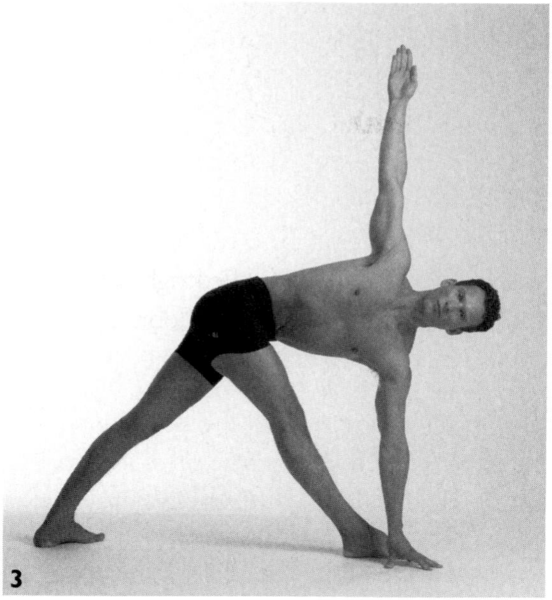
3

Be Aware:

Although Rotated Triangle utilizes the same starting position as the Triangle, it is not an advanced variation of the Triangle. Triangle is a side stretch in which the body is kept in one plane and forward bending or twisting is resisted. Rotated Triangle is a forward bend in which the hips, shoulders, and neck are deeply twisted. It is best to think of the Triangle and Rotated Triangle as completely different postures that are complementary and often practiced together.

Exercise caution in coming into Rotated Triangle, as its simultaneous forward bend and twist has the potential to strain the low back. Strength and flexibility in many muscles of the legs, hip, and trunk are required. Prepare the body with Triangle, Half Moon, Rotated Pyramid, Standing Runner's Stretch, and Lateral Angle. To twist safely and reap the benefits of Rotated Triangle, you must preserve the elongation of the spine. It is much more important to keep the spine elongated than it is to lower the hand to the floor. If you are unable to lower the hand to the floor while maintaining spinal elongation and other details of alignment, place a block on the floor by the inside of the foot and press your palm firmly into the block. As your flexibility increases, you can move the block to the outside of the foot and eventually remove the block entirely.

BELLY DOWNS

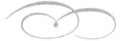

COBRA

(Bhujangasana)

1. Lie on your belly with the forehead on the floor. Reach the arms overhead and stretch your body to its full length using the support of the floor.

2. Place the palms on the floor under the shoulders, elbows touching the sides of the body. When the hands are positioned properly, the elbows point slightly upward. Bring the legs and feet hip-width apart or closer, with the tops of the feet on the floor.

3. Inhale and press the pubic bone, hip bones, and lower abdomen into the floor, stabilizing the core of the body. Use the press as a base to lift the head and then the torso by engaging the back muscles. Come up as high as you can without putting any weight on the hands, and pause there for several breaths.

4. Inhale and press gently into the palms, lifting the torso a few inches higher but keeping the lower belly on the floor and the elbows close to the sides. Elongate the spine by pressing the pubic bone down and lifting out of the waist. Open the chest and arch the spine back by pressing the sternum forward, rolling the shoul-

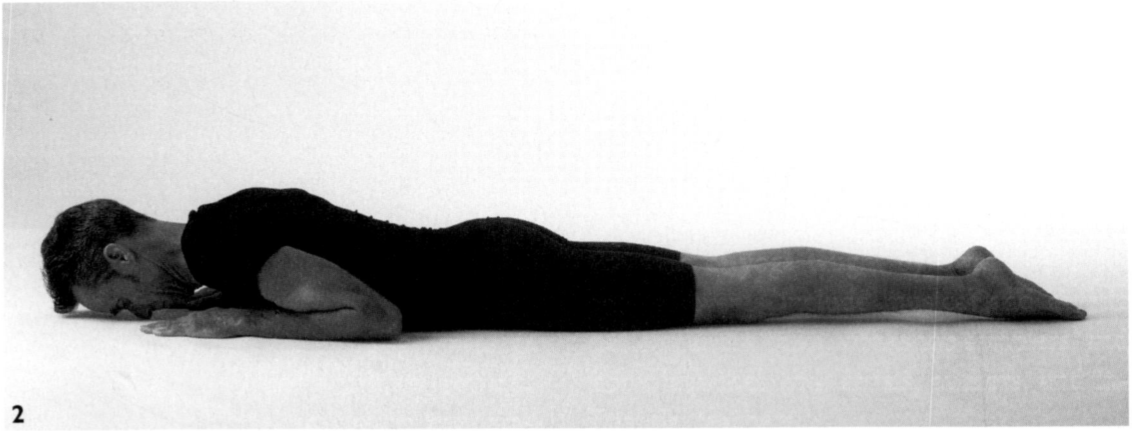

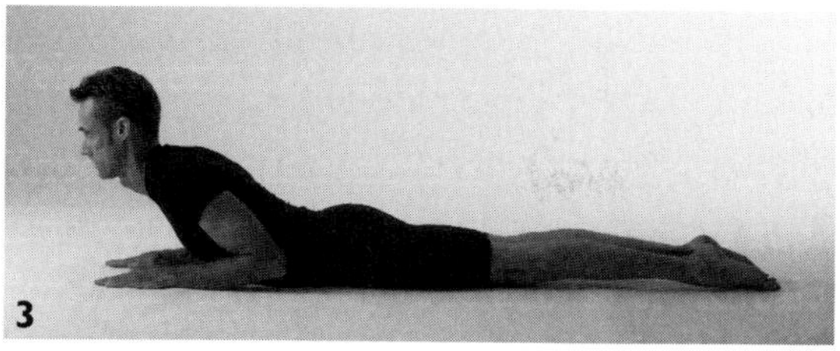
3

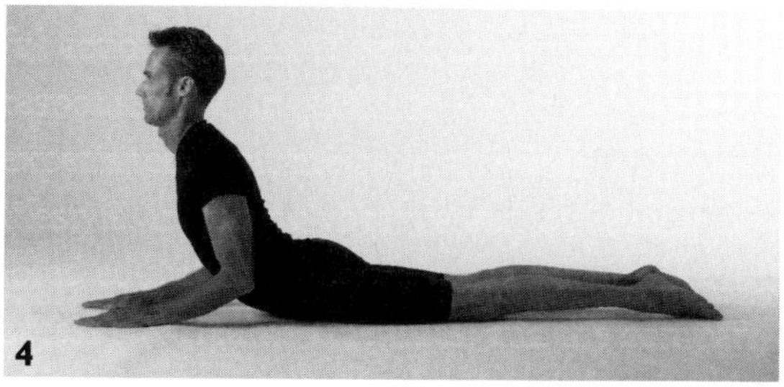
4

ders back and down. Keep the back of the neck long by slightly tucking the chin and extending through the crown. Breathe deeply as you hold.

5. The backward bend of the spine should be a smooth curve, without any sharp bend in the low back or neck.

6. To release, exhale and extend the torso forward and down to the floor. Turn the head to one side and bring the arms to the sides with the hands palms up.

Be Aware:

The press of the pubic bone and hip bones is the foundation of the Cobra, providing a solid base from which to engage the muscles of the back and lift the torso off the floor. The backward bend sought in Cobra is to the middle and upper back and not in the lower back or neck. If you feel compression in the lumbar spine, continue practicing Serpent and Sphinx to strengthen weak back muscles. If you want more challenge, try this enhancement. As you press the palms down, you can also pull back on them slightly. This will help you extend the sternum forward and facilitate a deeper opening in the chest.

DIAGONAL STRETCH

(Salabhasana)

1. Lie on your belly with the forehead on the floor. Reach the arms overhead and stretch your body to its full length using the support of the floor.

2. Keep the left arm overhead and slide the right arm down to the side, palm down. Bring the legs and feet hip-width apart.

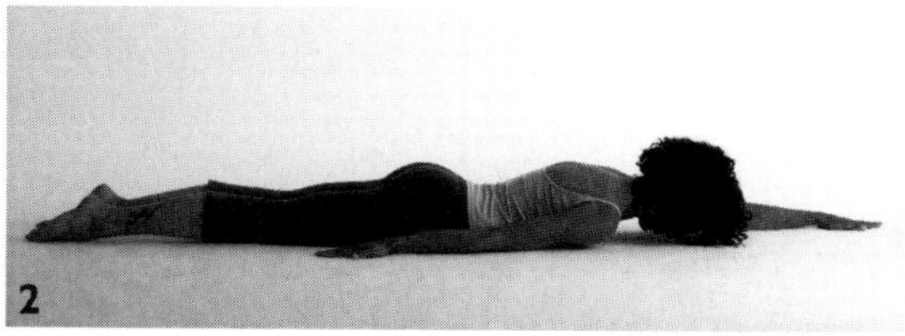
2

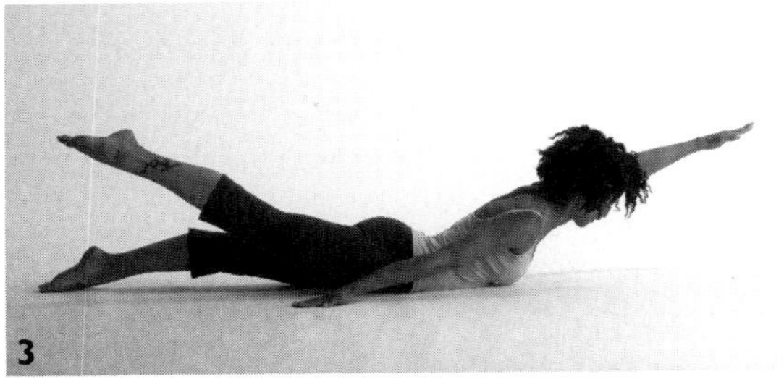

3

3. Inhale and press the pubic bone, hip bones, and lower abdomen into the floor. From that solid base, lift the left arm, right leg, and head. Keep the back of the neck long by extending through the crown. Press the left fingers away from the right toes, stretching diagonally across the back and elongating the spine. Breathe deeply as you hold.

4. To release, take a deep breath in. As you exhale, slowly lower the left arm, head, and right leg to the floor.

5. Reverse the position of the arms, bringing the right arm overhead and the left arm down to the side, and repeat.

Be Aware:
Diagonal Stretch is a great back strengthener that incorporates aspects of the Cobra, Locust, and Boat. By stretching diagonally across the spine, first one way, and then the other, it provides back muscles an opportunity to let go of tensions and return to a balanced muscle tone.

LOCUST SERIES

(Salabhasana)

1. Lie on your belly with the forehead on the floor. Reach the arms overhead and stretch your body to its full length using the support of the floor.

2. Bring the arms down to your sides, palms down. Stretch the chin forward, resting the chin on the floor and opening the throat. Rock from side to side, using the side-to-side motion to walk the arms under the body. Reach the hands down as low as you can, and bring the arms close together. Try to touch the elbows together near the navel. The insides of the

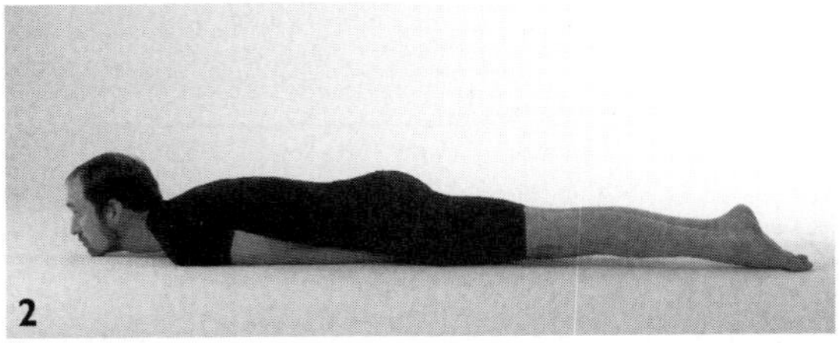

2

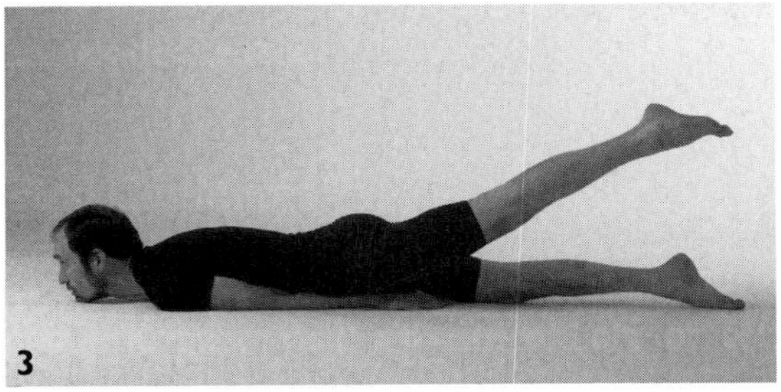

3

forearms also touch, running just inside the hip bones. The palms are flat on the floor with the pinkies touching. Bring the legs and feet together.

3. To come into Half Locust, bring your attention to the left leg. Take a deep breath in. As you exhale, press into the hip bones and slowly lift the left leg off the floor. Keep both hips pressed equally into the floor and the left leg straight. Press out through the toes to lengthen the leg, and up through the heel to lift the leg as high as you can without bending the leg or lifting the left hip bone off the floor. Keep the full length of both arms on the floor. Breathe deeply as you hold, relaxing into the massage of the abdomen by the elbows and forearms.

4. Exhale and slowly lower the left leg to the floor. Move directly into Half Locust on the right side.

5. To come into the Full Locust, take a deep breath in. As you exhale, press down on the hip bones and pubic bone and lift both legs off the floor. Engage the arm muscles by pressing down on the palms, and use this leverage to roll the body weight forward onto the abdomen and chest, lifting the hips off the ground. Keep the legs straight. Press out through the toes to lengthen the legs, and up through the heels to lift the feet as high as possible. Let the breath move freely in and out as you hold.

7. To release, exhale and slowly lower the legs to the floor and relax.

Be Aware:

With the arms underneath the body, Half Locust provides a powerful abdominal massage. Full Locust develops great strength in the muscles of the low back, abdomen, and thighs. Unlike most postures, Full Locust is entered into quickly on an exhalation. Move into it immediately upon lowering the left leg to complete Half Locust. When the legs have lifted and the weight has rolled forward onto the abdomen and chest,

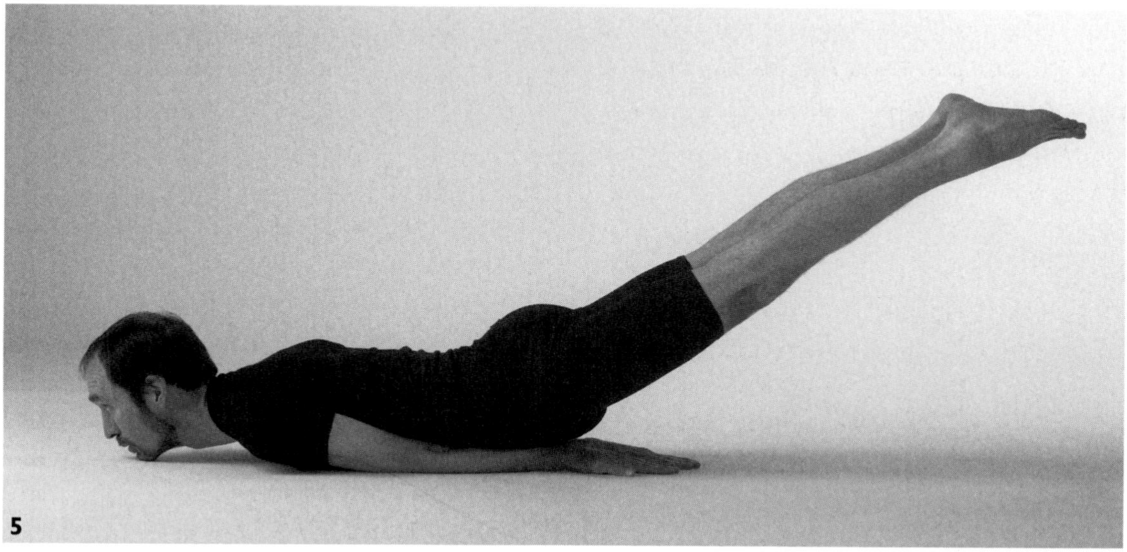

5

it is possible to sustain a flowing—if shallow—breath while holding. Because of the intense effort involved, it is important to let the body rest for a few moments after the Full Locust. Once the heartbeat and breath have returned to normal, move on to the next posture. Do not practice Full Locust if you have high blood pressure or a heart condition.

HALF BOW

(Ardha Dhanurasana)

1. Lie on your belly with the forehead on the floor. Reach the arms overhead and stretch your body to its full length using the support of the floor.

2. Keep the left arm overhead and slide the right arm down to the side. Bend the right knee and bring the heel of the right foot close to the buttocks. Reach the right hand back to clasp the inside of the right foot at the instep. The pinky finger will cross the foot just below the base of the toes. Press the pubic bone, hip bones, and lower abdomen down to stabilize the core of the body.

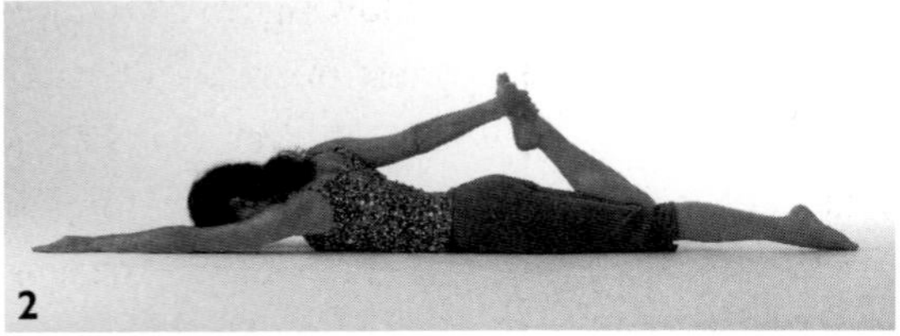

2

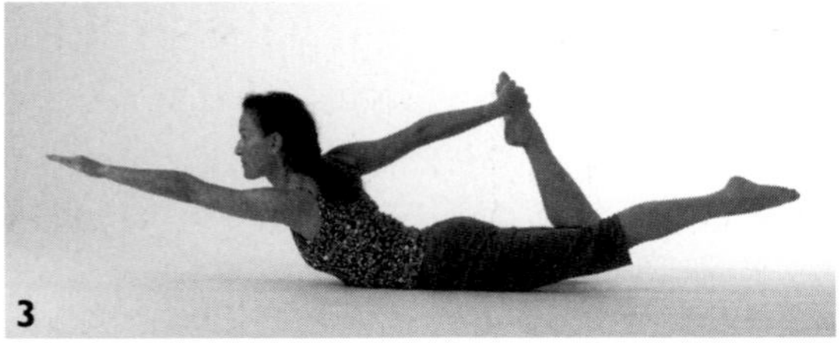

3

3. Inhale and press the right foot back into the hand, pulling the right shoulder back, lifting the chest, and lifting the right knee off the ground. Lift the left arm and leg off the floor, pressing the fingertips of the left hand forward and the toes of the left foot back. Keep the neck long by extending through the crown. Breathe deeply as you hold.

4. To release, take a deep breath in. As you exhale, slowly lower the arms and legs to the floor.

5. Repeat on the opposite side.

Be Aware:
Half Bow is another asymmetrical posture that works one side of the back, and then the other. This helps maintain the balanced muscle tone supportive of spinal alignment. Watch the tendency of the bent knee to swing out to the side, which avoids the leg and torso stretch. Keep the bent knee in line with the hip and shoulder.

BOW

(Dhanurasana)

1. Lie on your belly with the forehead on the floor. Reach the arms overhead and stretch your body to its full length using the support of the floor.

2. Bend both knees and bring the heels close to the buttocks. Reach the hands back one at a time to clasp the outside of the feet at the instep so the pinky fingers cross the feet slightly below the base of the toes. Press the pubic bone, hip bones, and lower abdomen down to stabilize the core of the body.

3. Inhale and press the feet back into the hands, pulling the shoulders back and lifting the chest and knees off the floor. Relax the muscles of the chest and press the sternum forward to open the chest. Keep the neck long by extending through the crown and gazing straight ahead. Breathe deeply as you hold.

4. To release, exhale and slowly release the press of the feet into the hands, lowering the legs, torso, and head to the floor. Release the feet and extend the legs.

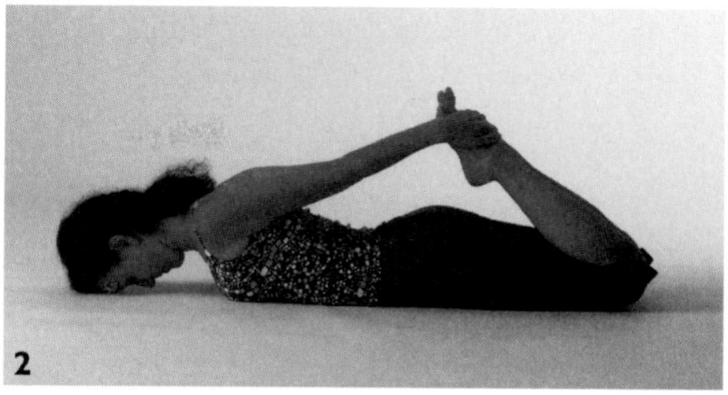
2

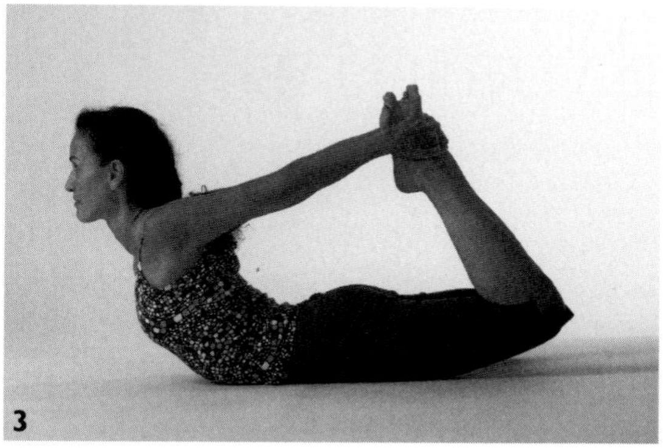
3

Be Aware:
Bow is the culmination of the belly down postures. Practiced properly, it does not strain the low back. The key is to emphasize the press of the feet into the hands while keeping the knees hip-width apart. The arms remain passive and the upper body relaxes, allowing the shoulders to be pulled back and chest opened. Although some muscular effort is required to lift the head, the overall experience is one of letting go into a stretch generated by the work of the legs. After Bow, you may want to wave or circle the feet to release tension from the low back. Then press into Child Pose, a great complementary posture for every belly down. Do not practice Full Bow if you have high blood pressure or a heart condition.

BACKBENDS

INVERTED TABLE

(Purvottanasana)

1. Come into a sitting position with the knees bent, feet on the floor in front of you and hands on the floor behind you. Adjust the feet so they are hip-width apart. Adjust the hands so they are shoulder-width apart, fingers spread wide and pointing away from the buttocks. Tuck the chin toward the chest.

2. Press into the feet and hands to lift the hips up. Press the pubic bone toward the ceiling to

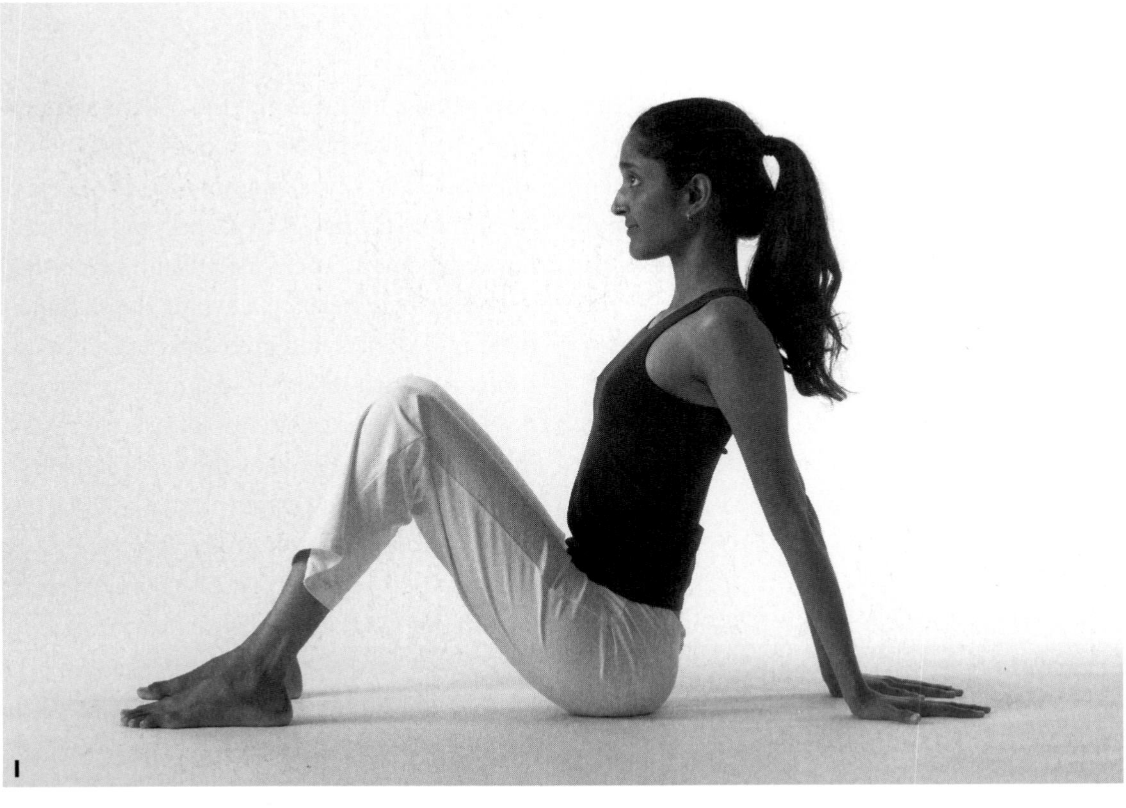

1

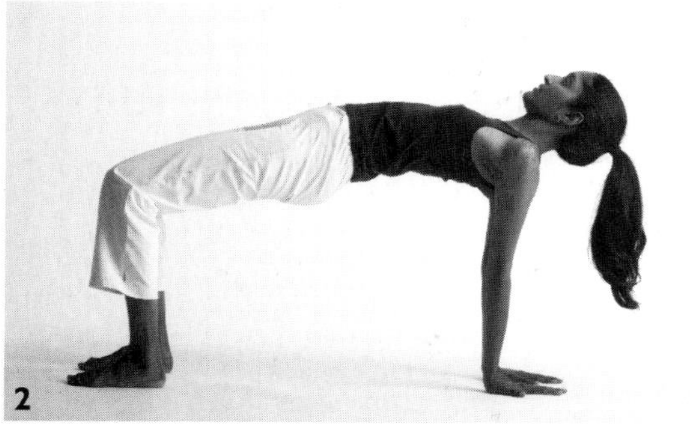

2

lift the hips as high as possible. Keep the chin slightly tucked and extend through the crown to elongate the neck.

3. To release, take a deep breath in. Exhale and lower the hips and buttocks to the floor.

Be Aware:
Inverted Table is only a mild backbend. More of a hip and chest stretch, it is included in this backbend section as a valuable preparatory pose for Camel and Wheel. The chin is tucked to protect the neck. Once you have come into the posture, you can gradually release the tuck, extending through the crown to keep the neck long and in line with the spine.

BRIDGE VARIATIONS

(Setu Bandhasana)

1. Lie on your back with the legs extended. Reach the arms overhead on the floor, and stretch your body to its full length using the support of the floor.

2. Bring the arms to the sides. Bend the knees, bringing the feet close to the buttocks, hip-width apart, and come into Bridge. Pause for a moment to breathe freely and let the body adjust to the posture.

3. Walk the feet together until they touch at the centerline of the body. Shift your weight onto your left foot, pressing it firmly into the floor as you extend the right foot upward. Keep the hips square and press the sole of the foot toward the ceiling. Breathe deeply as you hold.

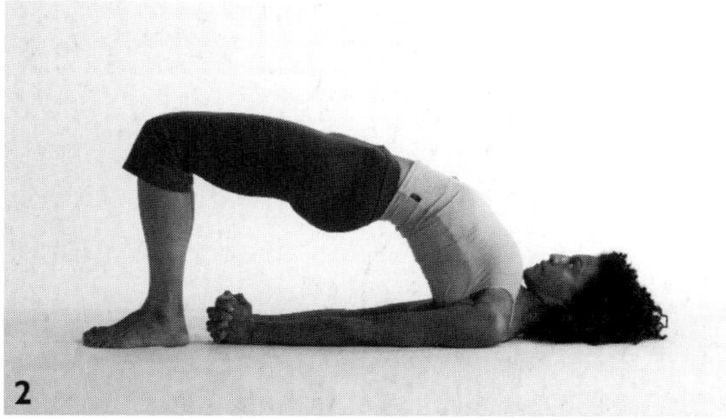

2

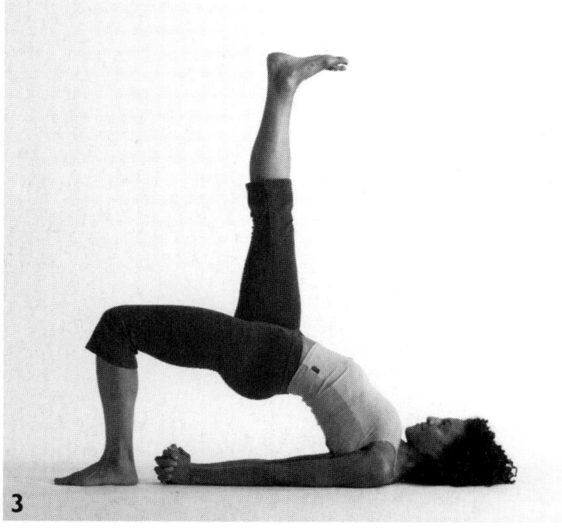

3

4. Lower the right foot, returning it to the floor at the centerline of the body. Shift your weight onto your right foot, pressing it firmly into the floor as you extend the left foot upward and come into the posture on the other side. Breathe deeply as you hold.

5. To come into the next variation, return to basic Bridge. Keeping the elbows on the ground, bring the heels of the hands to the sacrum, fingertips pointing out to hold the hips. Slide the right foot away from the buttocks until the heel rests on the ground. Then slide the left foot away until the heel rests on the ground. With the heels hip-width apart, point the feet. Breathe deeply as you hold. To release, bend one leg and then the other, returning to basic Bridge.

6. To release, take a deep breath in. As you exhale, separate the hands, slide the arms out to your sides, and slowly lower the spine and buttocks to the floor.

Be Aware:

Bridge is a versatile posture, with these variations offering distinct benefits. In the first, press one foot firmly into the floor and the other toward the ceiling. This strengthens the standing leg while stretching the opposite hip and leg. Some people like to lift the leg from basic Bridge, without centering the feet as detailed above. Experiment to see what works for your body. The second variation provides a profound sacrum press. At first, you may not be able to comfortably extend both legs away. Alternate extending one leg, then the other, until you can extend both. For a different Bridge handhold, see Wheel Pose.

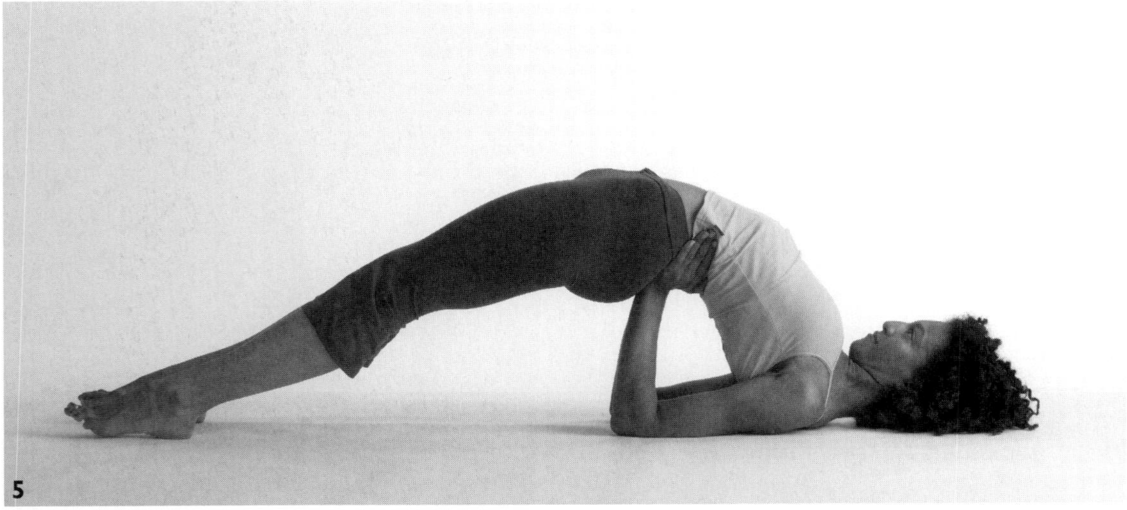
5

HALF CAMEL

(Ardha Ushtrasana)

1. Come into a kneeling position with the knees hip-width apart, buttocks lifted, and arms at the sides. The feet are on the floor directly behind the legs. Press the knees into the floor, level the pelvis, lift out of the waist, and extend through the crown to elongate the spine.

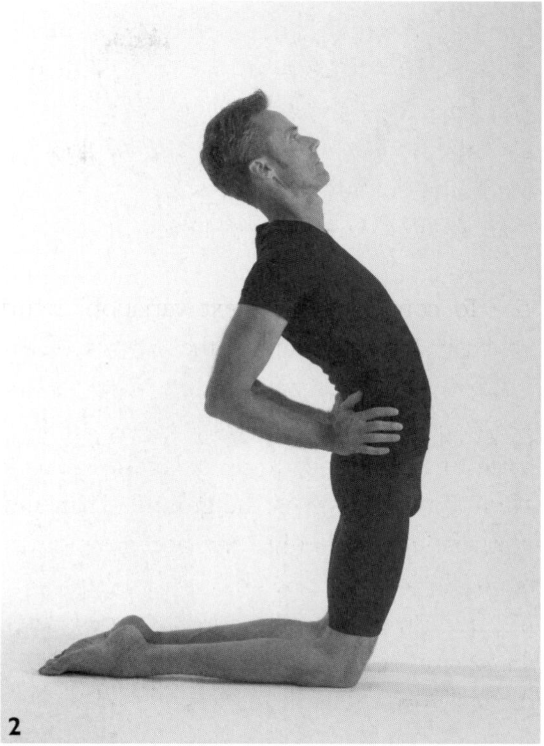
2

2. Bring the heels of the hands to the sacrum, fingers pointing out to the sides. Tuck the chin into the chest. Gently contract the muscles of the thighs, buttocks, and pelvic floor. Inhale and use the hands to press the pubic bone and hip bones forward, arching the spine back.

3. Reach the right hand back and down to grasp the right heel. Press the right hand down onto the heel to stabilize the position of the torso.

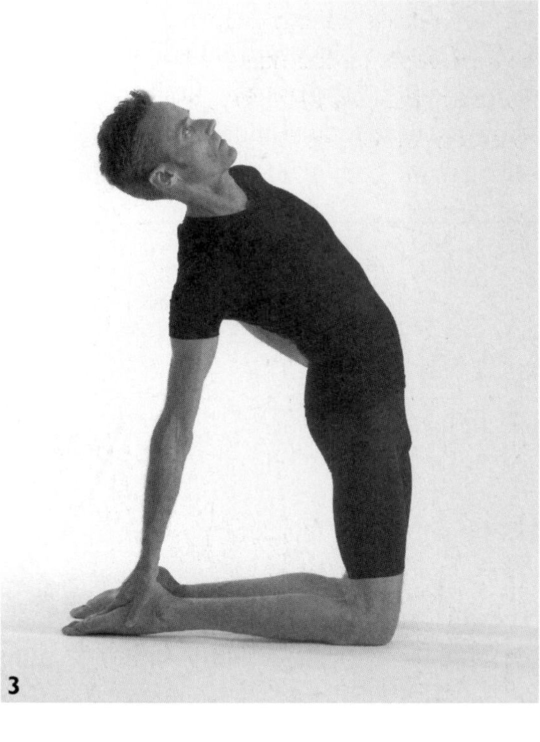
3

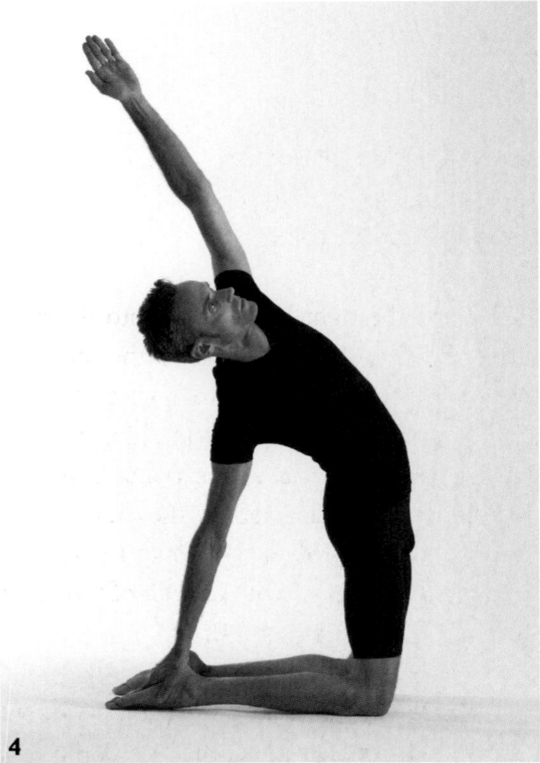
4

4. Lift the left arm overhead and behind you, pressing the fingertips away from the left hip. Allow the head to turn and gaze to focus on the ceiling to the right of you. Press the pubic bone and hip bones forward. Breathe deeply as you hold.

5. To release, inhale and return the left hand to the hip. Press the hips forward and release the right heel to bring the torso back to vertical.

6. Return both hands to the hips, and repeat on the opposite side.

Be Aware:
Often taught as a means to acquire the flexibility and strength required for Camel, Half Camel is a beneficial backbend and side stretch in its own right. Make sure to elongate the spine as detailed in step 1 before arching the spine back. If you find Half Camel challenging, just practice steps 1 and 2. Pressing the pubic bone and hip bones forward with the help of the hands provides a safe backbend. You can also practice Half Camel with the toes curled under and heels lifted for an easier stretch.

CAMEL

(Ushtrasana)

1. Come into a kneeling position with the knees hip-width apart, buttocks lifted, and arms at the sides. The tops of the feet rest on the floor directly behind the legs. Press the knees into the floor, level the pelvis, lift out of the waist, and extend through the crown to elongate the spine.

2. Bring the heels of the hands to the sacrum, fingers pointing out to the sides. Tuck the chin into the chest. Gently contract the muscles of the thighs, buttocks, and pelvic floor. Inhale and

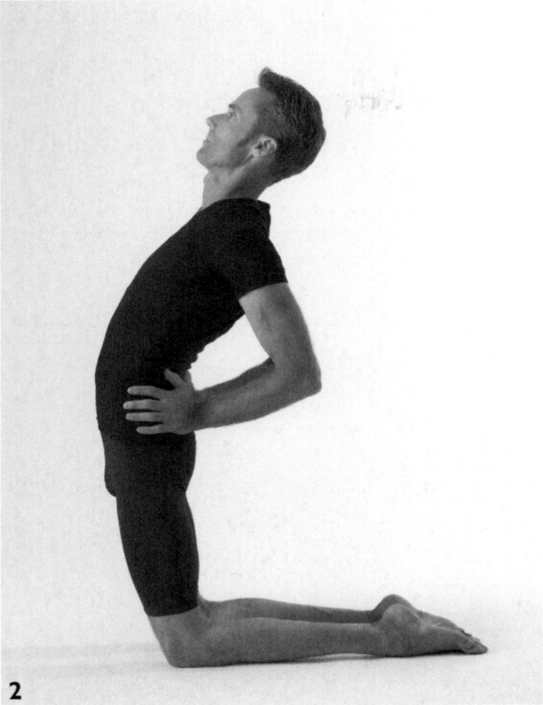

2

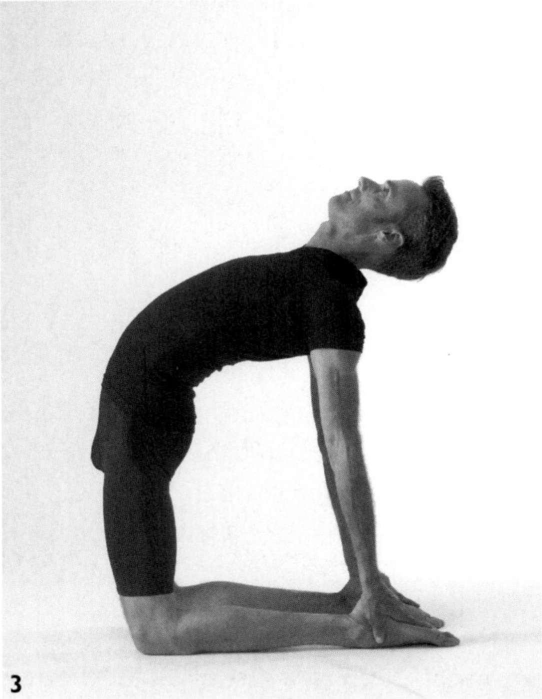

3

use the hands to help press the pubic bone and hip bones forward, lifting out of the waist and arching the spine back.

3. Reach the right hand back onto the right heel, and then the left hand to the left heel. Press the hands down and sternum up to open your chest and avoid overstretching the low back. Continue pressing the pubic bone and hip bones forward, keeping the chin tucked and extending through the crown to keep the neck long and in line with the rest of the spine. Breathe deeply as you hold.

4. To release, inhale and bring one hand, and then the other, to the sacrum. Press the hips forward to bring the torso back to vertical.

Be Aware:
Camel is an exhilarating backbend, and it is important to slowly work into the full posture to avoid straining the low back. If you have low back or neck sensitivity, proceed cautiously and only after mastering the preparatory belly down postures—Cobra, Locust, and Boat—as well as Bridge, Inverted Table, and Half Camel. Begin practice using Half Camel as a warm-up. Start Camel with the toes curled under and heels lifted. Keep the chin tucked to protect the neck, and refrain from dropping the head back.

As you become comfortable with the posture, emphasize the forward press of the pubic and hip bones and the lifting of the sternum. The sternum lift should be strong enough that it eventually takes much of the weight off the hands and heels. For an adept practitioner, the lifting of the sternum is so pronounced that the hold on the heels prevents the chest from flying up. An alternate way to release the Camel is to simply lower the buttocks onto the legs, coming into a kneeling posture, and then flowing into Child.

WHEEL

(Chakrasana)

1. Lie on your back with the legs extended. Reach the arms overhead on the floor, and stretch your body to its full length using the support of the floor.

2. Bring the arms to the sides. Bend the knees, bringing the feet close to the buttocks, hip-width apart, and come into Bridge. Pause for a moment to breathe freely and let the body adjust to the posture.

3. Work into your full expression of Bridge, lifting the hips high. You may want to reach down to clasp the ankles. Press into the feet, lift the hips, and use the handhold to pull the ankles, lifting the sternum toward the chin. Pause and breathe deeply as the body adjusts to this position.

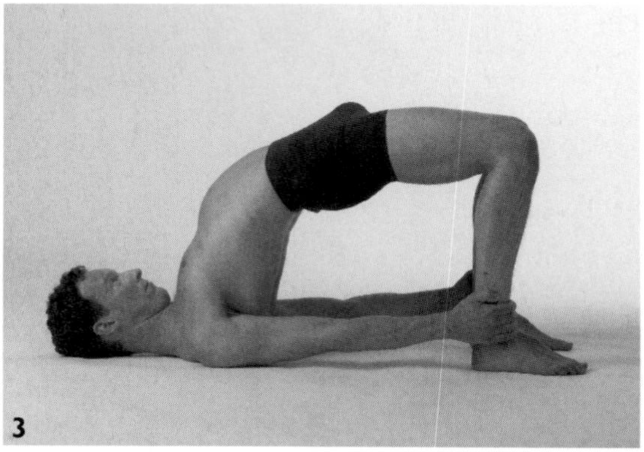

3

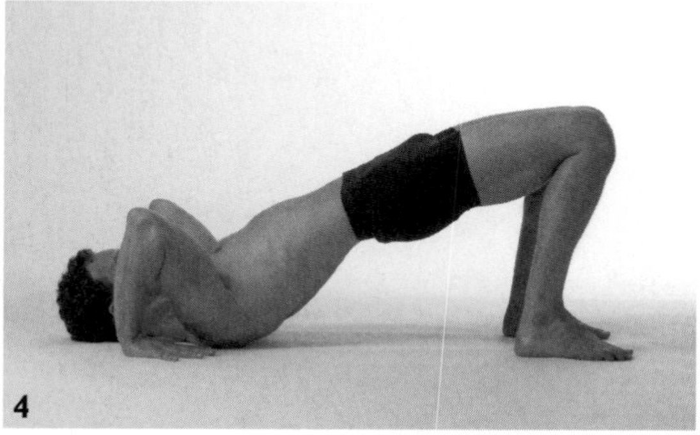

4

4. Bring the hands to rest palms down near the tops of the shoulders, elbows lifted and fingers pointing toward the feet. Spread the fingers wide.

5. Inhale and press into the roots of the fingers, straightening the arms and lifting the head off the floor. Lift the hips high and press the sternum toward the ceiling. Breathe deeply as you hold.

6. To release, take a deep breath in. As you exhale, slowly lower hips and buttocks to the floor. Bring the knees into the chest and gently rock from side to side to release the low back. Relax in Corpse Pose before moving on to the next posture.

Be Aware:
Wheel is the culmination of the backbends. It requires both the upper body strength needed to lift the torso off the floor and flexibility throughout the entire spinal column, particularly in the upper chest and back. Wheel is not to be practiced if you have low back sensitivity.

Steps 1–3 guide you into an advanced version of the Bridge. The ankle handhold helps you lift the sternum and bring the backward bend into the upper chest and back. This is necessary preparation, as attempting Wheel without upper spine flexibility is likely to overstretch the low back. Practice this Bridge variation for several weeks before moving on to the Wheel.

Although Wheel is a vigorous posture, work to isolate the effort, relaxing everything that is not essential to holding the hips and chest high. Let the breath flow and tension melt from the entire body. After releasing Wheel, you will find your entire body refreshed and exhilarated.

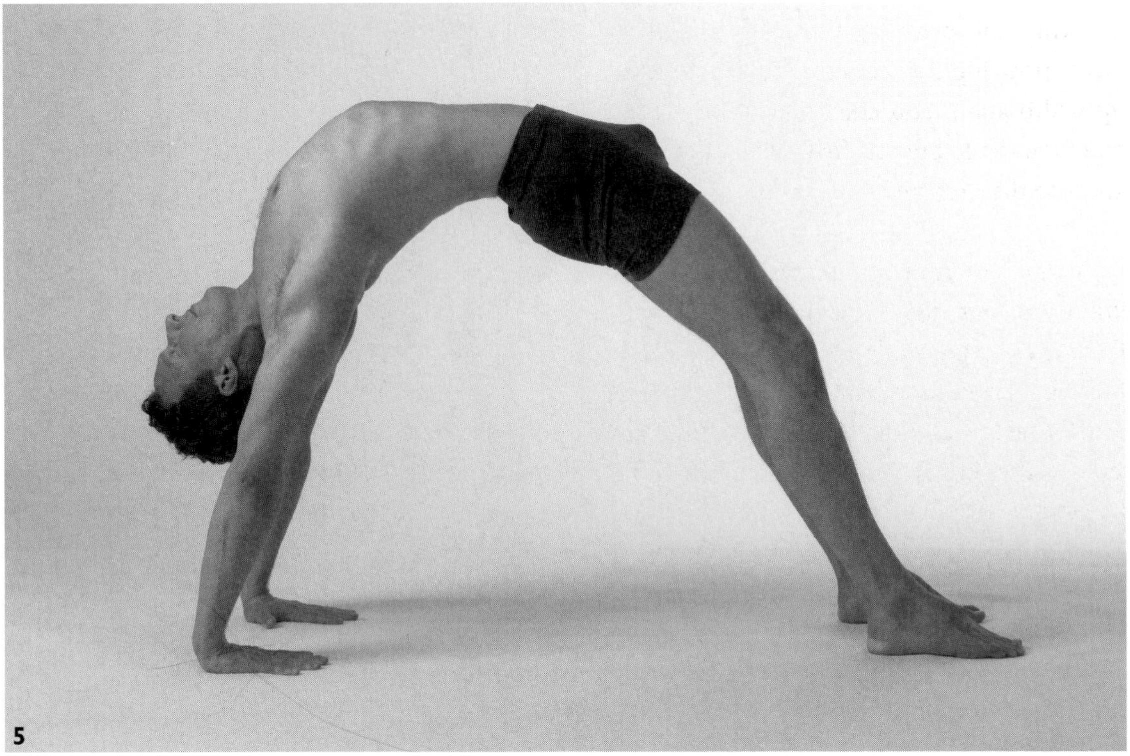

5

FORWARD BENDS

PYRAMID AND ROTATED PYRAMID

1. Step the feet as wide apart as your legs are long. Press into all four corners of the feet to engage the legs. Stabilize the core and elongate the spine. Bring the hands to rest on the thighs.

2. Take a deep breath in. As you exhale, lift the tailbone and hinge at the hips, coming forward with a straight spine, sliding the hands down the legs. Bend the knees as needed to avoid strain.

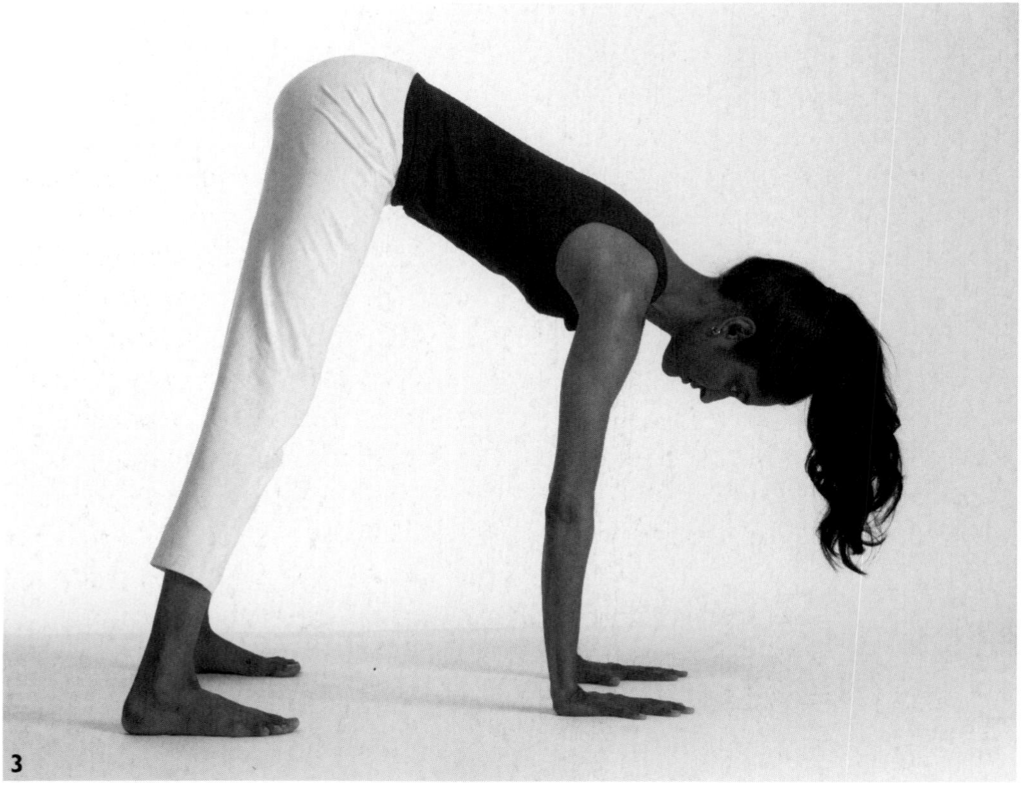

Let the breath flow freely as your body adjusts to this position.

3. Rock your body weight forward and reach the hands onto the floor about twenty-four inches in front of the toes. Continue to rock a few times forward and back, adjusting the position of the hands by feel until the weight is equally supported by hands and feet. The hands are directly under the shoulders. Spread the fingers wide and press down into the hands. Press the buttocks toward the wall behind you, opening the cheeks. Extend through the crown, focusing the gaze at a point on the floor slightly in front of the hands. This is Pyramid. Breathe deeply as you hold.

4. To come into the Rotated Pyramid, lift the left hand off the floor and place it on the outside of the right hand. Spread the fingers wide and press the left hand firmly into the floor. Exhale and sweep the right hand toward the ceiling, twisting the spine and opening the right shoulder joint. The eyes follow the movement of the right hand, eventually gazing at the raised hand. Breathe deeply as you hold.

5. Lower the right arm on an inhalation, returning to Pyramid. Lift the right hand off the floor, place it on the outside of the left hand, and come into Rotated Pyramid on the left side.

6. To release, return to Pyramid. Walk the hands back to the feet. Soften the knees and lift the torso back to vertical. Step the feet hip-width apart.

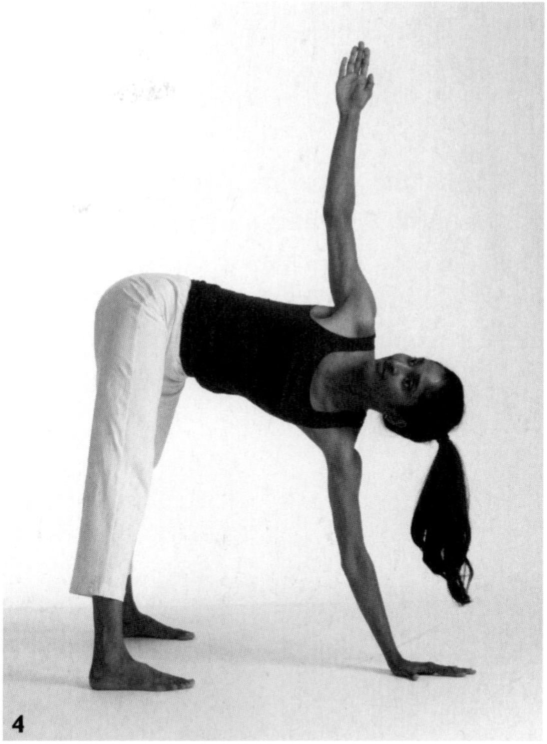

4

Be Aware:

Although they may appear similar, Pyramid and Downward Dog are very different postures. With the weight equally distributed between hands and feet, and the hands positioned directly under the shoulders, Pyramid is a very steady pose. Some yoga teachers describe the stretch that results from pressing the buttocks back as *opening the book of the buttocks.* Rotated Pyramid is a great preparatory posture for the Rotated Triangle. If you feel any tension in the low back, bend the knees before rotating the arm into the twist.

YOGA MUDRA

(Symbol of Yoga)

1. Come into a kneeling position, knees and ankles touching, palms resting on the thighs. Press the sitz bones down, the sternum forward, and extend through the crown. Inhale and lift the arms in front of you to shoulder height, pressing out through the fingertips to lengthen the arms.

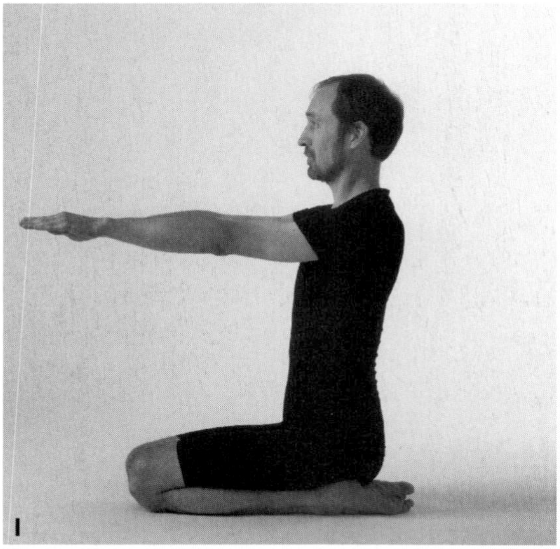

1

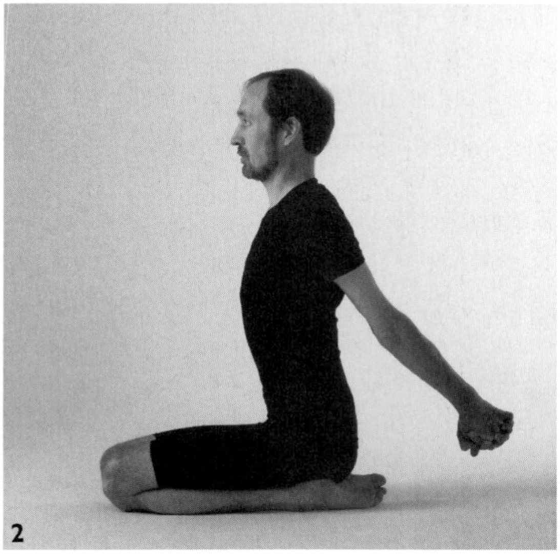

2

2. Exhale and circle the arms out to the sides and behind your back. Interlace the fingers and squeeze the palms together. Press the knuckles down and back to straighten the arms and draw the shoulder blades together. Press the sternum forward to open the chest.

3. Take a deep breath in. As you exhale, lift the tailbone and begin to hinge at the hips. Come forward with a straight spine, extending the torso over the thighs and knees. Continue to hinge at the hips, bringing the forehead to the floor. Press the knuckles toward the ceiling and the back of the hands toward the floor in front of you.

4. Breathe deeply as you hold.

5. To release, inhale and press the knuckles back, engaging the hips to bring the torso back to vertical. Release the hands and let them circle back in front of you, slowly lowering them to the knees.

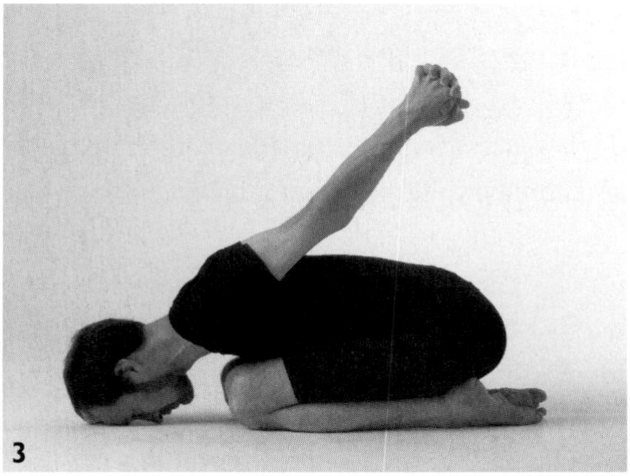

3

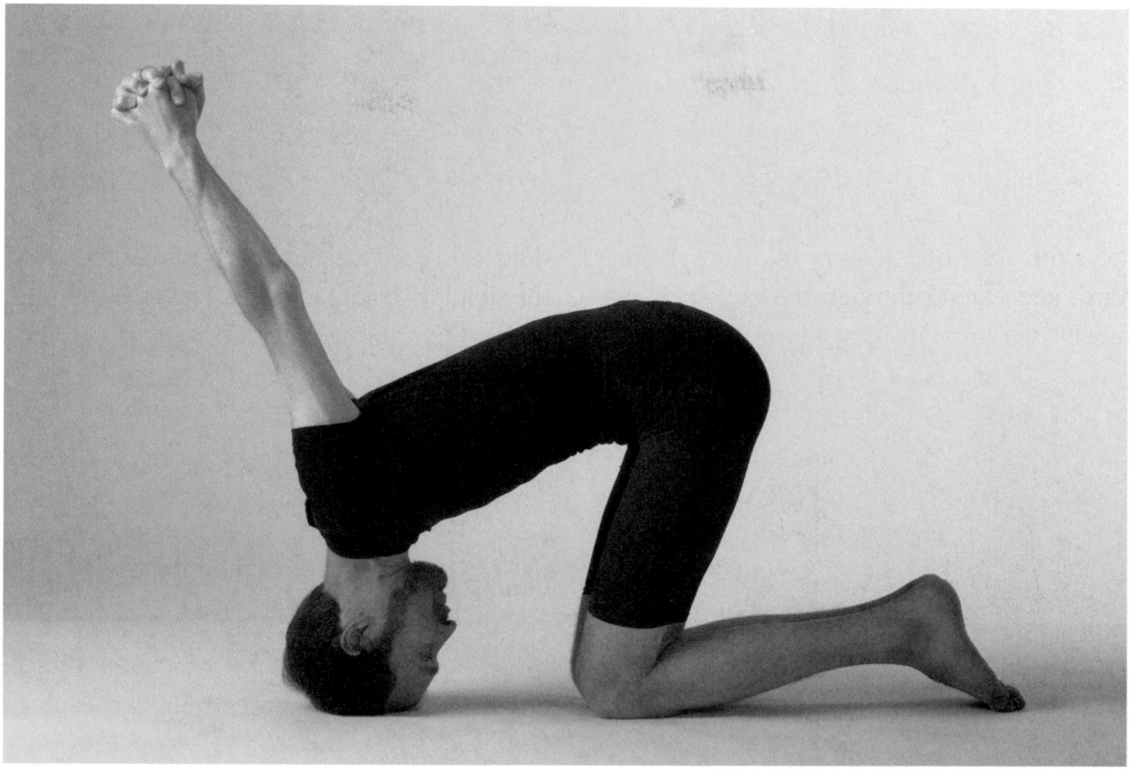

Be Aware:

The word *mudra* means *gesture,* and Yoga Mudra is a gesture of surrender in which you place the head below the heart. This posture is traditionally practiced slowly with great sensitivity to feeling, as a meditation on the need to accept life on its own terms.

If you want more challenge, come into the posture as above with forehead resting on the floor. Then in slow motion roll from the forehead onto the crown of the head, pressing the arms forward. A small portion of the weight of the upper body will come onto the crown of the head, and the buttocks will lift off the heels. Most of your body weight will remain on the knees and shins. Move slowly and gently so as to stretch but not strain the neck. Gently roll back down into the basic posture and release as described above.

CHIN TO KNEE

(Janu Shirshasana)

1. Sit with the legs extended. Bend the left leg and cross it over the right knee, positioning the left heel near the right hip. Square the hips to face forward. Rest the hands on the knee.

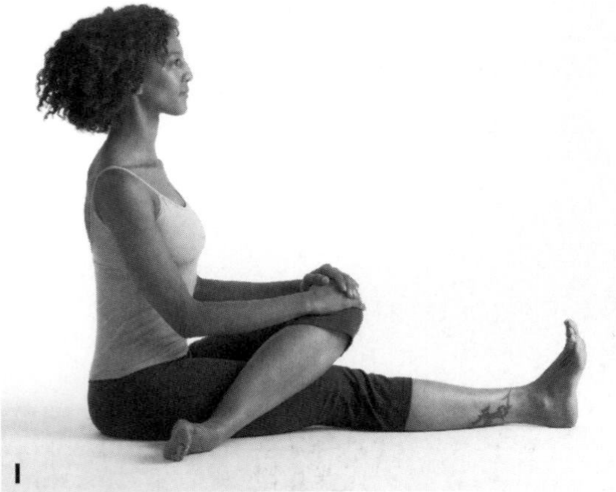

1

2. Press the sitz bones and both knees into the floor. Lift out of the waist, extend through the crown, and flex the right foot to engage the leg muscles.

3. Inhale and lift the arms overhead, shoulder-width and palms facing. Extend through the fingertips to further elongate the spine. Exhale and relax the top of the shoulders away from the ears.

4. Take a deep breath in. As you exhale, lift the tailbone and hinge forward, coming to your full forward extension with a straight spine.

5. Continue to extend through the crown, lowering the hands to rest on the shins or feet.

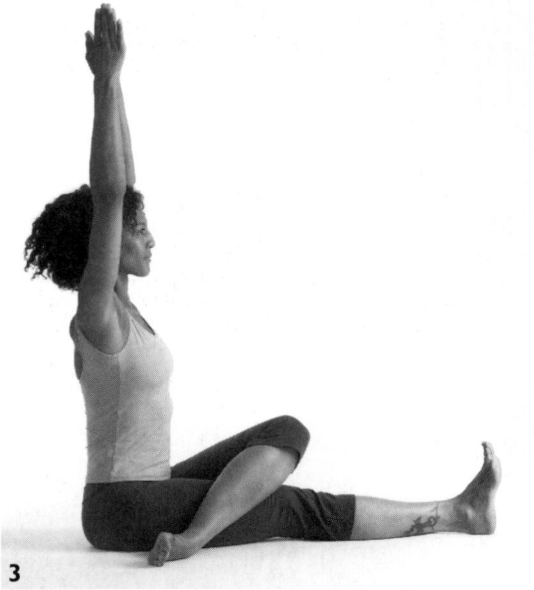

3

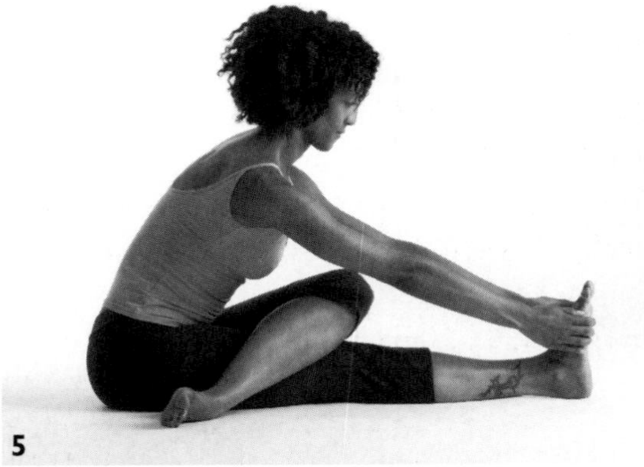

5

6. To release, bring the hands to palms down on either side of the extended leg. Rotate the hip joints to bring the torso back to vertical, hands sliding along the floor.

7. Cross the right knee over the left leg, and repeat on the opposite side.

Be Aware:

Chin to Knee provides a similar stretch to Great Seal, noticeably intensified by the crossed position of the knee. The same principles of alignment apply to both postures. If coming down with the arms overhead is a strain, slide the hands along the floor as you rotate the hips and come forward with a straight spine. As traditionally taught, the upper spine rounds and the chin rests just over the bent knee, which is where the posture gets its name.

SEATED ANGLE

(Upavistha Konasana)

1. Sit with the legs extended. Spread the legs wide apart and walk the hips forward to come to your maximum split. Bring the palms to rest on the floor in front of you. Press the sitz bones down, sternum forward, and extend through the crown. Press the heels away and flex the feet to engage the legs.

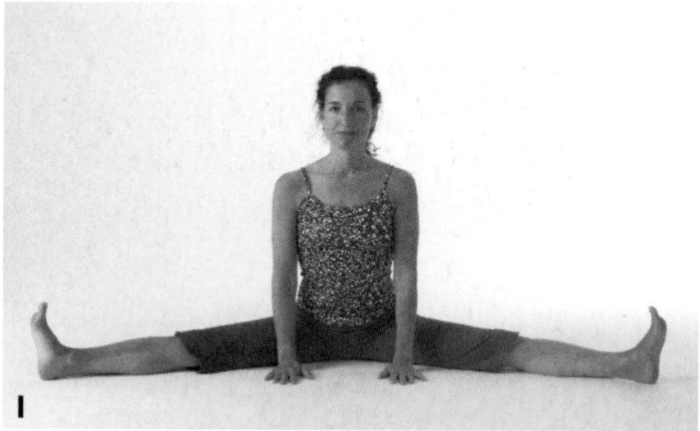

1

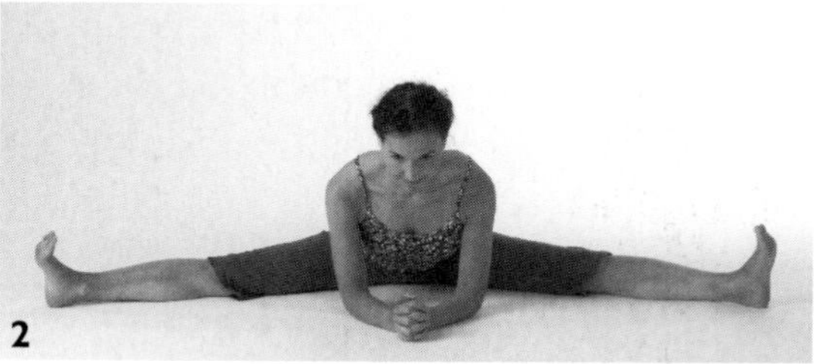

2

2. Take a deep breath in. As you exhale, lift the tailbone and begin to slowly hinge from the hips. Slide the hands as you come forward with the spine elongated. Move into the stretch gradually, stopping to breathe, relax, and feel at places of resistance or tightness. You should feel the stretch in the legs, hips, and pelvis versus the low back. Come down onto your forearms.

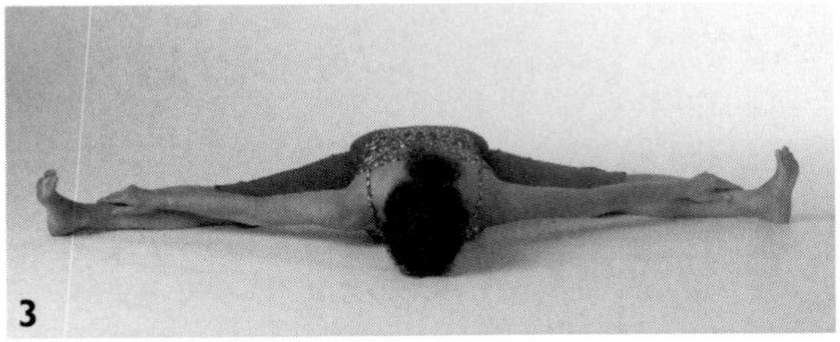

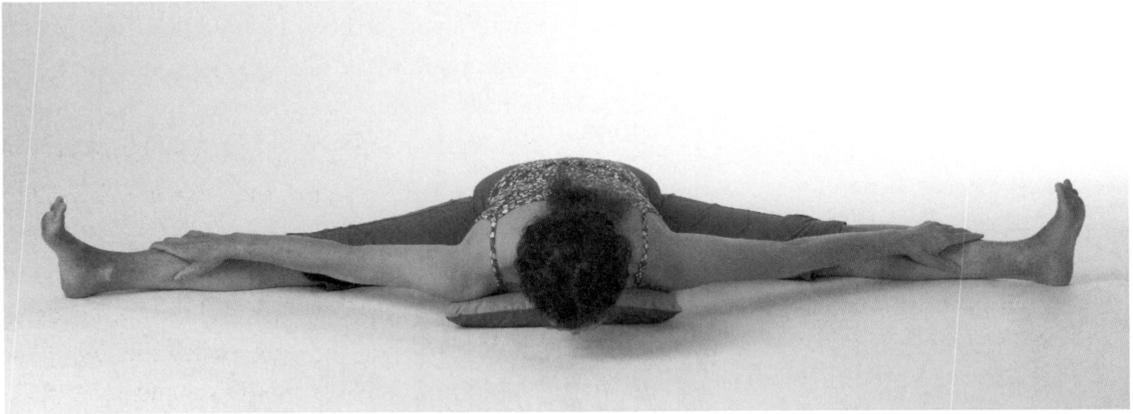

3. If you want more stretch, come to your full forward extension with a straight spine by rotating the hips and extending through the crown. If possible, reach the arms out to clasp the feet and allow the forehead and chest to rest on the floor. Breathe deeply as you hold.

4. To release, inhale and engage the hips to bring the torso back to vertical. As you come up, slide the hands along the floor, or walk the hands toward your body. Lean back and bring the legs together.

Be Aware:

Seated Angle is the culmination of the forward bending postures. With the legs rotated out to the sides, the torso is free to come forward to its maximum forward extension. Care must be taken to avoid rounding the spine, which can compress the lumbar vertebra. Elongate the spine and hinging at the hips to come forward with a straight spine. Press the hands into the floor to provide needed support to keep the spine from rounding. Emphasize long, slow exhalations that squeeze out residual air.

Move on to step 3 only after the regular practice of preparatory postures such as Standing Angle, Side Warrior, Great Seal, Posterior Stretch, and Frog. At first you may want to place one or more pillows on the floor in front of you. This will allow you to come partially into the posture, yet experience the relaxation that results when you can rest the chest and forehead on the floor.

TWISTS

HALF LOTUS TWIST

(Ardha Padmasasana)

1. Sit with the legs extended in a V. Bend the left knee and draw the sole of the left foot against the inside of the right thigh. Bend the right knee and draw the right foot close to the left foot. Use the hands to place the right foot on the left thigh. This is Half Lotus.

2. Press the sitz bones down. Elongate the spine by lifting out of the waist and extending through the crown.

3. Turn to look over the right shoulder, twisting the spine to the right. Reach the right hand behind the back to grasp the right foot, pinky near the ankle and thumb near the toes. Bring the left hand to rest on the right knee. This is Half Lotus Twist.

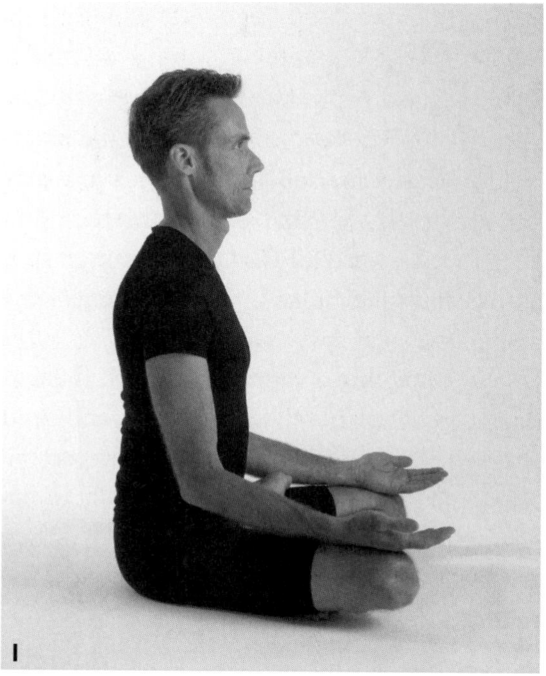
1

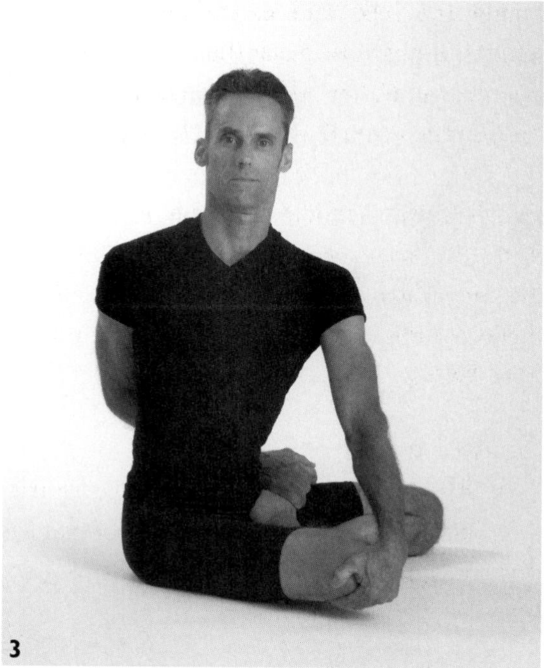
3

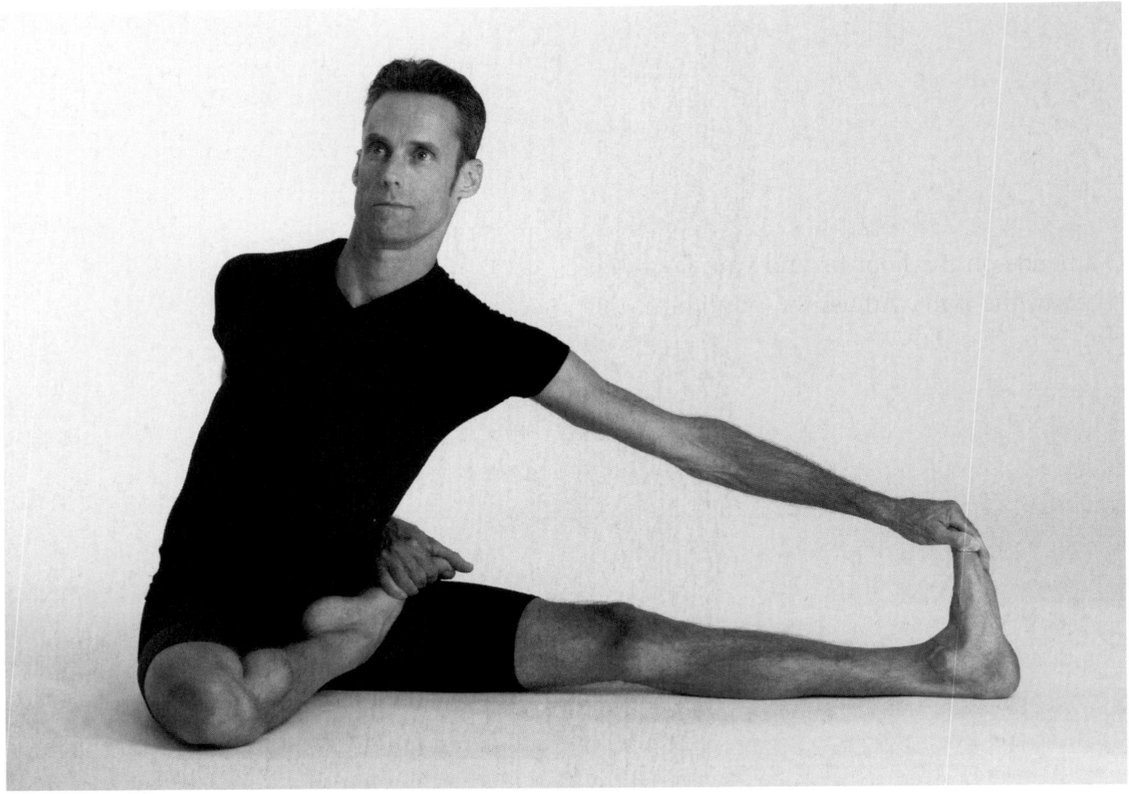

4. Continue pressing the sitz bones down and elongating the spine by lifting out of the waist and extending through the crown. Rotate the spine from bottom to top, eyes looking right. Breathe deeply as you hold.

5. To release, carefully uncross and extend the legs. Repeat on the opposite side.

Be Aware:

More detailed instructions to enter Half Lotus appear on page 399. To accomplish the hand-hold essential to Half Lotus Twist, you may have to reach the hand behind the back and then lean the torso forward. Once your grasp is secure, return the torso to vertical, elongate the spine, and come fully into the twist.

To come into a variation, sit with the legs extended. Keep the left leg extended, and bend the right knee to bring the right foot onto the left thigh in Half Lotus position. Follow the above instructions to grasp the foot. Then reach the other hand to hold the toes of the extended foot.

FOLDED LEG TWIST

(Matsyendrasana)

1. Sit with the knees bent, feet on the floor in front of you a little wider than hip-width apart, and hands on the floor behind you. Rock the knees to the right. Adjust the position of the feet so the left knee rests against the sole of the right foot. Press the right hip and both knees into the floor. Press the sternum forward to open the chest.

2. Sweep the left hand up and overhead, pressing the fingertips toward the ceiling to elongate the spine as the arm arcs overhead.

3. Bring the arm all the way down to rest on the floor, shoulder-width apart from the right hand. Press the hands into the floor and extend through the crown to further elongate the spine. Walk the hands to the right, twisting the spine, rotating the shoulders, and turning the head to the right. Breathe deeply as you hold.

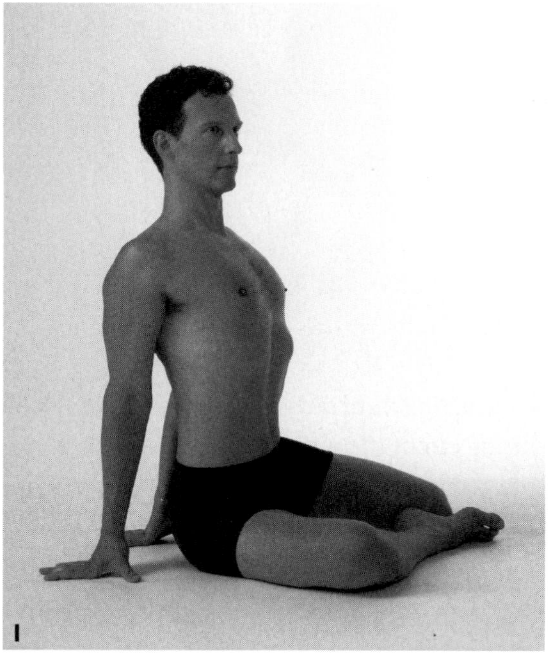

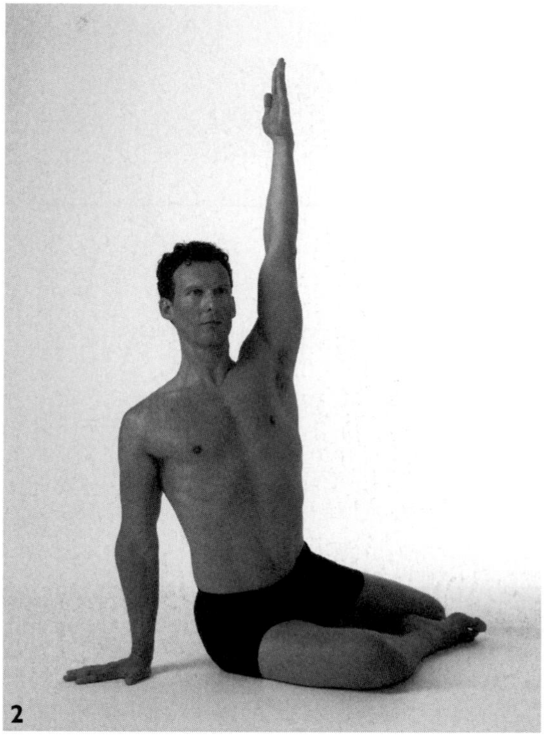

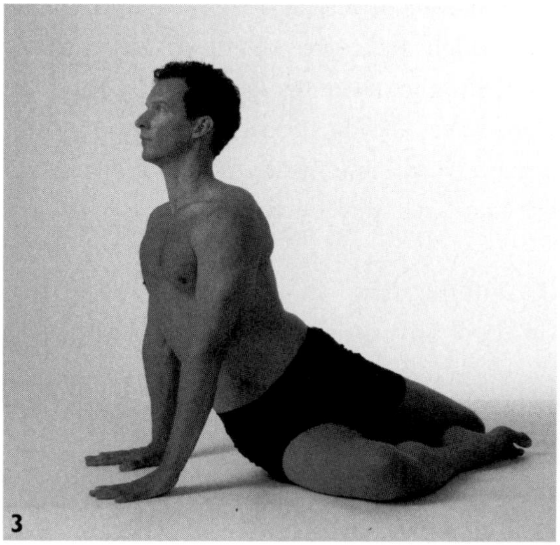

4. To release, walk the hands to the left, coming out of a full twist. Inhale and arc the left hand overhead and return to the starting position.

5. Rock the knees to the left, and repeat on the opposite side.

Be Aware:
Most twists elongate the spine from a vertical torso position. Folded Leg Twist provides a refreshing spinal twist from an angled position. Spinal elongation is accomplished through the press of one hip, both knees, and the hands into the floor. Some find that Folded Leg Twist provides a deeper release of the hips, shoulders, and neck than other spinal twists.

SEATED SPINAL TWIST

(Ardha Matsyendrasana)

1. Sit with the legs extended and hands resting on the floor at your sides. Press down through the sitz bones and extend through the crown of the head to elongate the spine.

2. Bend the left knee and bring the sole of the left foot to rest against the inside of the right thigh. Relax the muscles of the bent left leg, letting the knee rest on the floor. Bend the right knee, sliding the right foot up close to the body and interlacing the fingers around the knee.

3

3. Lift the right foot off the floor and place it on the floor outside the left knee. Allow the weight to rest evenly on both sitz bones. Use your hand strength to pull the sternum toward the knee, and elongate the spine by pressing down through the sitz bones, gently contracting the muscles of the pelvic floor, lifting out of the waist, and extending through the crown.

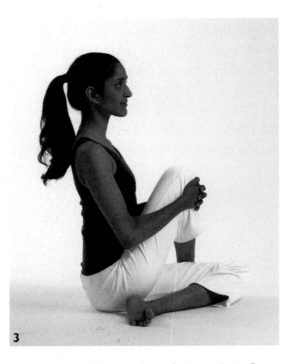

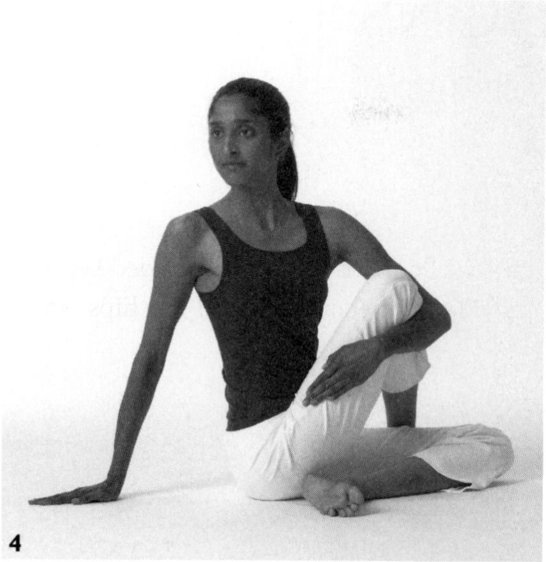

4

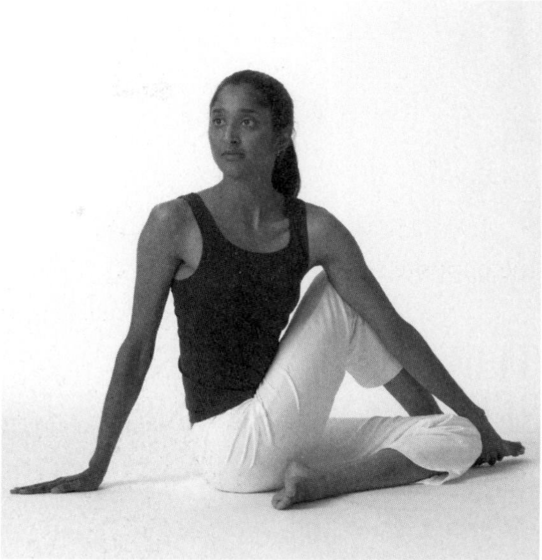

4. Wrap the left elbow around the right knee, placing the left hand on the outside of the right thigh. Raise the right arm up to shoulder height. Inhale and sweep the right arm to the right, following the movement of the hand with your gaze and twisting the spine. When you have twisted fully, lower the right palm to the floor behind you. Breathe deeply as you hold.

5. To release, lift the right arm back to shoulder height. Inhale and sweep the right hand back to center. Lower the right hand to the ground, and straighten both legs.

6. Repeat on the opposite side.

Be Aware:

Except for the leg position, this posture is identical to the Straight Legged Spinal Twist taught in Sun Series. Folding both legs provides a noticeably deeper twist and hip stretch. If you cannot wrap the elbow around the raised knee, simply hold the raised knee with the opposite hand. Once you have come fully into the twist, you may want to enhance the stretch by adjusting your arm position to hold the raised knee in the crook of the arm. If you want more stretch, come into the posture as described above, then reach the left arm down the outside of the right leg, hand clasping the foot.

INVERSIONS

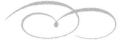

THREE-QUARTERS SHOULDERSTAND AND FISH

(Sarvangasana and Matsyasana)

1. Come into Half Shoulderstand. Let your breath flow as the body adjusts to this position.

2. Inhale and press the hips and pelvis forward, sliding the hands up to the mid-back. As the hands slide up, press the feet toward the ceiling to straighten the torso. Find a comfortable position in which you can hold, maintaining a slight angle between the legs and torso.

3. Adjust the hands so the thumbs grasp the outside of the ribs and pinkies are close to the spine. Let the majority of your body weight be supported by the elbows and shoulders, with no more than nominal weight on the back of the neck. Breathe deeply and hold in stillness, or explore slow motion micromovements with the legs.

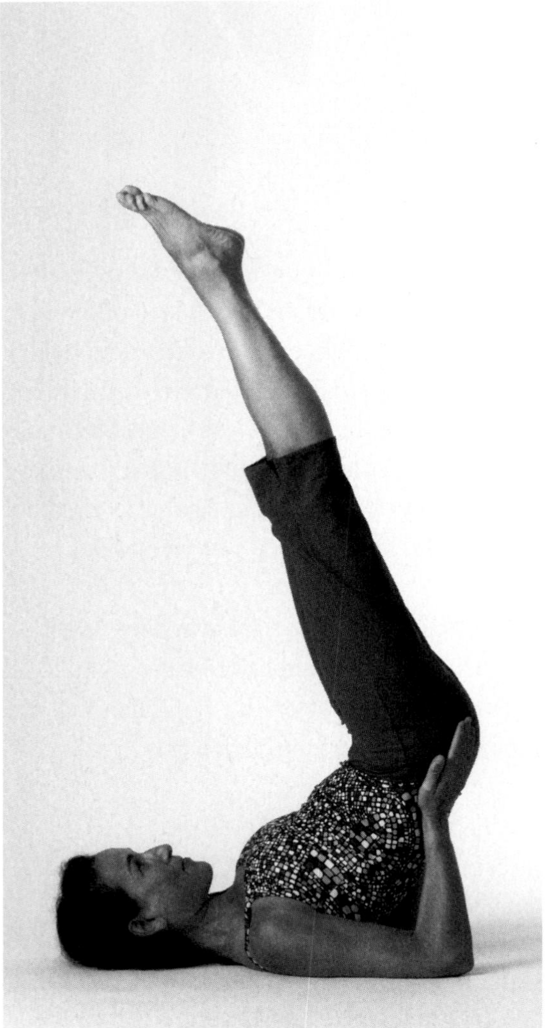

1

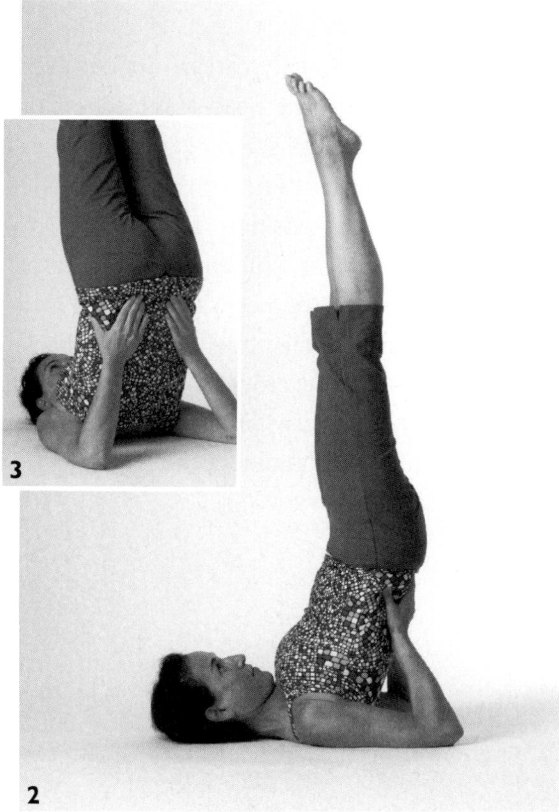
3

2

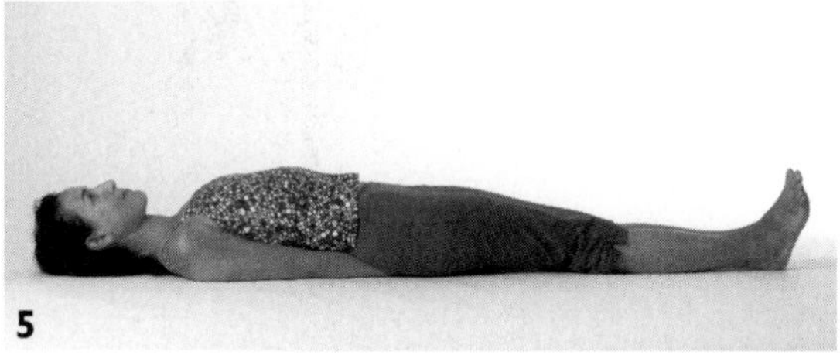
5

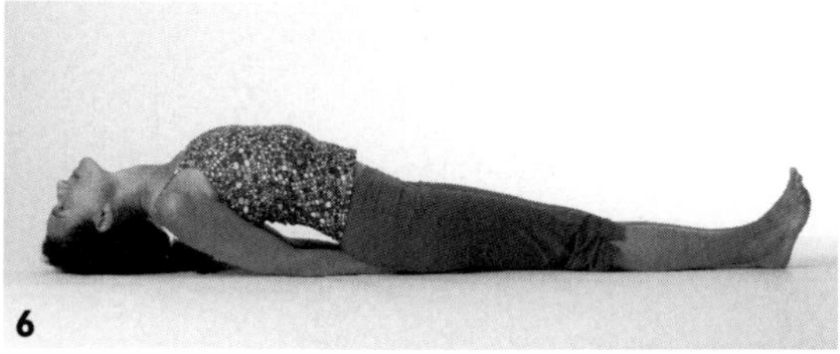
6

4. To release, slide the hands back down to the hips, returning to Half Shoulderstand. Take a deep breath in and out. Lower the knees to the chest, and let the hands slide across the buttocks as you gently roll out of the posture vertebra by vertebra, returning the legs to the floor. Rock the head gently from side to side to relax the muscles of the neck. Breathe, relax, and feel.

5. To come into Fish, walk the arms underneath the body. Reach the hands down as low as you can, and bring the elbows as close together as possible. The palms are flat on the floor with the thumbs touching. Touch the feet together, and press out through the heels to lengthen the legs.

6. Inhale and press the sitz bones and elbows into the floor. Lift the sternum toward the ceiling, arching the back and sliding the head along the floor until the upper back of the head—not the crown—rests on the floor. Keep the back of the neck long by slightly tucking the chin. The sitz bones and elbows support your body weight. Only the weight of the head is supported by the neck. Breathe deeply as you hold.

7. To release, press the elbows and sitz bones into the floor and gently slide the back of the head onto the floor. Bring the arms out from under the body to rest, palms up at your sides. Rock the head gently from side to side to relax the muscles of the neck. Breathe, relax, and feel.

Be Aware:

The classic Shoulderstand brings the torso and legs directly above the shoulders. While this provides a full inversion, it also brings significant weight to bear on the delicate cervical vertebrae, which presents a risk of injury, especially with long-term practice. In this variation, a slight angle is maintained between the legs and torso. This provides a powerful inversion, yet distributes the weight across a larger area, protecting the upper spine and neck.

Fish is the traditional complementary posture to Shoulderstand. Where the Shoulderstand brings the chin into the throat and lengthens the back of the neck, the Fish opens the throat and reverses the neck stretch. Where Shoulderstand applies a gentle pressure to the thyroid and parathyroid glands, Fish releases this pressure and allows maximum blood flow to these glands.

In Fish, be especially careful not to place excessive weight on the head and neck. Emphasize the press of the sitz bones and elbows, and the lift of the sternum, both of which slide the head into proper position. This "sliding" or "dragging" movement utilizes the support of the floor to protect the neck as it comes into proper position with the upper part of the back of the head—not the crown—resting on the floor. Practiced properly, Fish is beneficial for the neck and helps counteract the tendency to round the shoulders.

SITTING POSES

THUNDERBOLT

(Vajrasana)

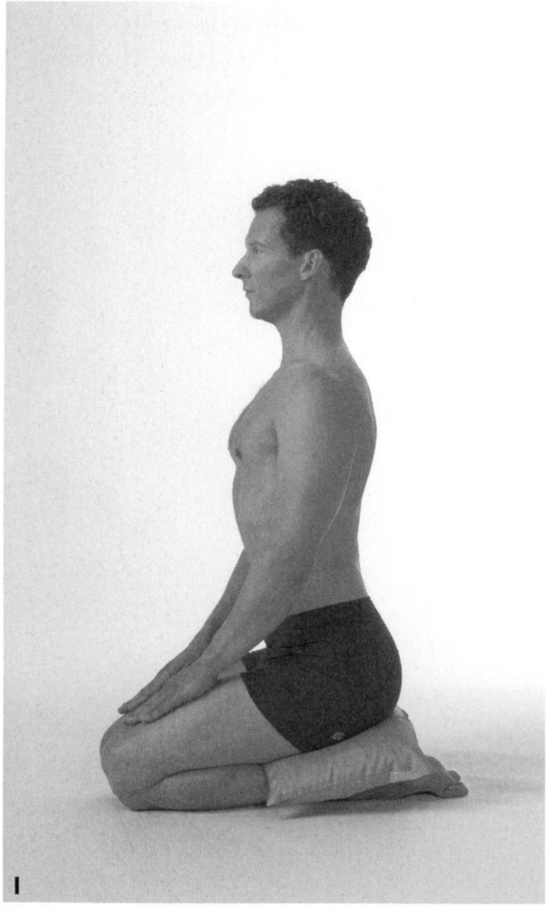

1

1. Sit on the heels in a kneeling posture. Adjust your position so each buttock rests squarely on a heel. Rest the hands palms down on the knees. Press the sitz bones down. Elongate the spine by lifting out of the waist and extending through the crown. Roll the shoulders back and down. Bring the chin parallel to the floor.

Be Aware:

Thunderbolt is a naturally erect sitting posture conducive to the practice of breathing exercises and meditation. If you experience discomfort in the knees, sit on a thick cushion, which reduces the bend required in the knees. If your calves feel pinched, lean forward and use the hands to roll the calf muscles outward, then sit back down. Once you get comfortable, holding Thunderbolt reinvigorates the feet, knees, and legs.

ADEPT'S POSE

(Siddhasasana)

1. Sit on the edge of a cushion or folded blanket with the legs extended in a V.

2. Bend the left knee and draw the sole of the left foot against the inside of the right thigh, heel just to the right of the pubic bone. The ankle is roughly centered at the midline of the body.

3. Bend the right knee and draw the right foot close to the left foot. Slide the last four toes of the right foot in between the left thigh and calf. The big toe remains visible and the ankles rest one on top of the other.

4. Rest the hands palms up on the knees. Press the sitz bones down. Elongate the spine by lifting out of the waist and extending through the crown. Roll the shoulders back and down. Bring the chin parallel to the floor.

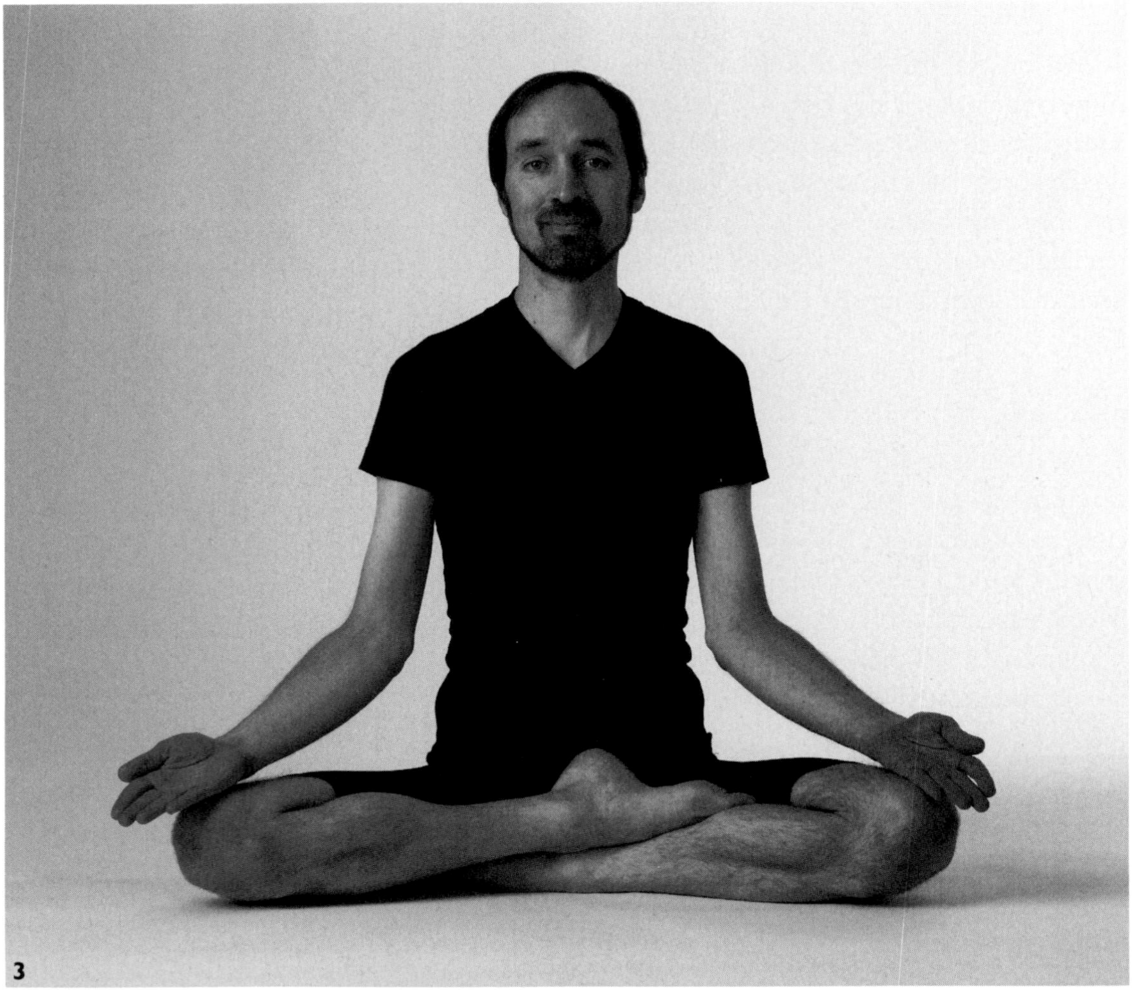

3

5. To release, carefully uncross and extend the legs.

Be Aware:
In Adept's Pose, the feet are placed in a position that over time becomes quite comfortable. The ability to sit comfortably relaxed and still is invaluable for the practice of meditation.In the classic Adept's Pose, the heel of the lower foot presses against the perineum. Pressure on this sensitive area of the body has the potential to cause nerve and vascular damage for men. In this variation, the heel rests just to the side of the pubic bone.

HALF LOTUS

(Ardha Padmasasana)

1. Sit on the edge of a cushion or folded blanket with the legs extended in a V.

2. Bend the left knee and draw the sole of the left foot against the inside of the right thigh, heel just to the right of the pubic bone. The ankle is roughly centered at the midline of the body. Bend the right knee and draw the right foot close to the left foot.

3. Bring your right hand to hold the outside of the right knee, and your left hand to hold the top of the right foot. Lift the knee and foot to place the top of the right foot on the left thigh, and lower the right knee to the floor.

4. Rest the hands palms up on the knees. Press the sitz bones down. Elongate the spine by lifting out of the waist and extending through the crown. Roll the shoulders back and down. Bring the chin parallel to the floor.

5. To release, carefully uncross and extend the legs.

Be Aware:
Half Lotus is another ideal posture for breathing exercises and meditation. Step 3 details the proper way to lift then place the knee and foot. Follow these instructions to avoid torqueing and potentially straining the knee.

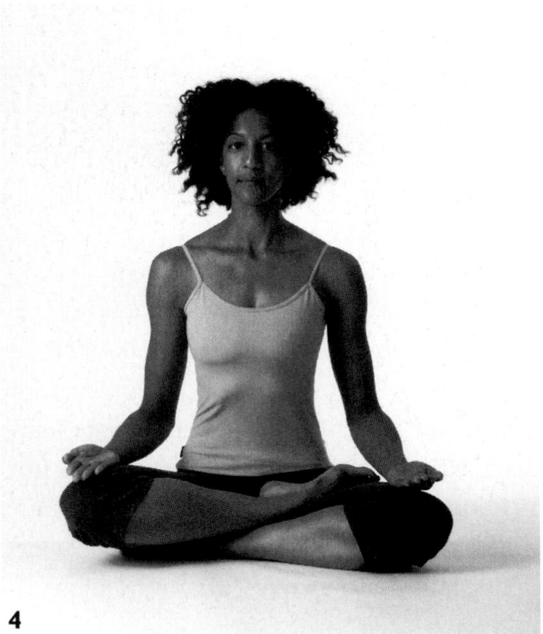

4

In Full Lotus, the feet rest on opposite thighs. Lotus requires a high degree of hip and leg flexibility. It is not uncommon for zealous yoga enthusiasts to seriously injure their knees by forcing into Lotus. If you want to learn the Lotus, master the hip-opening postures and seek the help of a qualified yoga teacher.

HERO

(Virasana)

1. Come into Table Pose. Cross the right knee over the left, splay the feet out to the sides.

2. Carefully sit back between the heels. Make any minor adjustments required for the weight to rest evenly on both sitz bones. Rest the hands on the opposite feet. Elongate the spine, press the sternum forward, and bring the chin parallel to the floor.

3. To release, bring the hands onto the floor in front of you and press back up to Table. Carefully uncross the legs, and repeat on opposite side.

Be Aware:
Hero is also called the "Seat of Tranquility" because of its ability to energetically balance the body. Hands rest on opposite feet, integrating upper and lower, and right and left sides. Given its intensive leg and hip stretch, a feeling of tranquility in this pose may initially seem unlikely. With regular practice it soon becomes a posture conducive to rest and meditation.

1

2

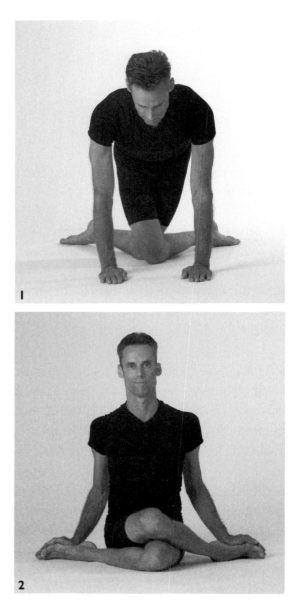

BLESSING

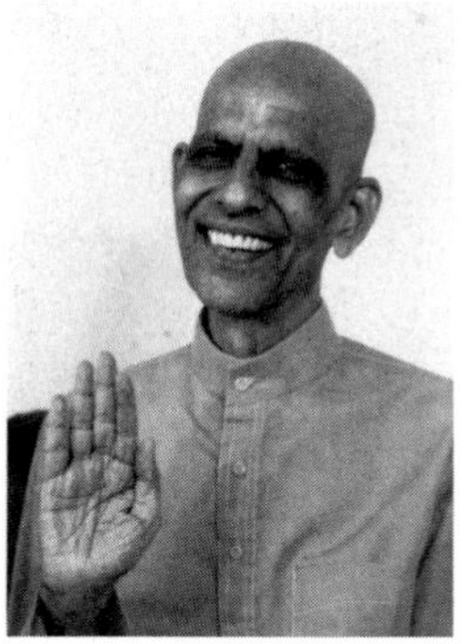

Swami Kripalu always concluded his public talks with the following prayer:

May everyone here be happy and healthy.

May everyone here be prosperous.

May no one be the least little bit unhappy at all.

My auspicious blessing to you all.

It is only fitting to end this book by wishing you well in that same spirit.

BIBLIOGRAPHY AND RESOURCE LIST

Books

Benson, Herbert. *The Relaxation Response*. Rev. ed. New York: HarperCollins, 2000.

Berner, H. C., ed. *Revealing the Secret: A Commentary on the Burning Lamp of Sun-Moon Yoga (Hathayoga Pradipika) by Swami Kripalu*. Merimbula, N.S.W.: H. C. Berner, 2002.

Cope, Stephen. *The Wisdom of Yoga: A Seeker's Guide to Extraordinary Living*. New York: Bantam Books, 2006.

———. *Yoga and the Quest for the True Self*. New York: Bantam Books, 1999.

Cope, Stephen, ed. *Will Yoga and Meditation Really Change My Life?* North Adams, Mass.: Storey Publishing, 2003.

David, Marc. *Nourishing Wisdom: A New Understanding of Eating*. New York: Bell Tower, 1991.

Devi, Nischala Joy. *The Healing Path of Yoga*. New York: Three Rivers Press, 2000.

Faulds, Danna. *Go In and In: Poems from the Heart of Yoga*. Greenville, Va.: Peaceable Kingdom Books, 2002.

———. *One Soul: More Poems from the Heart of Yoga*. Greenville, Va.: Peaceable Kingdom Books, 2003.

———. *Prayers to the Infinite: New Yoga Poems*. Greenville, Va.: Peaceable Kingdom Books, 2004.

Faulds, Richard, ed. *Sayings of Swami Kripalu: Inspiring Quotes from a Contemporary Yoga Master*. Greenville, Va.: Peaceable Kingdom Books, 2004.

Feuerstein, Georg. *The Yoga Tradition: Its History, Literature, Philosophy, and Practice*. Prescott, Ariz.: Hohm Press, 1998.

Jahnke, Roger. *The Healer Within: Using Traditional Chinese Techniques to Release Your Body's Own Medicine*. San Francisco: HarperSanFrancisco, 1997.

———. *The Healing Promise of Qi: Creating Extraordinary Wellness Through Qigong and Tai Chi*. Chicago: Contemporary Books, 2002.

Jerome, John. *Staying Supple: The Bountiful Pleasures of Stretching*. New York: Breakaway Books, 1998.

Lee, Michael. *Phoenix Rising Yoga Therapy: A Bridge from Body to Soul*. Deerfield Beach, Fla.: Health Communications, 1997.

———. *Turn Stress into Bliss: The Proven Eight-Week Program for Better Health, Relaxation, and Stress Relief*. Gloucester, Mass.: Fair Winds Press, 2005.

Levitt, Atma Jo Ann, ed. *Pilgrim of Love: The Life and Teachings of Swami Kripalu*. Rhinebeck, NY: Monkfish, 2004.

Migdow, Jeffrey, and James E. Loehr. *Breathe In, Breathe Out: Inhale Energy and Exhale Stress by Guiding and Controlling Your Breathing*. New York: Time-Life Books, 1999.

Muni, Swami Rajarshi. *Infinite Grace: The Story of My Spiritual Lineage*. Vadodara, India: Life Mission Publications, 2002.

———. *Yoga: The Ultimate Spiritual Path*. St. Paul, Minn.: Llewellyn Publications, 2001.

Ornish, Dean. *Dr. Dean Ornish's Program for Reversing Heart Disease*. New York: Ivy Books, 1995.

Pert, Candace. *Molecules of Emotion: Why You Feel the Way You Feel*. New York: Simon & Schuster, 1997.

Sarley, Dinabandhu, and Ila Sarley. *The Essentials of Yoga*. New York: Dell, 1999.

———. *Walking Yoga*. New York: Atria, 2002.

Schaeffer, Rachel. *Yoga for Your Spiritual Muscles: A Complete Yoga Program to Strengthen Body and Spirit*. Wheaton, Ill: Quest Books, 1998.

Stapleton, Don. *Self-Awakening Yoga: The Expansion of Consciousness Through the Body's Own Wisdom*. Rochester, Vt.: Healing Arts Press, 2004.

Weil, Andrew. *Spontaneous Healing: How to Discover and Embrace Your Body's Natural Ability to Maintain and Heal Itself*. New York: Ballantine Books, 2000.

Weintraub, Amy. *Yoga for Depression: A Compassionate Guide to Relieve Suffering Through Yoga*. New York: Broadway Books, 2004.

CDs and DVDs

Carroll, Yoganand Michael. *Pranayama: The Kripalu Approach to Yogic Breathing, Beginning Level Practice*. CD. Muddy Angel Studios, 2001.

———. *Pranayama: The Kripalu Approach to Yogic Breathing, Intermediate Level Practice.* CD. Muddy Angel Studios, 2001.

Cope, Stephen. *Kripalu Yoga Dynamic.* DVD or VHS. Kripalu Center, 1998.

———. *Yoga for Emotional Flow.* 2 CDs. Sounds True, 2003.

Foust, Sudhir Jonathan. *Art of Relaxation.* CD. Kripalu Center, 2001

———. *Energy Awareness Meditations.* 2 CDs. The Relaxation Company, 2003.

Green, Ann, and Todd Norian. *Partner Yoga.* DVD or VHS. Kripalu Center, 1999.

Kronlage, Rebekkah, *Kripalu Moderate Yoga.* CD. Kripalu Center, 2004.

Lundeen, Sudha Carolyn. *Kripalu Yoga Gentle.* DVD or VHS. Kripalu Center, 1998.

McRae, Sudhakar Ken. *Sadhana: The Daily Practice of Yoga,* vol. 1 & 2. CD. Peace of Mind Center for Yoga & Meditation, 1997 and 1999.

———. *Sadhana: The Daily Practice of Meditation.* CD. Peace of Mind Center for Yoga & Meditation, 2000.

Peirce, Rudy. *Gentle Series.* 4 CDs. Yoga for Body, Mind, and Soul, 1997.

Weintraub, Amy. *Breathe to Beat the Blues.* CD. Yoga to Beat the Blues, 2003.

ACKNOWLEDGMENTS

Kripalu Yoga took birth in a volunteer community that spanned three decades and inspired members to selfless service and the co-creation of a shared work. As a result, a great multitude of people from Kripalu's past, some directly and others indirectly, contributed in important ways to the creation of this book. While honoring past contributions, it is important to acknowledge the individuals currently moving Kripalu Yoga into the future. This is an attempt to do both.

One group that deserves special credit is the ashram's teaching faculty. For many years, this creative powerhouse went largely unrecognized due to a shared ethic of not serving from a place of ego and the ashram custom of attributing all teachings to the guru. Not only did these individuals source a potent body of transformative teachings, a portion of which appear in this book, they also touched and transformed the lives of thousands. Most people closely associated with the ashram received and used a Sanskrit name. For greatest name recognition, both Sanskrit and English names appear below, with the proviso that only a minority continue to use the names they were known by in the ashram. Special thanks to:

Shivanand Thomas Amelio, Kiara Kate Andrews, Snehadip Doug Anzalone, Ketul Wayne Arnold, Umesh Eric Baldwin, Vasanti Lenore Baldwin, Devanand Christopher Baxter, Jhanvi Sara Berg, Preksha Deborah Binder, Rajiv Jordan Blank, Vasudev Daniel Bowling, Balbhadra Kim Brady, Rupkumar Carlos Bulnes, Rupa Erin Burch, Megha Nancy Buttenheim, Anandi Susan Camp, Anamika Coleman, Rameshvari Fern Corbett, Kapil Bruce Cornwall, Nina Dawe, Vidya Carolyn Dell'uomo, Shankari Michelle Deschamps, Praphul Paul Deslauriers, Paritosh

Coldon DeWeese, Rambha Susan DeWeese, Chidanand Ron Dushkin, Varsha Barbara Edison, Karuna Laighne Fanney, Asita Deidre Fay, Jyoti Kate Feldman, Taponidhi Joel Feldman, Puja Sue Flamm, Deb Foss, Ganga Alison Gaines, Vihari Michael Gamble, Vinai Tom Gillette, Shobhana Constance Goldberg, Angira Ann Greene, Sumitra Joyce Hammond, Kunti Kathy Jackman, Anuradha Linda Jackson, Baladev Mike Karpfen, Malti Patricia Karpfen, Atmadev Michael Keane, Kiran Steven Keith, Ulka Melissa Keith, Arti Karen Ross-Kelso, Hansaraj Mark Kelso, Naresh Ron King, Nisharani Melanie Armstrong King, Nataraj Dan Leven, Atma Jo Ann Levitt, Narendra Kent Lew, Dashrath Endel Maadik, Menka Donna MacLeod, Sudhakar Ken McRae, Sanat Kumar Steve Marshall, Jutta Martin, Ramadevi Frances Mellon, Ramakrishna Peter Mellon, Durga Renee Mendez, Vivekenand Richard Michaels, Prabhakar Jeff Migdow, Ragunandan David Milam, Swati Laurie Moon, Suketa Susan Moore, Bhavani Lorraine Nelson, Jayadayal Dean Niles, Manu Todd Norian, Nijanand Will Nuessle, Savita Char Nuessle, Latika Janice O'Neill, Amarish Michael Orlando, Vasudha Joyce Orr, Lila Osterman, Devakanya Deva Parnell, Indrakshi Joyce Peirce, Navanit Russ Poole, Pandavi Anna Poole, Vandana Heidi Pramhas, Bhumi Harriet Russell, Dayashakti Sandra Scherer, Vrajmala Peggy Schjeldahl, Nateshvar Ken Scott, Niti Patricia Seip, Chitra Linda Smith, Premshakti Mary Stout, Nilu Ramsey Stuart, Vimala Phyllis Swackhammer, Shalini Ellen Towler, Gitanand Gray Ward, Sukanya Christine Warren, John Willey, Shila Janet Wilson, Anup Robert Wing, Lata Olivia Woodford, Priyanath Mark Yeoell, and Satyavati Kathryn Yeoell. Apologies to those undoubtedly missed in my attempt to recollect our shared history.

Special acknowledgment is due to the senior teachers who contributed written materials to this book. These include Maya Breuer, Yoganand Michael Carroll, Stephen Cope, Diana Damelio, Sudhir Jonathan Foust, Aruni Nan Futuronsky, Shantipriya Marcia Goldberg, Devarshi Steven Hartman, Rebekkah Kronlage, Michael Lee, Sudha Carolyn Lundeen, Konda Mason, Rasmani Deborah Orth, Rudy Peirce, Dinabandhu Garrett Sarley, Don Stapleton, and Amy Weintraub. Heartfelt gratitude to poet Danna Faulds, who not only lives with the gusto and grace with which she writes but also showers me with the gifts of her open heart daily. This book would not exist absent her individual contribution and the support offered me.

The ashram also was full of karma yogis, people who accomplished prodigious amounts with a clarity of focus and heartfelt generosity that inspired everyone. Although impossible to come up with a credible list, I would like to acknowledge a few who inspired me, and by so doing spark the memory of readers to recall many others. My thanks to Atmaram Kevin Kelly, Chandrakant Ernest Heister, Satyajit Moose Foran, Surabhi Leeah Foran, Saguna Toni Kenny, Nilima Carol Lew, Parimal Joel Levitan, Premal Cliff Nelson, Shankar Michael Risen, Sneha Karen Jegart, Sona Sheila Fay, Sukumari Betty Jo Goddard, and Indumati Paulette Slattery.

This book would not be possible without the contribution of Yogi Amrit Desai, the originator of Kripalu Yoga, and his wife, Urmila Desai, a yogini in her own right, along with their children, Pragnesh, Malay, and Kamini, who made many personal sacrifices to start and serve the ashram community.

This book bridges Kripalu's past with an exciting future, and another group whose service merits recognition is Kripalu's post-ashram board of trustees. Beyond shepherding the organization over, under, around, and through a host of gnarly predicaments, these friends ignored conventional wisdom to let me take on the task of writing this book at a time when my administrative responsibilities made that seemingly impossible. I can say with intimate knowledge that Kripalu owes its current existence to Jalesh Carl Bendix, Pier Paolo De Angelis, Marc David, Michael Lee, Manumati Betty Davis-Drewery, Nilam Al Meyerer, Tracey Roach, Niranjan David Sands, Adam Albright, Maya Breuer, Connie Chen, Jerry Colonna, Govinda Ron Dyer, Michael Gliksohn, Natavar Eric Knudsen, Hansa Carol Knox Johnson, Konda Mason, Justin Morreale, Jason Newman, Susan Piver, Michael Potts, Diane Utaski, Ramajyoti Vernon, and Al Weis.

For the past two years, Kripalu has been led by the dynamic duo of Dinabandhu Garrett Sarley, Kripalu's president, and Ila Sarley, Kripalu's chief operating officer, who both embody the vitality and skillfulness of a life of yoga. With them every step of the way is Patrick O'Shei, whose return to the organization as director of Kripalu Center operations inspired me personally and heralds an era in which Kripalu's high aspirations are matched by sound business principles. Serving alongside these three are Denise Barack, Jake Beauvais, Raya Buckley, Stephen Cope, Nina Dawe, Lorna Dolci, Jack Edwards, Elena Erber, Aruni Futuronsky, Jennifer Gigliotti, Shobhana Constance Goldberg, Devarshi Steven Hartman, Cathy Husid, Lee Johnson, Amber Kelly, Peter Lamb, Stephanie LaRoche, Callie Lockwood, Holly McCormack, John O'Neill, Paul Protzman, Tom Rocco, Bill Stoll, Grace Welker, and Jennifer Young.

Along with leaders and department heads, Kripalu has always been a place that recognizes the essential contribution made by the countless staff and volunteers who do the work day in and day out. To every soul who has shouldered tasks and gone about the business of serving the worthy cause that is Kripalu, asking little in return, I bow my head low.

In addition to the efforts of its professional and volunteer staff, Kripalu has always enjoyed the support of donors who believe in Kripalu's mission to uplift society, as we like to say, "changing the world one heart at a time." Space does not allow me to list individuals, but I would like to thank each and every one, especially Peter Alfond, who recently initiated a $2 Million Matching Gift Campaign that is still in process. This is a way you can support Kripalu's mission—one scholarship and brick at a time. As Dorothy Cochrain, the head of our Leadership Giving Committee, likes to say, "Generosity flows naturally from an awakened heart."

Very special thanks to all the Kripalu Yoga practitioners and teachers who entrusted me with their personal stories. Each and every reader will agree they make the text worth reading. I only wish there was space to include every courageous story of healing and transformation. To many who endured having their carefully written story whittled down to a sliver of its former glory, thanks for seeing the bigger picture. The eyes of readers will also enjoy the artistic photos that grace this book's pages. Credit for those goes to photographer Paul Conrath, Kripalu's Creative Director Elena Erber, photographer assistants Dorothee Brand and Josh Samuelsen, makeup and clothing wizardress Ramona Kelly-Hornstein, photo shoot coordinator Maureen Fayle, and models Chaya Heller, Jim O'Leary, D. Kavitha Rao, Monique Schubert, Brad Waites, Alexis Barth, Maya Breuer, Antonette Marchand, Andy Marston, Susan Maul, John Mole, Devika Tsoumas, and Sally Walkerman. Kripalu photographer Mary Schjeldahl took the cover shot, as well as a set of early photos that proved crucial to organizing the book.

I imagine that behind the authors of most books of this nature are parents who spent many an hour scratching their heads in wonder and worry over the life path their child was traveling. After all these years, my parents still scratch their heads in wonder. It is fulfilling, however, that worry has been replaced with trust. No wayward son could be blessed with better parents than mine, John and Kay Faulds, and I love them dearly. As for my siblings, I must begin with an apology for the inattention and absences entailed not only in writing this book, but in living the life required to undertake the task. Truth requires that I admit the same applies to many friends, particularly Lawrence Noyes, Len and Ling Poliandro, Marc and Meryl Rudin, and Marianne Spitzform. Special thanks to my sister, Karen Copenhaver, and her husband, Martin, in whose Vermont getaway the first draft of this book was written. Spirited encouragement to my nine-year-old niece, Natalie Faulds, who has joined the ranks of yoga enthusiasts and will receive the first copy of this book.

This experience has taught me that writing is only one step in the process in producing a book. Lots of heavy lifting has been done by the Bantam team, most notably Toni Burbank, whose editorial skills are legion and whose heart is larger still. Big thanks to art director Glen Edelstein, Kelly Chian, Susan Hood, Melanie Milgram, Robin Michaelson, and Julie Will.

This is—hopefully—my last task to bring this book to print. I want to end where I began, with a prayer that arose to keep me company along the way, with a tiny addition:

Salutations to the supreme spirit, divine beings, past masters of yoga, and my deepest and truest self. May the ancient wisdom of the Kripalu tradition be expressed in a contemporary format accessible to all—*and lived!*

INDEX OF POSTURES AND EXPERIENCES

KRIPALU CENTER FOR YOGA & HEALTH

Exploring the Yoga of Life

Kripalu Yoga is only one facet of what's happening at Kripalu Center. Swami Kripalu embraced the world's wisdom traditions, and in this same spirit Kripalu Center promotes all approaches that help people cultivate physical health, nurture emotional wellness, draw spiritual sustenance, and return home with tools that provide inspiration, energy, and integration. At Kripalu, we believe this nonsectarian yoga of life can do more than uplift us as individuals; it can serve as the foundation for a revitalized society and planet.

Workshops, Retreats, and Trainings

Located in the heart of the scenic and culturally rich Berkshire region of Massachusetts, Kripalu Center welcomes 25,000 people a year to its extensive curriculum of experiential workshops and personal retreats in yoga, holistic health, self-care, creative expression, personal growth, spiritual practice, intuitive development, physical fitness, integrative weight loss, nutrition, and more.

To participate in a Kripalu program is to enjoy an in-depth immersion experience offered in a vibrant, holistic environment. Along with the country's leading teachers, our integrative approach incorporates yoga practice, healthy diet, inner focus, outdoor experiences, artistic self-expression, the company of like-minded people, and an emphasis on providing you with practical skills to take home. Enjoy exquisite panoramic views, woodland trails, meditation gardens, a labyrinth, and a lake-front beach. Indoor amenities include a wellness center, saunas and whirlpools, and a well-equipped fitness room.

Professional Trainings

More than 500 holistic professionals are trained every year by the Kripalu Yoga teacher certification programs, the Kripalu School of Massage, and the Kripalu School of Ayurveda. There are more than 6,000 Kripalu Yoga teachers around the world and 35 Kripalu-affiliated yoga studios. Our yoga and massage programs offer 200-hour certification and 500-hour certification. Sallie Mae loans and scholarships are often available. Many Kripalu programs qualify for Continuing Education Credits (CECs) for professionals in fields such as social work, counseling, nursing, and massage.

Kripalu Yoga Teachers Association (KYTA)

KYTA is a professional association of more than 2,000 certified yoga teachers from all traditions and styles of yoga. KYTA supports its membership in exploring the depth and breadth of yoga, and it provides a wealth of practical information and marketing support for yoga teachers. Membership benefits include newsletters, audio CDs, inspirational and educational material, discounts on Kripalu programs, access to group insurance coverage, online support, and professional conferences.

Healing Arts

Kripalu has long believed that yoga, massage, and various forms of bodywork are powerful allies on the path of healing, growth, and transformation. Kripalu's wellness center specializes in healing modalities designed to bring the body, mind, and spirit into wholeness. We heartily agree with the wealth of medical research proving that a wide range of complementary and alternative therapies reduce stress, foster deep relaxation, enhance blood circulation to organs and glands, stimulate energy flow, decrease pain, improve sleep, and promote overall well-being. We offer treatments from both Western and Eastern traditions, including touch therapies, energy work, Ayurvedic treatments, acupuncture, and skin care. The endeavor to heal the body cannot be separated from restoring the mind and spirit, and we also offer a number of self-discovery and transformative sessions. All our therapists are highly skilled professionals who bring a depth of training, experience, and presence to their art of hands-on healing.

Conferences and Special Events

Kripalu brings together leading thinkers in conferences, experiential symposia, and other special events. Conferences on important topics and themes are a regular part of our program calendar. We also host an annual Yoga and Buddhism conference, a gathering for yoga teachers of all traditions, and an annual practice retreat for those exploring the path of yoga taught by Swami Kripalu. Special events include musical and artistic performances, talks, workshop samplers, and book launches with artists, authors, and influential teachers.

Volunteering at Kripalu

Kripalu provides hundreds of short- and long-term volunteer opportunities. Volunteers support the day-to-day operations of Kripalu Center in a work environment built on skillful action, authentic communication, and self-responsibility. In addition to an active work experience, volunteers experience a holistic lifestyle, including yoga classes, a specially tailored educational curriculum, a nutritious diet, access to Kripalu's amenities, and the company of like-hearted individuals. Kripalu's volunteer programs are an empowering opportunity to embrace self-development in community, based on the principle of *seva*, a Sanskrit word meaning *service*.

Institute for Extraordinary Living

Directed by Stephen Cope, the Kripalu Institute for Extraordinary Living was created to investigate what it means to be *jivan mukti* or "a soul awake in this lifetime," one of the central archetypes of the yoga tradition. The institute's mission is to study, promote, and embody states of optimal living through methods gleaned from the contemplative traditions as well as contemporary scientific inquiry. We are particularly interested in human flourishing and thriving, as reflected in qualities such as resiliency, creativity, mastery, authentic power, and happiness. The institute provides a forum for researchers, practitioners, and laypeople to develop and learn practical methods for cultivating the experience of "full aliveness" and transmitting that to families, communities, society, and the world.

Scholarships and Grants

Kripalu is committed to making its services available to people from all backgrounds and social classes. Since 2002, the Teaching for Diversity program has awarded thousands of dollars in grants each year to yoga teachers who provide classes to special populations, such as AIDS survivors, inner-city children, at-risk teens, prison inmates, senior citizens, and impoverished populations. We also provide partial scholarship assistance to hundreds of people a year attending various Kripalu programs. Scholarship applications can be obtained by e-mailing scholarship@kripalu.org.

History of Kripalu Center

In many ways, Kripalu's history parallels the evolution of yoga in America. In the late 1960s, Indian-born Amrit Desai taught yoga to a growing number of students in the Philadelphia area. In 1972, Yogi Desai and a handful of dedicated students established a small, residential yoga center in Sumneytown, Pennsylvania. It rapidly expanded to nearby Summit Station, Pennsylvania, before moving to Lenox, Massachusetts, in 1983.

From its inception, Kripalu Center was staffed by a committed group of yoga enthusiasts who formed the nucleus of an intentional yoga community or *ashram*. Yogi Desai was the guru and spiritual leader of the ashram, which eventually grew to offer a broad curriculum of yoga, holistic health, and self-discovery programs to the public. Developed and taught by ashram residents, these programs were the outgrowth of practices carried on within the community. Yogi Desai's guru, Swami Kripalu, came to the United States in 1977 and spent the last four years of his life at the ashram. Although he continued his life of intensive yoga practice, Swami Kripalu's presence galvanized the growth of the ashram community and inspired thousands to regular yoga practice.

Kripalu Center continued to expand in size and influence until 1994. Yogi Desai was an international figure in yoga, and the ashram was considered an exemplary spiritual community with two Lenox facilities staffed by 325 hardworking residents. The sexual relationships with female disciples that led Kripalu's board of trustees to call for Yogi Desai's resignation as spiritual director are well-known. Less understood is the intimate and trusting context of the guru/disciple relationship that caused these and other abuses of power to occur as a deep spiritual betrayal. These were difficult times for all concerned.

Even as he fell from his pedestal, Yogi Desai served as a catalyst for the evolution of the Kripalu community. The myth of the omnipotent guru was shattered, forcing the entire community to a higher level of individuation and self-empowerment. With the bloom of the resident community fading, the ashram gradually disbanded. Kripalu Center restructured itself as an educational nonprofit organization, hired a portion of its formerly volunteer staff, and extended its program offerings. Kripalu has the distinction of being the first, and possibly the only, yoga center in North America to make a successful transition from a traditional guru-disciple structure. Today Kripalu Center is much more than a program and retreat center. It is a university for the whole person, a place where everyone can experience the state of body, mind, and spirit integration that is yoga and shift the consciousness from which we live our lives.

In addition to participating in all Kripalu Center has to offer, you can play an important role in furthering its mission. It is only through the generous support of individuals, corporations, and private foundations that Kripalu can provide program scholarships and reach out to share the gifts of yoga with diverse populations. As a federally tax-exempt organization pursuant to section 501(c)(3) of the Internal Revenue Code, all gifts and grants to Kripalu are tax-deductible.

Find Out More

To receive a program catalog or learn more about Kripalu, visit www.kripalu.org or call 800-741-7353.